SOCIAL ORGANIZATION OF MEDICAL WORK

SOCIAL ORGANIZATION OF MEDICAL WORK

ANSELM L. STRAUSS,
SHIZUKO FAGERHAUGH,
BARBARA SUCZEK, AND
CAROLYN WIENER

WITH A NEW INTRODUCTION BY ANSELM L. STRAUSS

Routledge
Taylor & Francis Group
LONDON AND NEW YORK

Originally published in 1985 by The University of Chicago Press.

Published 1997 by Transaction Publishers

Published 2017 by Routledge
2 Park Square, Milton Park, Abingdon, Oxon OX14 4RN
711 Third Avenue, New York, NY 10017, USA

First issued in hardback 2017

Routledge is an imprint of the Taylor & Francis Group, an informa business

Library of Congress Catalog Number: 96-53073

Library of Congress Cataloging-in-Publication Data

Social organization of medical work / Anselm L. Strauss ... [et al] ; with a new introduction by Anselm L. Strauss.
p. cm.
Includes bibliographical references and index.
ISBN 1-56000-968-3 (pbk. : alk. paper)
1. Hospitals—United States—Sociological aspects. 2. Industrial sociology—United States. 3. Social medicine—United States. I. Strauss, Anselm L.

RA965.S54 1997
362.1'042—dc21 96-53073
CIP

ISBN 13: 978-1-138-53286-1 (hbk)
ISBN 13: 978-1-56000-968-9 (pbk)

To
R.B.
who understands this
all too well

Contents

In the beginning was *Work*. The Universe had to be made by someone or something: but by which God or which combination of natural forces we do not yet know. As for the Garden, it was not inevitable that Eve should eat the apple; it could have been Adam, and even the Serpent could not be said to have embarked on his career of villainy before he worked at tempting someone to eat the apple. So Work—or Act—is primary.

—Anonymous, 5th century B.C.

Marx was quite right in emphasizing the primacy of work but—transfixed by his images of human exploitation and engaged in a life/death struggle with Ricardo, Malthus, et al.—tripped into the mud puddle of a non sequitur. Work *is* primary; may lead to a division of labor in which exploitation reigns; may lead to many alternative divisions of work and many modes of relationship.

—Anonymous, 20th century

But in every case a study of the concrete situation—whether Flaubert, Valery, or the foreign policies of the Gironde—ends up bringing Sartre back to its deap-seated structural context. His research moves from the surface to the depths, and so links up with my own preoccupations. It would link up even better if the hourglass could be turned over both ways—from event to structure, and then from structure and model back to event.

—Fernand Braudel, *On History*

Introduction to the Transaction Edition

The reprinting of *The Social Organization of Medical Work* more than a decade after its first publication, and during a time when hospitals are being drastically curtailed, calls for some explanation.

This book is one of a long line of qualitative research studies that greatly enhanced understanding of health care institutions and practices. Those studies are regarded as classics of medical sociology, and they include such well-known works as Howard Becker's and Blanche Geer's *Boys in White*, Julius Roth's *Timetables*, Fred Davis' *Passage Through Crisis*, the monograph by Barney Glaser and Anselm Strauss, *Awareness of Dying*, the various writings of Eliot Freidson, and the influential concept of "negotiated order" coming out of the Strauss et al.'s *Psychiatric Ideologies and Institutions*. These monographs—mainly utilizing fieldwork, that is, "ethnographic" methods—coming directly out of Chicago style sociology, brought medical sociology into international prominence. They also underlined the importance of this specialization for providing intellectual stimulation to other sociological specialties. In addition, they, understandably, reflected the growing prominence and concern everywhere in the industrialized nations with matters of health and illness. What is additionally interesting about these and other studies, early and later, is that they helped to form the basis of an increasingly strong rationale for qualitative research in the face of a quantitatively oriented twentieth-century social science.

The Social Organization of Medical Work, which appeared in 1985, was a continuation of this tradition but also focused on some different topics and was an illustration too of a team approach to fieldwork itself. Concerning that third point, Steve Barley has observed to me (Strauss) that the use of a team was and perhaps still is an unusual form of doing an ethnographic study. The team consisted of three sociologists (Barbara Suczek, Carolyn Wiener, and me) and also a sociologically trained nurse researcher (Shizuko Fagerhaugh). The study could not possibly have been done by one field-worker/analyst, considering that the team members studied so many sites, observed and interviewed so many types of physicians, nurses, allied technicians, administrators (and even hospital architects), and studied work done around a great diversity of medical equipment and that used an immense variety of "supplies." This research team met virtually every week for a conference, at which one or another would report some of what they had observed or heard. Just as important, we turned the conferences into analytic sessions, working out patiently and in some detail an evolving theoretical structure. What helped the analytic and presumably the interpersonal process was that the team members had been my students. They were trained in "grounded theory" methodology and procedures, a point I mention because this monograph does not constitute the usual ethnographic study. Rather the team used standard (sociological) ethnographic methods to collect data, but its main intent was to use these data to develop grounded theory about a set of important sociological issues.

Among these were the following. We were above all interested in types of work, for the study of health and illness had always been, for me and my students, primarily a substantive ground for studying "the sociology of work." In this sense it was a continuation of the dual focus, begun in the study of dying in hospitals, on work and the organization in which the work took place. This later book centers around discussions of work in general and of universally found types of work: work with equipment, comfort work, sentimental work, and so on. Another theoretical issue addressed was how the work is carried out over time and space, which resulted in an elaboration of the concept of "trajectory." This is a central category in the book, helping to bring together a vast number and many types of work, tasks, and workers in some measure of coordination—or "articulation," as we called this working together with common if also divergent aims. A third theoretical focus was how a great many professional and technical specialties worked with different types of equipment and supplies—a contribution, we hoped, to the sociological study of technology. Still another concern was how a venerable institution (the hospital) was responding to the amazing proliferation of medical, nursing, and technical specialties in terms of its emergent contemporary social organization—the issue of "social order" spelled out for a major institution. And finally, though seemingly this was more substantive a focus, we were interested in how such an institution organized its work in terms of a predominant medical ideology of a battle against acute disease, against the reality of clients who were, in fact, mostly bedded down with long-term ("chronic") diseases for which pragmatic and often highly technical and successful procedures had been developed but for which a comparable ideology of chronic illness was pretty much lacking. In this sense, we thought of, and wished to document and analyze, an institution somewhat out of step with "reality." There are many more theoretical issues taken up in the extensive last section of the book.

What we did not foresee was the radical change in the American health care "system" in the last decade, including the "downsizing" of hospital staffs, the vastly increased number and severity of regulations governing the operation of hospitals, the disappearance and mergers of hospitals, the enormous growth of competition among them, their changing relationships with HMOs and clinics, and other such drastic changes in this institution. In an unpublished paper we did foresee the radical impact of regarding health care in terms of an industrial model, but could scarcely predict those specifics of the new model.

But thereby hangs a personal tale, specific to this book and its republishing. Twice in my sociological career I have had a hand in publishing books about institutions that were about to change drastically, and "downward"—one was the state mental hospital and the other was the medical hospital. This has meant a radically lessened interest in those institutions, and so in the studies that have described or analyzed them. But the other part of this tale is that sociologists probably read and purchase books largely in terms of substantive rather than theoretical interests. *Social Organization of Medical Work* surely has enough theoretical subjects, and rather enduring and general ones, to profit anybody who is interested in such theoretical matters. But I read its reception as having been basically a substantive one. It has never been translated into a foreign language; presumably the American hospital is too local a phenomenon to be of much interest even to foreign social scientists. Though the initial publication was extremely well received and its sales were quite good, in time as the institution changed and declined, its sales slacked off drastically enough so that the University of Chicago Press dropped it from its list. (This surely reflects the increasingly straitened circumstances and commercial policies of the hitherto stalwart university presses.) Irving Horowitz and Transaction quickly moved to suggest that the book be republished. We authors are all grateful for that, and for this eminent scholarly press' recognition that the book is more than a description of a rapidly vanishing past or nostalgic reminder of things that were. We are still proud of this book, and think of it, as said earlier, both as continuing a celebrated tradition and as addressing important social science issues, ones with clear implications for an improved health policy, in an age where HMOs, clinics, physicians in their private offices, kin at home, and patients everywhere are increasingly confronted with long-term, usually incurable, illnesses.

Anselm L. Strauss

August 1996

Preface

This book has dual messages. Both pertain to the primacy of work for shaping the divisions of labor which form around it, as well as the experiences and careers of the people who do the work, and for influencing the very structure of the organizations in which work takes place. The first message is meant to reach social scientists who may have no particular interest in the work done on hospital wards but are deeply interested in the topic of work as such and in how it may be studied, analyzed, and theorized about. The second message is addressed to readers who are vitally concerned with caring for hospitalized patients—who are working on, around, and with sick people.

In the most general sense, that latter message consists of this: the work of physicians, nurses, and associated technicians has been radically and irrevocably altered by today's prevalence of chronic illnesses—the illnesses that bring patients into contemporary hospitals—and by the technologies developed to manage them. But how, in detail, has that work changed and what are some of the experiences of those who do the work of managing those illnesses—including the patients themselves?

We bring a sociological perspective to bear on that question. Our perspective has been shaped by many years of observation in hospitals, these in turn preceding the four-year observational and interview study on which this book is based. The research reported on here was done on many different types of wards, in seven hospitals in the Bay Area of San Francisco, and the interviews done there were supplemented by others done with physicians, nurses, various technicians, architects, bioengineers, innovators of medical technology, who worked elsewhere, that is, not at the sites where the major portion of our research was carried out. Some of our answers to the question posed above about the changed character of medical work will be quite different from those commonly given, or assumed, by health workers themselves. Part of the respective difference is due to our sociological perspective, which trains us to look at the same events and yet see them differently. Part of the difference is doubtless due to the fact that however familiar we are with the work of health professionals, we do not engage in the work ourselves (although one author is a nurse with long professional experience). Nevertheless, we would be surprised and disappointed if those readers who actually do the work did not recognize themselves in our account and generally (if not always specifically) agree with it. One of the crucial tests of sociological research is that those who have been studied recognize themselves in the research report itself; if they do not, this should warn the researchers that they have simply imposed their own views of reality on what they have studied—a fault not uncommon among social scientists, but one that field researchers are less likely to have than those who collect their data through less direct means than using their own eyes and ears and being present when both the mundane and extraordinary events under study are occurring (Schatzman and Strauss 1973).

We are very aware that many of the issues we shall discuss in this book are among "the most heated, debated, and hysterically criticized" aspects of health care[1] today—"dehumanized," "overtechnologized," "technically oriented doctors," "hospitals like factories," "fragmentation of care" among them. Our perspective on such issues is to understand how such debate and heat comes about, given the conditions under which health practitioners work today and under which health care is given and received. The assumption behind this seemingly less passionate stance is a standard social science one, namely, that reform without prior understanding can only lead to ineffectual reform, or even to measures that will make matters worse—a not unusual outcome of much reform action. So while we are deeply concerned about these issues, we believe that this book has something to contribute to future health policy considerations.

Turning now to the primary message of this monograph and to our social scientist audience: that message is a complex one. One of its aspects is that work with and on human beings has characteristics not

[1]To quote one of our knowledgeable colleagues, Rue Bucher (personal communication), University of Illinois, Chicago, Illinois.

present when the material worked on is inanimate. Of course, everyone recognizes that the human material—as in "service work"—reacts to the workers and to the work itself (as "cooperative," "recalcitrant," "denying," etc.). Quite as important, perhaps, in many kinds of work with humans is that the worked-on can participate in the work itself; they are indeed either implicitly or explicitly part of the divisions of labor. (This is so even when the work setting is highly technologized and the work itself profoundly affected by the technology.) The implications of that infrequently recognized phenomenon are most important for the sociology of work. A second point that will be emphasized is that work can profitably be studied in terms of features not yet captured by traditional or current social science classifications and analyses. In this monograph, we shall analyze in considerable detail several different *kinds* of work, and their relationships, that go to make up the bundle known as medical-nursing care. Among the types of work discussed at length are: machine work, safety work, comfort work, sentimental work, and articulation work. Other types discussed less extensively in the last chapter include error work, body work, information work, and negotiative work. A third approach to work will emphasize the primacy of work over the division of labor itself, over workers' careers, over the organizations where work takes place. We do not mean that the influence is all one way—of course, it is not—but remarkably little writing in the sociology of work begins with work itself (except descriptively, not analytically) but rather focuses on the divisions of labor, on work roles, role relationships, careers, and the like. A concerted *analytic examination of work itself* ought to provide a needed corrective to more traditional approaches, which, however effective, still leave important issues untouched or unresolved. Our last chapter will address some of those issues directly, but they will not be disregarded elsewhere in the book.

Throughout we have taken pains to spell out linkages between the more detailed (microscopic) aspects of work and the larger structural (macroscopic) conditions, and in chapter 9 we have addressed the issue of their interaction—the issue touched on so vividly by the historian Fernand Braudel in the quotation at the beginning of this book (Braudel 1980). One proviso: the medical scene about which we are writing is located in specifiable place and time, so neither our description nor interpretation is meant to be universal. This is contemporary medicine, about 1946–85, in the United States. Relevant literature and also personal observations made overseas confirm that what we found is more or less true everywhere in the industrialized nations of the world, with local modifications as in the United States itself. In the Asian developing nations, we have seen combinations of western medicine operating in tandem with or embedded in a context of alternative conceptions of health, illness, and medicine. (That phenomenon is not really foreign to Americans, either, but it is less obtrusive, to use the western medicine–oriented practitioner's term.) So in those countries, the substantive detail written about here requires more qualification for varied conditions than in the United States. We have been explicit about that: after all, things were different and will be different again.

For support of the research on which much of this book is based, the authors are greatly indebted to the Health Resources Administration, Bureau of Manpower, United States Public Health Service, Division of Nursing, Grant #NU-00598. We are indebted to the staffs of the following Bay Area hospitals where we did extensive fieldwork: Alta Bates, Herrick, Letterman, Mt. Zion, Presbyterian, Stanford, and University of California, and to St. Bartholomew, London, with special thanks to Helen Collyers.

Our thanks also for their various contributions to this book—for data, ideas, reading of the draft manuscript—go to Diane Beeson, University of California, San Francisco; Robert Broadhead, University of Connecticut, Storrs, Connecticut; Rue Bucher, Department of Sociology, University of Illinois, Chicago; Wolfram Fischer, University of Muenster, West Germany; Berenice Fisher, New York University, New York, New York; Elihu Gerson, Tremont Research Institute, San Francisco, California; Roberta Lessor, School of Nursing, University of California, San Francisco; Evelyn Peterson, School of Nursing, University of South Dakota; Fritz Schuetze, University of Kassel, West Germany; Leigh Star, Department of Social and Behavioral Sciences, University of California, San Francisco, and Tremont Research Institute, San Francisco; Steven Wallace, Department of Social and Behavioral Sciences, University of California, San Francisco; Irma Zuckermann, Department of Social and Behavioral Sciences, University of California, San Francisco. We are especially grateful to Barney Glaser for his valuable consultation on the research and to Rue Bucher for her careful reading, editing, and general commentary on the next to final draft. Finally, our very special thanks go to Sally Maeth for her patient and persistent secretarial assistance and to the Department of Social and Behavioral Sciences, UCSF, which contributed additional secretarial funding after our grant money ran out.

1

Chronic Illness, Technology, and the Hospital

To understand properly the work of managing illness today, one needs first to understand a few salient features of the larger context within which the work takes place. Its features include (1) the contemporary prevalence of chronic illness, (2) images of acute care, (3) medical technology and its impact on hospitals, and (4) the hospital as a set of work sites. These will be discussed briefly in this chapter, but their implications for the kinds and organization of medical work will be evident throughout the book.

Prevalence of Chronic Illness

With regard to issues of health and illness, mankind is passing through a new era in its long civilized history. Though hardly as dramatic as the arrival of the atomic bomb or as well noted as the current population explosion, there is unquestionably something startlingly new about the biological condition of a considerable, and increasing, portion of the earth's population: namely, the prevalence now of the *chronic* rather than acute illnesses. There is a fateful paradox here: although the chronic illnesses are prevalent, and that has been recognized by some observers for two or three decades (Mayo 1956, p. 9), neither the general public nor the health professionals, as we shall see, recognize anything like the full implications of this for training, care, insurance, indeed for the health institutions themselves. We are just beginning to pass into a period when chronic illness per se (rather than specific or categorical chronic diseases) is referred to, thought about, acted upon as a general reality. This seems to be no less true in England, Sweden, and other medically advanced nations than in the United States (Gerson and Strauss 1975, Strauss and Glaser 1975).

Until the late 1930s, in industrialized countries, as in third-world countries today, the prevailing and often terrible afflictions were due to bacteria and parasites—the so-called acute diseases. A dramatic change took place when antibiotics and various improved immunological measures turned out to be so effective against many of the infectious and parasitic diseases. Those diseases still reign in the less fortunate countries, but in the highly industrialized ones (especially the United States, Canada, the Soviet Union, Japan, and in Europe) what people are sick from mostly are the chronic illnesses. They include the cancers, arthritis, and a great host of others that are currently incurable. Men and women have always suffered from these, of course, but they never were the prevalent illnesses. These now constitute the equivalent of plagues and scourges of yesteryear. They are what bring people to the doctor's office, the clinic, and into the hospital: they are what people in developed nations mostly die from.

Among the prominent characteristics of chronic illness (Gerson and Strauss 1975, pp. 2–18) are that they (1) are long term, (2) are uncertain, (3) require proportionately large efforts at palliation, (4) tend to be multiple diseases, (5) are disproportionately intrusive upon the lives of the ill and their families, (6) require a wide variety of ancillary services if they are to be properly cared for, (7) often imply conflicts of interpretation and authority among patients, health workers, and funding agents, (8) mainly require primary care, and (9) are expensive to treat and manage.

The Imagery of Acute Care

In the *hospitals*—the special focus of this book—the personnel still tend to think of themselves as treating patients who are acutely ill. This can only mean, however, that their clients are suffering from an acute phase of one or another chronic disease. What can be accomplished with these patients is, in common parlance, mainly "checking the progress of the disease," "getting them back on their feet," "slowing up the inevitable," and so on. Most personnel would certainly agree that they were not engaged in cure in the old-fashioned sense of curing pneumonia. Nevertheless, they tend to think of chronic patients as those so incurably ill that they belong in nursing homes or other specialized warehousing institutions. That is why one sociological researcher recently found that hospitalized stroke patients seemed, from the staff's viewpoint, to be out of place (Hoffman 1974).

While the hospital's organization has been radically changed by the incurable, long-term illnesses of its clients, this acute-care mentality, derived from the previous era of the acute illnesses, still profoundly colors the operations of the hospital. Even nursing home care is, aside from its housekeeping functions, modeled along notions of medical care. Indeed, federal regulations emphasize just those aspects of care.

Impact of Medical Technology on Hospitals

The diagnosis and treatment of the chronic illnesses have contributed to the widespread use of a great array of drugs, rapidly increasing numbers and types of machinery (clinical laboratory tests are now thoroughly dependent on machinery), and, of course, various surgical and other procedures. In the United States, as in other industrialized nations, a considerable industry has evolved for manufacturing and supplying drugs, machines, and other elements of these technologies (Fagerhaugh et al. 1980). New occupations are growing up around the servicing and utilization of this machinery (bioengineers, safety engineers, respiratory therapists, physiotherapists, radiology technicians), and many of the medical specialties are centrally dependent on its use. The larger hospitals are speedily becoming machine-dependent, as the various specialty wards press to fulfill their respective technological requirements. (Since our own recent research has been centered especially on medical machinery, we shall emphasize, in this section, its impact especially—although, of course, much of that machinery is utilized in conjunction with drugs.)

Halfway Technology

Before we discuss the impact of the foregoing trends on hospitals and on medical care, it should be noted that despite the growth of this technology—and the obvious success of some of it—a governmental commission has aptly dubbed it as only "halfway technology." The term has been popularized by Lewis Thomas (1974), who notes that this technology constitutes medical intervention applied after the fact, in an attempt to compensate for the incapacitating effects of disease (or to postpone death) whose course one is unable to do much about. This technology is located in varying amounts and kinds in hospitals, clinics, doctors' offices, and increasingly in the homes of the chronically ill. Medical technology has prolonged lives, but it has also made both the professionals and the patients more dependent on technology throughout the course of long chronic illnesses. Patients cycle through the hospital, to the clinic or doctor's office, to their homes, and back again to the hospital during acute episodes—and again to their homes.

So, articulating the care given in hospitals, clinics, and homes has become a major problem. The technological explosion and its effect both on the organizational structure of health care and on the work of health professionals, in turn, have affected the kind and quality of patient care—that is, of medical, nursing, and technical *work*.

Medical Specialization and Technology

A special feature of medical specialization and technological innovation is that the two are simultaneously parallel and interactive, creating an impetus to further technological innovation and specialization. Medical specialization leads to technological innovation: the technological innovation then leads back to production through industry (drug, machine, supplies, etc.). Then, through the utilization of technology, with reports feeding back to industry, technological improvements are made and often with great rapidity. All of this results in increasingly sophisticated medical specialties and their associated work.

In turn, this expansion of specialized departments and services in hospitals requires (1) the expansion of physical facilities, (2) the reallocation of workers and the integration of new skilled personnel into a continuously changing division of labor, and (3) the establishment of complex relationships among a multiplicity of hospital services and departments. Understandably, those developments have had profound impact on hospital organization, including that of even the smaller hospitals, for the rate of technological migration to smaller hospitals and their associated communities is also rapidly rising. That diffusion is furthered by the increased role of industry in medical technology and its perceived need for expanding the market; the spread of trained personnel from large research and training centers who are seeking opportunities to practice their skills; the prestige requirements and the competition of hospitals for attracting patients and physicians; and the demand that services and resources be distributed equitably among all citizens. Thus, the impact of technology on hospital structure and work in smaller hospitals parallels that felt by the personnel in larger institutions, differing only in rate and intensity.

Technology and Its Impact on Chronic Care

Increased technological specialization and complex bureaucratic health structures together have resulted in two additional important developments: first, the fragmentation of chronic care, with increasing possibilities that continuity of care will go awry, accompanied by accusatory cries of dehumanization; second, the incorporation of new workers and roles to remedy the effects of fragmented care and dehumanization.

During patients' hospitalizations, they are frequently moved to and from specialized machine areas where machines are used to do tests, monitor the course of diseases, or provide treatments. Patients are also being moved according to the acuity of disease, from acute to intermediate to rehabilitation wards or back to acute and intermediate wards as their condition changes. In addition, a constant stream of workers comes and goes, performing tasks *on* patients. The scheduling of work for diagnostic tests and monitoring of illness status, treatments, and general nursing care is complex; there is a high likelihood that schedules will go awry since each machine area and patient care unit has its own schedules and contingencies. For example, in any specialized service or patient care unit there may be a machine breakdown for which staff are unable to command immediate repairs, or a key staff member may be tied up elsewhere, or a higher priority "emergency" may suddenly develop. When multiple services are scheduled for a given patient, there is a high probability that his or her total schedule will go awry—two meals missed in a row, delays in meeting requests. As a consequence, patients become angry, anxious, and discomfited—making for accusations of negligence or of depersonalization. Health professionals are becoming more cognizant of the untoward effects of fragmented care and are working toward remedying the situation by adding liaison nurses and fashioning new roles like that of the "primary nurse" (Mundinger 1973) or "primary doctor" (Andreopolous 1974) and "patient advocates" (Hamil et al. 1976). But given the organizational considerations outlined earlier, remedying the situation is shatteringly difficult.

The Hospital as Multiple Work Sites

A useful way of conceiving of the hospital is as a large number of work sites. A walk around the different floors and sections of any fairly large or complex hospital gives one an astonishingly varied visual experience. Over here is the X-ray department—familiar to us all—with its huge mobile machines, its shielded area where the radiologist or X-ray technician pulls switches while the patient lies or stands immobile under or in front of a machine, having been carefully positioned by the technician, while other patients are lined up in a nearby area, usually in wheelchairs, each waiting to be worked on. Not far away is the cardiologist's terrain, where a single patient is hooked up to a complicated cardiac monitoring machine, operated by another kind of technician:

the patient is sitting, standing, or walking on a treadmill machine, the technician is carefully operating the equipment and keeping an eye on the patient; meanwhile, a physician is looking at the unwinding printout, interpreting what the patient's heart is doing during his or her performance. Down in the basement is the central supply department; no patients are in sight, but low-salaried personnel are doing numbers of tasks related to sending supplies up to the clinical wards.

Upstairs, on the main floors of the hospital, are a variety of wards, each visually and often spatially different to the visitor's quick glance. The postoperative recovery room is heavily staffed with highly skilled nurses who carefully, minute by minute, monitor their relatively few and initially unconscious patients, who in turn are hooked up to multiple machines. Nearby is the intensive care unit (ICU) with its relatively few beds, with patients largely nonsentient who are relatively exposed to each other, its battery of machines for monitoring each patient's vital signs, its one-to-one ratio of nurse to patient, its floating population of easily accessible physicians, its auxiliary specialists like respiratory technicians, its frequent patient crises and quick gathering of staff for fast action. In the cancer ward, the work pace is much slower ("we take our cues from the patient"): some patients are dying, others are there for X-ray treatments or chemotherapy and are suffering from varied degrees of physiological and psychological distress—so the nurses are doing much comfort care (medical and psychological) with most patients, while working on their own threatened composure and overinvolvement with the patients.

In short, a hospital consists of variegated workshops—places where different kinds of work are going on, where very different resources (space, skills, ratios of labor force, equipment, drugs, supplies, and the like) are required to carry out that work, where the divisions of labor are amazingly different, though all of this is in the direct or indirect service of managing patients' illnesses.

Decades ago the hospital was much less differentiated. Of course, there has long been a division between surgical and medical sections, though in many hospitals in developing countries there often is little difference to be seen between such sections. The hospital included servicing departments like X ray and pharmacy but had nothing then like the complex array of wards that reflect today's explosion of medical specialization or the immensely varied chronic illnesses found in the contemporary hospital. If one focuses only on the clinical wards, however, it is easy to miss the similar explosion in the number and variety of support and servicing departments like transport, physical therapy, respiratory therapy, nutrition, safety, equipment repair, bioengineering, echotherapy, EKG, and even a full-scale clinical laboratory for doing the host of diagnostic tests ordered from the various clinical wards. Hospital administration, too, has proliferated into its own specialist sections, though in this book we shall hardly be concerned with them, except as they touch on the hospital's clinical work. In general, the administrators do not enter directly into that work but their policies, decisions, and operations affect the resources available to the various wards, which typically compete vigorously for those finite resources.

A closing reminder: the hospital's many and varied workshops operate directly or indirectly in the service not merely of managing illnesses, but of managing illnesses that are overwhelmingly chronic in nature. The careers, stakes, and satisfactions of the personnel aside, that is what clinical-oriented work in the hospital is all about.

2
Illness Trajectories

A distinction central to the analysis presented in this book is that drawn between a course of illness and an illness trajectory.[1] The first term offers no problems to the reader since everyone has experienced an illness that did not merely appear but developed gradually over time, getting worse and then perhaps clearing up. To the knowledgeable medical, nursing, and technical staffs, each kind of illness has its more or less characteristic phases, with symptoms to match, and often only skilled intervention will reverse, halt, or at least slow down the progress of the disease. *Course of illness* is, then, both a commonsense and professional term. In contrast, *trajectory* is a term coined by the authors to refer not only to the physiological unfolding of a patient's disease but to the total *organization of work* done over that course, plus the *impact* on those involved with that work and its organization. For different illnesses, the trajectory will involve different medical and nursing actions, different kinds of skills and other resources, a different parceling out of tasks among the workers (including, perhaps, kin and the patient), and involving quite different relationships—instrumental and expressive both—among the workers.

[1]This distinction was first utilized in B. Glaser and A. Strauss 1967, but the analysis of trajectories was not then focused on some of the more subtle features of types of work, as in the current monograph. See also Fagerhaugh and Strauss 1977 and Strauss and Glaser 1975.

A concept like trajectory is necessary for sociological understanding of illness management. It protects the researchers from being confined by the perspective of the health workers themselves—minimizes the dangers of simply appreciating or criticizing the "natives" as judged essentially from within their own framework. At the same time, this concept is rooted in close observation (seeing, hearing, interviewing) of health workers and so, we hope, does justice to their viewpoints. So much so, that those studied ought to recognize themselves in our account of them and their work, and not disagree with the major thrust of that account—a requisite for our kind of research. But the concept is above all a means for analytically ordering the immense variety of events that occur—at least with contemporary chronic illnesses—as patients, kin, and staffs seek to control and cope with those illnesses. Of course, all work—industrial, commercial, artistic, domestic—involves a sequence of expected tasks, sometimes routinized but sometimes subject to unexpected contingencies. It may be that trajectory fits the organization of those kinds of work also.

But there are two striking features of health work shared only with certain other kinds of work. One consists of the unexpected and often difficult to control *contingencies* stemming not only from the illness itself, but also from a host of work and organizational sources as well as from biographical and life-style sources pertaining to patients, kin, and staff members themselves. A second and crucial feature of health work is that it is "people work." The product being worked on, over, or through(!) is not inert, unless comatose or temporarily nonsentient. Two things follow: (1) the patient can react and so affect the work; (2) the patient can participate in the work itself, that is, be a worker. The latter point is equivalent to saying that the product is not only worked on or over but also sometimes with. As will be seen, both major features (contingencies and people work) of illness trajectories affect the various specific kinds of trajectories, and differentially so along their various phases. Taken together, both features insure that trajectory work harbors the potential for being complex and often highly problematic.

Further Sources of Problematic Complexity: Chronic Illness and Technology

Two other sources—the prevalence of chronic illness and associated technologies for dealing with it—make for complicated and often highly problematic trajectories. In brief, their combined impact is as follows. Some kinds of technology (like the machinery, drugs, and various procedures used for kidney dialysis patients) are producing new trajectories (Plough 1981). Until the health professionals gain experience with the novel twists and turns of the illness and with it and the regimen's impact on other bodily systems, and with the organization of work to manage all of that, the resulting trajectories can be difficult indeed, as the history of dialysis treatment has shown. At the other end of the age scale: babies saved in the sophisticated ICNs may develop disabilities and systemic illnesses—some not known until somewhat later—that are not necessarily curable and their extent is still not at all known (see chap. 9, and Wiener et al. 1979).

Improved technology has also produced a lengthening of trajectories. By this we mean that although the technology (for example, open heart surgery) keeps ill persons alive, and may even improve them symptomatically, they then face uncertain futures regarding both the physiological consequences of the surgery, drugs, etc.—including drastic impact on other bodily systems—and in the organization of work to manage regimens and attendant life-styles. Even without the creation of such related physiological disturbances, the lengthening of the trajectory poses new medical, organizational, and biographical problems: for example, the diabetics who, now living longer, encounter end-of-the-trajectory complications that neither they nor often their physicians dreamed of.

Since many patients suffer from multiple chronic illnesses (whether related systemically or not), their respective regimens need to be balanced carefully or else there are physiological aftermaths that result in unexpected and sometimes uncontrollable kinds of physiological, and so work-related trajectory, developments. (We offer a case a few pages below, which serves as a poignant illustration.) Sometimes the balancing is hampered by lack of knowledge of, say, the side effects of new drugs or even older ones used with a given patient; or by the staff's own focus on a primary trajectory to the virtual exclusion of others regarded as secondary; also of their lack of knowledge that the patient has other illnesses.

Advances in halfway technology utilized in the service of managing difficult chronic illnesses result in unexpected contingencies during the acute illness period—as when experimental or relatively new drugs, or familiar ones used with specific patients, produce unexpected physiological occurrences that amount essentially to new phases in the illness and its attendant work. Surgical nurses have remarked to us about avant-garde surgery that in postsurgical phases it is difficult even to assess "what is going on" and to what degree the surgery has been successful. Because "everything is so new," they literally do not quite know what to expect or how to evaluate it. Complicating much trajectory work, also, within the hospital especially is that new microphases and the lengthening of trajectories bring in the services of multiple departments, involving the work of their respective technicians and specialists, some of whom are struggling with new phenomena.

The hospital staffs increasingly recognize that patients need to be taught requisite skills for handling drugs and equipment and for doing various therapeutic procedures when at home. So something else is being added to the trajectories, in the last days or hours before the patient leaves the hospital. In the days or weeks afterward, the patient may be visited and worked on by visiting nurses, social workers, respiratory therapists, and other kinds of health professionals.

It is easy to see that the complexities of trajectory work are added to by the host of new specialists (medical, nursing, and technical) who are working on the patient's illness and having to relate to each other and to each other's work. These health workers are in various degrees experienced or inexperienced. Worse yet, since many specialties are quite new, their practitioners are essentially finding their way in their work on the patient's illness.

In a very real sense, contemporary medical efforts not only are producing new chronic illnesses and phases of illness —and the associated trajectory work—but are also producing new kinds of chronically ill people. They are predominantly older persons, of course, but also include the ICN "graduates"—sometimes referred to by staff as "damaged goods"—and, in fact, people of all ages. Naturally, the interplay of life cycle and life-styles with the purely physiological conditions is immensely varied; said another way, so are the trajectories.

Trajectories, Routine and Problematic: Case Illustrations

Despite all the conditions that further the problematic character of trajectories, of course, many are relatively routine. Certain illnesses and their possible developments are well known, as are the impact of therapy and the resources and organization needed to control those illnesses. In the pages below and in later chapters, we shall be discussing trajectories that run the full range from quite routine to highly problematic—totally out of control or partly out of control. It should be useful for readers who are little acquainted with hospital work if first they are provided with some images of trajectory work through the presentation of two case illustrations drawn from our research. The commentary on these cases will be minimal, just enough to highlight a few features of trajectories and trajectory work that will be addressed in later pages.

Chapter 2

1. We begin with a case that illustrates such phenomena as: (*a*) multiple trajectories, (*b*) emergency (acute) hospital care, (*c*) initial steps in diagnosing or mapping of a major trajectory (heart failure), (*d*) the complexity of the division of labor, including that among trajectory managers as well as among various technical specialists from different departments, and (*e*) the several kinds of work involved in trajectory management.

The patient, Mr. Einshtein, was hospitalized for possible congestive heart failure. He had had a myocardial infarction eight years previously when he was 57 years old, but had since lived quite a normal life except for self-administered medication to control angina. Einshtein had recently experienced much more angina but attributed it to the action of cold weather, which had always affected him somewhat, for he had been on an extended visit to Australia during its winter season. His chronic bronchitis was also "acting up," for he was coughing up much more phlegm daily than usual. (Before hospitalization he did not realize that his increased coughing was intimately tied with a malfunctioning heart.) Ten days before hospitalization, he had a checkup by his internist who discovered, through a routine blood test, that he had mild anemia. A barium X ray was then ordered to check for possible blood loss in the colon. The internist awaited this report before moving to his next diagnostic tactic of taking a bone biopsy. Meanwhile, the internist knew that the patient had appointments the following week with both his cardiologist and his respiratory specialist. Besides the anemia, a possible cardiac flare-up, and difficulty with his lungs, Einshtein had, some months before, developed such severe neck pains that he now could only sleep sitting up, despite being put on home traction by an orthopedist.

The cardiologist and the respiratory specialist, seen on successive days, both suspected congestive heart failure (a heart "gallop" and considerable edema had now appeared) and so hospitalized him speedily. For three or four days he was given intense, virtually emergency care. A host of laboratory tests were ordered—Einshtein giving freely of blood, urine, and so on—EKGs were taken at the bedside, he was sent to be X-rayed and then for an echocardiogram procedure. Cardiologist and respiratory physician worked closely together, each in his own province, but essentially the lungs took immediate precedence. So the lung problem was attacked by giving antibiotics and by utilizing the services of physiotherapists and physical rehabilitation technicians who trooped in and out of Einshtein's room, giving mist and bronchosil treatments and pounding Einshtein's rib cage area in an effort to loosen his phlegm and clear his lungs of it. All those respiratory treatments went on undiminished—and ultimately had a successful outcome—during the two weeks of his hospitalization. After the first days of emergency treatment the respiratory physician moved into the background—the cardiologist moving into the foreground—evincing this by manner and less frequent face-to-face monitoring of the patient.

Einshtein's cardiologist was actually new to this case, had indeed never seen him until just before the hospitalization, Einshtein having switched from another cardiologist. One reason for Einshtein's choice of this cardiologist, recommended by the internist, was that he reasoned that all of his physicians (internist, cardiologist, respiratory specialists) could work together, for they were associated with the same hospital and knew one another. During the first days of hospitalization, the cardiologist awaited the results of various tests including the echogram both to verify the suspected congestive heart failure and to locate which section of the heart was most affected and with what degree of damage. He attacked the edema with a diuretic, but within three or four days changed to a second diuretic when it became clear that Einshtein's body had overreacted to the first one. Meanwhile the nurses were making frequent checks of the patient's blood pressure, which was quite low and unstable, while keeping careful watch over his urine output. When the diagnosis of congestive heart failure became clear, then the cardiologist moved to the forefront in the patient's management. He informed Einshtein of the diagnosis agreed on by all three physicians involved in the case; he put him on isodil every three hours to prevent angina and explained that a couple of days later he was going to treat the heart failure with the drug apresoline, which, by affecting the vascular system, would allow the heart to function more strongly because of the lessened resistance. He explained that if this worked, then the dosage of apresoline eventually would be increased. Patient and physician discussed the impossibility of predicting accurately "how far back" the patient would come: a wait-and-see attitude was necessary, and indeed it would be many months before the outcome would be known. The cardiologist also explained the necessity of cutting down on sodium to lessen edema and had a representative of the dietary department visit with the patient and explain the low-sodium diet.

Meanwhile, for his neck pains the patient was doing some trajectory management himself, as well as making some operational decisions, which affected at least temporarily the cardiac and lung trajectories. He requested pain medication so that he could sleep at night and was allowed it. He asked for a large chair and several pillows, and each night surprised each new night nurse by sleeping in that chair; only at the very close of his hospitalization did he discover, through experimentation, that he could now sleep fairly comfortably by raising the movable bed so that his head was about eighteen inches above normal sleeping position. Most evenings he requested back rubs from whatever nurse was on duty, and they were cheerfully given, in part no doubt because he accompanied each request with "at your convenience, when you aren't too busy."

Einshtein's pain management occasionally interfered with the respiratory management; sometimes he made choices in favor of the former at the possible expense of the latter. For instance, proper placement of his body during the rib-pounding and stimulation of his lung area called for having the lower part of his body raised above the upper part, but since this increased his neck pain markedly, he persuaded the physical therapists to do their work while he lay flat. Again, he was supposed to "posture," that is, lie on his side and cough, but sometimes he delayed posturing, or omitted it, because lying down hurt too much. Paradoxically he also learned how to attack the immediate respiratory problem—coughing up the phlegm, which was sometimes very difficult or wracked him—by putting together bits of information garnered over several days of querying the seven or eight different respiratory technicians who arrived at his bedside. Nobody thought to coach or query him about possible difficulties in coughing—he was just supposed to do it. The wracking cough, of course, interfered with the cardiac regimen of resting as much as possible, so by better management of the coughing he was, in however minor a way, contributing to better management of the cardiac trajectory.

Once he played a more prominent part in the cardiac drama. The cardiologist had cut down drastically on the diuretic dosage because it was contributing to too low a blood pressure; but hours later a nurse gave the old, stronger dosage. Einshtein, groggy at the time, did not immediately notice the familiar pill, but minutes after swallowing it queried the head nurse—who got flustered, called in the intern, who in turn apologized for the error and ordered an IV, explaining that it would be necessary now to counteract the diuretic with a twenty-four-hour intravenous drip.

About four days after hospitalization, Einshtein's internist reported the barium X ray was negative and did a bone biopsy to check out another possible source for the anemia. And he ordered iron pills to counteract the anemia. Einshtein would continue to take this medication for many months.

The internist, long familiar with his patient, assured him from time to time that the cardiologist was on top of things. The cardiologist also contributed measurably to relieving Einshtein's anxiety by relatively unhurried visits, clear explanations, and after several days by responding to questions about potential progress and limits to complete recovery, anticipated posthospital phases, expected length of the recovery period, and, during one session, about the possible effect of congestive heart failure on longevity. The cardiologist also carefully explored the patient's life-style and expressed a wait-and-see attitude about whether and how much it would have to be altered. In fact, though he did not reveal his suspicion, he had real doubts about how much recovery was possible. Einshtein discovered this only three months later through his internist who told him that the cardiologist was happily surprised at the rate and degree of recovery.

As the day of leaving the hospital approached, the cardiologist carefully explained to Einshtein the home regimen to be followed and answered questions about alternative treatments considered and reasons for discarding them; he also explained how the drug therapy would be altered depending on "how things turn out," for the next weeks would be essentially an experimental, drug-juggling period. The chief respiratory therapist turned up and talked about home mist treatments. A physical therapist taught Einshtein a set of breathing exercises. A dietician carefully explained the rules of a low-sodium diet, leaving a list of sodium values found in ordinary food and loaning a book on cooking without salt that might be useful. The intern, who had taken a deep interest in this case and clearly had been instrumental in some of the daily operational medical decision making, dropped in for a ceremonial farewell. Then Einshtein's wife, who had performed many functions while he was in the hospital and would do varied trajectory work in the months to come, called for a cab and took him home.

There he would be subject to the cardiologist's provisional program of juggling drug dosages and would carry out the respiratory regimen faithfully. As for his management of the neck pain, he asked his internist to recommend a reputable acupuncturist and switched to another orthopedist, who recommended physiotherapy. Within two months, Einshtein's neck pains had so diminished that he was finally able to posture properly and sleep lying down so that he could get the full measure of rest required by his cardiac condition.

2. Next is a case illustrating a trajectory which is highly problematic from everyone's point of view: physicians, nurses, and patient. Some features of this case that stand out are: (*a*) the multiple trajectories, (*b*) the multiplicity of trajectory managers and the confusion over coordination of their efforts, (*c*) the number of medical and technical departments drawn upon as resources, (*d*) the sheer difficulty of predicting outcomes of the medical interventions and the difficulty of deciding which to utilize, (*e*) the patient's active role both in reacting to

staff decisions and making her own daily decisions, and (*f*) the cumulative impact on everybody, including frustration because of great difficulty in gaining and maintaining control over the various courses of illness, anger and upset over the patient's "uncooperative" behavior, conflict and resulting anger among the staff members themselves, and dismay and upset over the issue of dying.

Mrs. Price, 45 years old, was hospitalized for the fourth time (Fagerhaugh and Strauss 1977). She had been diagnosed as having lupus erythematosus two years previously. As a result of her lupus, she now had (*a*) pericarditis, (*b*) pleuritis (both of which caused pain), (*c*) cerebritis, which caused some personality changes and a tendency toward tremors and convulsions, and (*d*) chronic obstructive lung disease from the lupus and her heavy smoking. As a result of the steroid treatments she also had (*e*) gastric ulcers and (*f*) cushingoid syndrome.

She was readmitted to the hospital because of continued chest pain. The lupus specialist suspected a pleuritic flare-up from the lupus and recommended hospitalization at the university hospital for reevaluation and readjustment of the steroid drugs. During her first three days of hospitalization, the house staff was busy evaluating her illness status: this involved innumerable blood studies, an electrocardiogram, and chest X rays. Meanwhile, she was having increased chest pain. By the seventh day she developed abdominal pain, which increased during the next week. All early tests for the source of that pain were negative. On the seventh day she became very nauseated. Continuous intravenous infusions were started because she was developing fluid and electrolyte imbalances. With continued nausea the house staff decided that gastric suction would relieve the discomfort, but she objected because in the past she could not tolerate the gagging caused by the tube. Therefore, antinausea drugs were added to her drug list. Dr. Ambrose, a gastrointestinal specialist, was next consulted about her abdominal pain. He suspected pancreatitis and recommended a barium X ray and gastric analysis tests. To accommodate the possibility of painful pancreatitis, extra pain drugs were ordered whenever an uncomfortable test was done.

With the appearance of numerous new symptoms the nurses began monitoring Mrs. Price's vital signs more closely. On the fourteenth day a definitive diagnosis was made: she had developed a huge gastric ulcer. A chest X ray also showed broken ribs. Both were attributed to the steroids, and yet they could not be stopped because the lupus would then get out of control. Everyone was upset by this news, as well as by the general deterioration of the patient's condition. The nursing staff had long since been upset over the patient's uncooperativeness concerning medications; indeed, some nurses recollected experiences with her during her previous hospitalizations.

Immediate treatment problems were posed. The medical choices were limited. In the patient's current physical state she was a poor surgical risk. Yet the size and location of the ulcer, unless immediately treated, had dangerous consequences: there could be erosion of the ulcer into the peritoneal cavity or it could cause pancreatitis, both potentially fatal or at least extremely painful.

Numerous specialists were consulted. After much debate, the decision was made to radiate the stomach to knock out the acid-producing cells and so prevent further extension of the ulcer. The radiation dosage would be low so that other organs would not be compromised. Concurrently, hyperalimentation treatment (special intravenous feeding through a tube placed in the subclavian vein, located in the neck) would be started to overcome malnutrition. The physicians explained to the patient the limited choices, why the treatments were necessary, and that the radiation dosage would be extremely low. Mrs. Price agreed reluctantly because she was very frightened of the radiation; later she wanted to stop it but was finally talked into continuing it by her husband, who was a physician.

In the ensuing twelve days, her nausea increased and she had several days of diarrhea, each related to the radiation. She would frequently resist the treatment, either because she felt too ill or because she doubted the wisdom of the therapy. Some days she would be persuaded by the staff, but increasingly she resisted. Or she would agree in the morning but change her mind in the afternoon. Finally the staff in desperation gave her intravenous tranquilizers just prior to the test to make her sleepy and less resistant.

Over the weeks innumerable specialists streamed in and out with no one person coordinating the patient's care. After considerable discussion, pushed by the house staff, a decision was reached: house staff and the gastrointestinal specialist would together be the major coordinators, and all new orders issued by the attending staff would be discussed first with the house staff. The nursing staff sighed in relief because at least the "mess" would be under control. However, the coordination continued to break down from time to time. One physician in particular would telephone the nursing desk with orders based on his past experiences with the patient. This created much tension within the house medical staff.

Blood studies next indicated a low hemoglobin count as a result of the ulcers as well as the lupus; a blood transfusion was given. The nurses were becoming increasingly weary of daily hassles with the patient who wished to delay various treatments.

On the twenty-seventh day the patient developed tremors of the hands and legs. She became very anxious since this was seen as a possible forerunner to convulsion, but because of her great anxiety the staff had difficulty making an assessment of her actual condition. They decided to wait and see. Mrs. Price thought immediate action was called for and again phoned an attending physician who ordered drugs without consulting the house staff, which angered them. The tremors did subside a few days later.

Because of continued nausea, all drugs were administered by injections—some thirty a day. The injection sites were becoming fibrous knots and so the nurses were concerned not only about the poor drug absorption but also about the possibility of infections because of the high steroid dose.

On the thirtieth day, Mrs. Price developed joint pains and swelling of her hands, elbows, feet, and knees—all symptoms of lupus. The steroids were adjusted. In a few days the symptoms subsided. On the forty-first day, X rays showed no decrease in her ulcer's size. There was much troubled discussion among the staff. The patient was blamed for her uncooperativeness in taking the antacids and for her chain smoking, which had increased the gastric secretions. The patient, of course, was very upset. She remarked to the researcher: "I knew all along the radiation wouldn't work. All I probably got out of the radiation is kidney damage."

During the next days there was much discussion about the next course of treatment until a decision was reached: the only alternative was a subtotal or total gastric resection. There were surgical risks but without intervention there would be danger of peritonitis or pancreatitis and hemorrhage. With surgery she might live several more years. She was informed of the recommendation, the staff realizing her decision to accept surgery would be a difficult one.

For the next three weeks, she agonized over whether or not to have the surgery. Her husband thought it the only alternative. The psychiatrist thought that the patient, if discharged home, would "drive the husband crazy" and that she would not consent to a nursing home. So surgery, the staff reasoned, should be done.

Over the next days the patient talked about dying to her husband, to the psychiatrist, and to the social researcher. The three had many discussions among themselves about her sad dilemma and how to help her. The staff now had difficulty in talking about as well as interacting with her.

By the fifty-eighth day, she was wavering on whether to have the gastric surgery, though it was becoming more evident it was required. She frequently stated now that she had been saved from death twice and didn't know if she wanted to be saved again. She would take her chances with no surgery and so hemorrhage and die. She was weary of all the uncertainty and the pain. She was talking more about wanting to commit suicide, too. The psychiatrist consulted with a suicide expert, who thought the probability of her seriously considering suicide was low; still the staff could not dismiss this possibility. As a precaution, her clothes were taken home and money and drugs were removed from her purse because she was talking about taking a taxi and jumping off the bridge.

On the sixty-seventh day the X rays showed an increase in the size of the ulcers. There was total agreement among the physicians, including the psychiatrist, that a gastrectomy was required and should occur while the lupus was stable. For the next seven days she agonized over whether to have a gastrectomy. The surgeons and psychiatrist tried to answer as best they could any questions she might have. She consulted other attending physicians. They all agreed a gastrectomy was essential. Her husband backed them. A relative also persuaded her the surgery would be the only solution. She finally signed the consent slip for surgery. She was transferred to a gastrointestinal surgical unit. The surgery was successful, and the patient was weaned finally from the hard drugs but not without considerable interactional difficulties between staff and her. Indeed, the purely physiological (surgical-pain trajectory) orientation of the surgical staff maximized the interactional difficulties. On the one hundred and twelfth day, she was discharged, free of her ulcers but, of course, still having to live with her lupus.

Control and Contingency

It is the interplay between efforts to control illness and contingencies, whether expected or not, that make for the specific details of various trajectories. Only under quite routine conditions is control over the medical process and product like that exerted over industrial processes. Although the latter can be tremendously complicated in sequence and great in range of resources and division of labor utilized, nevertheless, once the trial-and-error period of "working out the bugs" is completed, then the number and range of interfering or upsetting contingencies are minimal. Managing illness trajectories is more like the work of Mark Twain's celebrated Mississippi River pilot: the river was tricky, changed its course slightly from day to day, so even an experienced, but inattentive pilot could run into grave difficulties; worse yet, sometimes the river drastically shifted in its bed for some miles into quite a new course. As Mrs. Price's case illustrates, the physician's and staff's management may be even more complex and the outcome of their work even more fateful than the pilots. Some of the various contingencies may be anticipated, but only a portion of them may be relatively controllable, while some contingencies are quite unforeseeable, stemming as they do not only from the illnesses themselves but from organizational sources. In some instances, contingencies may also stem from sources external to the hospital.

As the pages below will suggest, a helpful image of what goes on with relatively problematic trajectories is this: efforts to keep the trajectory on a more or less controllable course look somewhat gyroscopic. Like that instrument, they do not necessarily spin upright but, meeting contingencies, they may swing off dead center—off course—for a while before getting righted again, but only perhaps to repeat going awry one or more times before the game is over. Sometimes, though, the trajectory game finishes with a total collapse of control, quite like the gyroscope falling to the ground.

At any rate, the interplay between control and contingency challenges the very idea of illness (and trajectory) management per se. As a term, "management" does not catch anything like the full complexity of this work, its medical outcome, or the consequences for all who are working at it. For that reason, we need to add to management two other ideas. One is that "managing" the problematic trajectories is better understood as "shaping" them, that is, handling the contingencies as best one can, although being far from fully in control of the trajectory. (This point will be discussed again later.) The second idea is that trajectories are also experienced. Unless we are inclined to think only of the social and psychological impact on patients and kin, it is necessary to recognize that staff members can be affected profoundly by their work on particular trajectories. Together the three terms, managing, shaping, and experiencing, give a much more adequate picture of what happens when trajectories are complex and problematic.

Diagnosis and the Trajectory Scheme

Diagnosis is the health professional's term for the beginnings of trajectory work. To do anything effective, other than just treat symptoms, the illness has to be identified. Once that is accomplished, the physician has an imagery of the potential course of the illness without medical intervention. The physician also has a mapping of what the interventions might be, what might happen if they are effective, and what resources are required to make them. In effect, he has then what might usefully be termed a *trajectory scheme*. This may not be filled out in all its details—probably it rarely is—but it does involve an imagery of sequences of potential events and anticipatable actions.

The point can be brought home by remarking that twenty-five years ago one of the authors of this book, while making field observations of physicians in a teaching hospital, noted that with difficult cases they frequently were not prepared to make definitive diagnoses, but would say, "we will wait and see"—that is, wait until more symptoms had appeared that would fall into a more interpretable gestalt. Then they would know what they were dealing with and what sequences of actions they needed to take. Physicians still do this, despite the enormous increase in the diagnostic means available and the great improvements in their effectiveness in specifying a patient's illness and the current phase of its developing course. Such improved diagnostic means allow for greatly improved *locating* of the specific illness and the *mapping* of anticipatable tasks.

The initial diagnostic work is, of course, only the beginning of the trajectory work. Chronic illnesses often insure that the first phases in trajectory work are done by patients themselves. Characteristically they notice certain new occurrences affecting their bodies, often disregard these for a time, and then, growing concerned or alarmed, they visit a physician. The latter may offer a tentative diagnosis, or an incorrect diagnosis, or even decide "nothing is really wrong," or counsel a wait-and-see period. Continued symptoms may lead the physician to consultations with colleagues but alternatively may lead the unsatisfied patient to make the rounds of several physicians (and/or alternative care practitioners) in search of a diagnosis with associated therapy that can control the disease or at least its symptoms. (Hence the anger evidenced by patients whose cancers or other illnesses had been fatefully misdiagnosed by one or more physicians before correct identification.) A *diagnostic search* of varying duration, then, made by either patient or physician can sometimes precede a diagnosis upon which everyone agrees.

The difference between the patient and the physician is that the latter has more experience both in diagnostic search and in judging the reliability of his diagnostic means. In urban centers today, physicians may need to be very careful in assessing that reliability, since clinical laboratories, X-ray centers, and the like may vary in the quality of their work. Thus, an experienced and skeptical oncologist:

> I think you just learn to know who you can trust. Who overreads, who underreads. I have got X rays all over town, so I've had the chance to do it. I know that when Schmidt at Palm Hospital says, "There's a suspicion of a

> tumor in this chest," it doesn't mean much because she, like I, sees tumors everywhere. She looks under her bed at night to make sure there's not some cancer there. When Jones at the same institution reads it and says, "There's a suspicion of a tumor there," I take it damn seriously because if he thinks it's there, by God it probably is. And you do this all over town. Who do you have confidence in and who none.

But the diagnostic reliability is not at all foolproof, and physicians who are increasingly at the mercy of the work of the clinical laboratory workers and other diagnostic technicians do not necessarily find it easy to judge their diagnostic reliability; nor because of their own busy practices do they have sufficient time to judge that reliability accurately. Asked by the researcher how a physician can judge the results of a CAT scanner, the physician quoted above answered:

> I don't believe them anyway: I see them all myself. I make them show me. And even so, not being an expert in it, they can pull the wool right over my eyes. But at least I've seen the actual readout they get from the scanner. Most guys don't have the time to do that, or make the time. I think you tend to take what you get. Though they can become expert enough to know when somebody's saying, "I think this is bigger." This takes a lot of time, it really does, to spend the time to go over them.

The question of laboratory or technician error, then, is at least occasionally a real possibility. Error may arise not only from misinterpretation, but from machine error, too, since some machines at least have to be calibrated carefully or the test results that they produce may be inaccurate. (See chap. 3 and 4.) Moreover, while a physician obviously can rely on the laboratory not to err in sending the right report for the right patient, he cannot always be absolutely certain. There is some irony, then, associated with today's diagnostic procedures, since the very increase in resources for diagnostic accuracy has made the physician more dependent on those resources for accuracy in interpreting and reporting test results.

It is worth noting, too, that with chronic illness, diagnostic locating and mapping do not necessarily occur just once, at the outset of therapy. Quite aside from monitoring an illness and the effect of interventions—phenomena to be discussed later—the physician may believe an illness is relatively in check. Later, the appearance of other symptoms may be read by him or another physician as requiring a new diagnosis, involving another illness, or forcing him into a diagnostic search that leads eventually to rediagnosis of the original illness.

> I've got a patient who had a melanoma four years ago, which was excised from his nose. Then about a year later it recurred in a node in his neck. It was a bad form of a bad tumor. Yet going over it, we wouldn't find any evidence it had spread at all. Seven months ago he developed a pain in his back, and his doctor saw him, and because of his history of cancer got some X rays of his spine, but found nothing. And he developed all the symptoms of a disk, was put on bed rest and got better, then finally got worse again. Eventually, not as soon as one might have hoped, but eventually, he came for a bone scan, and the scan showed a red-hot lesion in his sacrum. It was very hard for them to believe that meant cancer, except that's really what it means. Unless you've got a clear-cut fracture. So they took tomograms of it and showed destruction of a couple of the bony processes of the sacrum. He's got a metastic melanoma. Well, the state of the art is such that if they had not really been very reluctant to find out that this guy had cancer, they'd have done a bone scan six months ago and found the cancer.

However, even if this oncologist had been seeing the patient regularly, a kind of rediagnosis would have been attempted once suspicious symptoms appeared or old ones increased: the physician needs to know just where the disease course is now.

This suggests, in fact, that even for the initial diagnosis many chronic illnesses require not only that an identification be definitive but also that the *location* along the course of the disease be made as specific as possible: Where is the lesion, tumor, or deterioration of vertebrae? What kind? How large or how much? Impinging on what? Remaining static or getting worse? And at what rate? Such questions hint at an additional paradox that attends the diagnostic search. Often the physician now enjoys multiple options for getting the desired diagnostic specificity. But some tests cost more, cause the patient more pain or discomfort, are potentially more dangerous, or are of still debatable efficacy. The physician will balance those considerations and what they mean for the patient against the generalized rule that the more specific a diagnosis, the more potentially effective can be the prescribed treatment.

For the sociologist, the medical term "treatment"—based on diagnosis—translates into a plan of action involving: (1) things to be done to control present or anticipatable developments in the disease course (X-ray treatment, use of specific medications, EKG monitoring, blood pressure monitoring, types of surgical intervention) and (2) those things to be done in some sort of sequence (3) by specified or assumed kinds of personnel (even by specifically designated persons). This is the *trajectory scheme* touched on earlier: it includes not only the physician's visualization of potential disease developments, but also foreseeable actions in relation to those events. Implicit, and sometimes explicit, in that visualization is the coordination of those actions, which usually involve many different kinds of technicians and specialists, and often several different hospital departments.

Complexities of Organizing Therapeutic Action

The complexities of organizing therapeutic action derive mainly from two sources. The first is the problematic character of so many trajectories. As will be noted directly below, if the illness course is well understood and no untoward contingencies arise, then the stereotypical picture of a single physician instituting therapeutic plans and having them carried out successfully is a realistic picture. If the trajectory is problematic, however, then that classic image of medical work can be very far from accurate. The second source for the complexities of therapeutic action is the number and range of tasks *as well as* the organization of those tasks, so that even relatively routine expectable trajectories can develop unanticipated complexities around organizational issues. These, in turn, can profoundly affect the organization and efficacy of therapeutic action. In the next pages, some of these complexities will be discussed.

Trajectory management is relatively routine for courses of illness that turn out to be relatively standard—they are all well known and the physician and staff members have had much experience with them. Hospital wards are equipped to handle routine cases with some efficiency, using standard operating procedure: the needed machinery is on the ward, the desired medications are on hand or easily obtainable, the nursing staff understand the procedures, and the head nurse has had much experience in coordinating the scheduling and timing of various resources or services needed from other departments. Indeed each ward tends to have what we would term its characteristic "shape" (Strauss, Schatzman, Bucher, Ehrlich, and Sabshin 1964*a*), for it has its characteristic types of illness, which are handled there—and though complex, the requisite tasks are well understood and their larger organization relatively worked out. An example would be a recovery room for postcardiac surgical patients, where the latter are initially in parlous conditions, where the clusters of tasks require highly skilled nursing and physician staff, but where the routines are well laid out even for handling emergencies and the organization for all that is nicely coordinated. The chief physician, as the main trajectory manager, can count on all that organizational machinery for handling—hopefully without undue hitches—anticipatable routine cases, through the first days of postsurgical recovery. By contrast, if a patient is placed on a ward into whose shape he does not fit at all—that is, the staff have little or no experience with his illness, have no experience with the equipment used on him or with medications ordered for him—then the routine trajectory turns into a nonroutine and, also, often highly problematic one. Worse yet, difficult cases become even more problematic under these "out-of-shape" conditions.

Cases that are, on diagnosis, viewed as potentially problematic will require a more complicated order of task organization and coordination. To begin with, the physician may not be able to foresee clearly the course that the illness will take, or perhaps its rate of development, with or without medical intervention. Or the disease course may be relatively recognizable, but the impact of experimental drugs or procedures (old ones not being effective) are not well known. He can, however, visualize some of the tasks to be done and rely on the ward personnel to carry them out, but they and he know or suspect that other resources (specialists, departments, treatments) may have to be called upon as unanticipated developments occur to supplement the more usual standard operating procedure of the ward. In extreme cases (as with Mrs. Price) whole clusters and sequences of tasks are unanticipated, and a great deal of ad hoc organization is required to get them decided upon and to get them done.

To back up a bit, however, the initial diagnosis leads the physician in charge of the case to considerations of medical intervention, of treatment. Here again, modern medical technology—however "halfway"—is likely to offer several initial *therapeutic options*. Breast cancer, for instance, can be treated with surgery, radiation, or chemotherapy, and there are several types of each; they can be used singly, in combination, and in different sequences. Which options to choose? The physician's experience may lead him to one choice or another; so may his medical or social ideologies; his set of beliefs about surgery or particular kinds of surgery, or about various drugs or machine treatment, or his more socially tinged convictions about womanhood and about sexual relations. Considerations of cost, convenience, availability, speed of impact, skill, risk, discomfort, and psychological impact on the patient will also be balanced.

In managing more-or-less standard cases, the physician will not need to search for viable options, since he will know most of them. For more problematic cases, he may institute a *search for options* other than those he has already had experience with, utilizing literature and collegial consultations. House staff may be involved in both the search and the decisions about which options shall be tried. Typically the physician will anticipate certain outcomes from medical interventions, some undesirable (drug side effects), and will alert the nursing and physician house staff to monitor for those effects and, if they appear, to stand ready with countermeasures.

There may also arise, however, some of those unanticipated contingencies discussed earlier. When they appear, the responsible physician may not have ready options to utilize as countermeasures. Again, he may institute a search for options, or house staff (even nursing staff) may press alternative courses of action on him. So while one physician may make the *option decision*, others may also be involved in that decision. Moreover, at these unexpected *option points* whoever is present may sometimes need to make strictly *operational decisions*, needing to choose one or another option quickly, without consulting the physician—providing that the danger to the patient is perceived as great and immediate. In that event, the trajectory management is further diluted or, necessarily, shared. (One example is the incident in the Einshtein case, when the cardiac patient discovered the nurse's error concerning his diuretic medication, alerting then the head nurse, who in turn called the intern, who made a quick decision to counter the potentially dangerous contingency with an intravenous drip.)

Each new contingency, whether large or small, requires some choice of alternative lines of action in order to get the trajectory into the best possible manageable order, that is, to keep the gyroscopic shaping of the trajectory as successful as possible. Again, we say "trajectory" rather than simply refer to the illness course, because so much more is involved than the illness itself. For example, the physician may not only order a procedure changed but request that a specific skilled person carry it out. Moreover, at crucial option points, several persons with somewhat different stakes in the case may be weighing, and pressing their respective views on, various possible options.

One important implication of that last sentence is that, under conditions of contemporary hospital practice, it is not always a simple matter to say who is in charge of managing the trajectory. In routine cases, the principal physician is primarily responsible for visualizing the trajectory: for ordering, evaluating, and acting on diagnostic tests; for laying out the lines of work that need to be done; for utilizing the ward's organizational machinery. When the course of illness becomes problematic, however, when things get out of hand, when other physiological systems go awry, when other chronic illnesses impinge on the primary one—and even begin to take priority—then the trajectory management begins to get shared with other medical specialists. And as the case of Mrs. Price has illustrated, these specialists may disagree or their orders may conflict, so that problems of coordination can play havoc with house staff and, not incidentally, also with patient care. Lack of coordination amounts to a blurring of the division of labor, with untoward consequences then flowing from unclear or disagreed upon conceptions of responsibility.

On the other hand, the specialists may work well together, sharing in the *shaping* of the trajectory. It is important to understand that with complex trajectories, this shaping, which involves a complicated division of labor, may be parceled out not only among several specialists, including a psychiatrist, but may also involve the efforts of kin. Patients themselves may enter this process at key option points, entering as intensely interested parties or being invited in by the physicians, who may even press them to make certain decisions when the options are very risky, or their potential psychological or biographical impact is great. But they may enter as intensely interested parties who weigh the option criteria differently from the physicians. Their own option searches may lead them to propose and even to insist on consideration of alternative options (see chap. 9). One patient with severe respiratory disease whom we followed closely in and out of the hospital was astonishingly and successfully assertive in his own trajectory management, pressing his physician repeatedly on all kinds of issues, but one of his major controlling strategies was to know the whole range of pharmaceutical possibilities and to utilize them with or without his physician's knowledge.

An additional complication is that precedence in the trajectory management is directly affected by the existence of multiple illnesses. As the case of Mr. Einshtein illustrated, when the lungs were under control and the cardiac condition was specifically diagnosed, then the management shifted from respiratory to cardiac specialist, while the internist stayed in the background managing the minor and noninterfering condition of anemia. If, however, the illness that brought the patient into the hospital affects another—or starts another—then the first can drop into a position of secondary importance, at least for a while, the other taking precedence. Usually this means that the chief trajectory manager, until illness priorities change again, will be another medical specialist.

One feature of highly problematic trajectories, especially when there are several deeply interested parties or even trajectory managers, is what might be called *trajectory debates*, which involve not merely technical but also ideological issues. As the trajectory (or trajectories) goes badly awry, many voices are heard, some soto voce, but some loud and clear, expressing different views on why the illness is out of hand, why the new symptoms or illness have appeared, what alternative lines of action ought to be taken, who ought to be brought into the act and who pulled out, and so on. In every highly problematic trajectory whose unfolding we have watched over the years, we have observed this kind of debate, exemplified, of course, by Mrs. Price's case. The debate encompasses not only the medical specialists, but most of the ward's personnel—sometimes right down to the nursing aides who may express themselves publicly, too—and the arguments and attempt at persuasion take place in conferences, at the nursing desk, in the corridors, and inevitably, since the patient is involved, passionate arguments occur in the sick person's room, too. Since particular decisions about options at critical points can profoundly affect the shape of the trajectory (and the patient's life!), it is worth thinking of those decisions as, in the profoundest sense, potentially very fateful. A poignant scene drawn from our field notes should make this point graphically and, not incidentally, illustrate how some of the operational decisions made on the floor can be quite invisible to the main physician himself. The action takes place on a cardiac recovery ward; the central figure is an elderly, very ill, lady scheduled for surgery the next day.

> She is now sitting up in bed, glasses on her nose, writing on a clipboard, absorbed in her writing, struggling with it. Her daughter is at her right, helping to hold the clipboard. The physician is at her left, the nurse hovering. When the patient finishes writing, the nurse takes the clipboard and puts it on the bedside table. As she leaves the room, I follow her and ask what this scene is all about. The nurse draws me further into the hall, and with some passion tells me the patient has been facing whether to die or to go through another operation. She has had three previously. (She is now bleeding into her lung.) The nurse had told her that it was her own option to decide. Now the daughter is angry at the nurse for saying that; but the nurse questions whether it makes sense for the patient to go on. She added that I could see the patient's note later if I wished. It said approximately that: I have decided to die. It's up to God. Doctor Smith says that I have only a fifty-fifty chance, and that makes no sense.
>
> Then I glanced back into the patient's room. The daughter and the physician were still at the bedside in their respective positions. The patient was looking from one face to the other, but had now agreed to the operation (the daughter had persuaded her), smiling through her tears at the physician. Both he and the daughter then disappeared down the hall together.

> Then a young resident began to enter the room, saying something to the nurse. She swept him back into the hall. He said the tube now in her is not long enough to reach her lungs; that the blood then will flow from one lung to another. He wanted to put a new tube in. The nurse angrily said "no," that this woman had just been through "a dramatic scene." Nothing doing! The resident then said at least they could shove the tube down a bit further, since there was about one centimeter left, and that could make the difference. He led her over to the X ray to show her the patient's film and to point out that if they didn't get the tube lower, the right lung would look like the left lung before tomorrow's operation, if there was one. She reluctantly agreed.
>
> Immediately after, the nurse having cued the resident to the patient's live-or-die dilemma, the two of them entered her room and stood opposite each other at the bedside. The nurse said gently but passionately to the patient that the decision was up to *her*; and the young physician agreed. . . . The next afternoon when I returned to the ward, the nurse said sadly that the patient had died in surgery.

The drama reflected in the field note concerns dying, but, of course, many decisions concerning the choice of options do not actually confront that dire issue. Yet those choices represent a fateful shaping of the trajectory and ultimately may have profound impact on the patient's life. In seeking to control highly problematic trajectories, the very choice of some options early in the trajectory closes off others, leading to developments that force confrontation with other sets of options, whose selection again may later foreclose on options that might earlier have been feasible. The biographical and medical consequences may be momentous.

Now, we shall conclude this section on the complexities of organizing therapeutic action by reiterating that for even relatively unproblematic trajectories, let alone highly problematic ones, the term *shaping* is quite as applicable as managing the trajectory. A single physician may, in fact, hold fast to the managerial helm, handling the case in a very organized and brilliant fashion. Nevertheless, because (1) he is not doing all the work himself and because (2) the work involves the organization of countless tasks, it follows that even the principal trajectory manager is supplemented by numerous other persons (including patient and kin) who are helping to shape the full evolution of the trajectory. Some patients elect to die rather than struggle on and others can in an emergency prevent their own immediate deaths because they know their own physiological reactions and the personnel do not. (We observed this once.) These are simply dramatic instances of how trajectories get shaped rather than simply managed.

While the more technical management entails primarily medical and organizational skills, the total range of trajectory work requires different additional types of work that help to shape the entire trajectory. Each of these types of work will be discussed in later chapters, but first it will be useful to look at trajectories in terms of the *clusters and sequences of tasks* that constitute the details of trajectory work. One ought not to be unduly surprised if the discussion is reminiscent of the Shakespearean "For want of a nail, a horse. . . . a kingdom was lost," since tasks can pile on tasks and errors or failures that require additional corrective tasks can occur significantly at any point (see chap. 13). The next pages, then, will focus on more microscopic details of trajectory work, touching also on the variants of work involved other than the purely medical and technical. They will also bring out some of the organizational underpinnings necessary for carrying out that work and those tasks.

Trajectory Phases, Arc of Work, and Task Sequences

Since trajectories extend over time, they have *phases*. The physician's and staff's trajectory scheme includes visualization of some of those phases—more accurately for routine than for problematic trajectories. When the trajectory manager anticipates these phases, he or she has in mind certain things that will need to be done per phase, beginning with the diagnostic period and moving along through various therapeutic steps. The physician in his or her trajectory scheme visualizes what might be termed an *arc of work*, that is, the overall work that needs to be done to control the illness course and get the patient back into good enough shape to go home. The arc of work may not be completely visualized by the physician, and, indeed, the physician may hold in abeyance precisely what further work is required until after initial steps are done, until "we see how things work out"—until the actual phases are known. Under those conditions, the total arc of work will evolve more slowly, as the trajectory manager senses or calculates what needs to be done next. And in problematic trajectories that go quite awry, even temporarily out of control, the total sequencing of work may be known only after the case is finished. (The case of Mrs. Price exemplifies the evolution of unanticipated phases, unanticipated sequences of work, and an arc of work that could only be known post hoc.)

At any rate, during each phase it will be decided that certain things need to be done: monitor cardiac output, get another X ray, continue the dialysis sessions, monitor the postsurgical condition, and so on. Any point at which it is decided to do those things we call a *trajectory sequence point.* The term is apt because at each point a different cluster of tasks is required; they will change partially or totally at the next sequence point. But the term is less important than our recognition that the cluster of tasks (E. C. Hughes [1971] calls them "bundles of tasks") have both a sequential ordering *and* an organizational base that allows their being carried out.

The physician ordinarily does not concern himself with the organizational and operational details of carrying out the orders, the supervision and articulation of those tasks fall under the province of various technicians and nurses and, where specialized tasks are done, such as X ray or brain scanning, other medical specialists. If there is some defect in organizational arrangements, then there will be difficulty in adhering to the sequence and its timing, as will be illustrated below. The resource base includes the proper skills, a sufficient work force, appropriate equipment, necessary drugs, enough time, and so on. Some of the resources will be allocated to and found on the ward itself; others must be drawn from other departments and sometimes from outside the hospital itself, like repair services for equipment or the electricity to run equipment.

To give some concreteness to the foregoing abstract statements and to convey additional points that pertain to organizational functioning, we present four short case histories with an accompanying commentary. They will bring out some of the diverse and interlocking types of work involved in trajectory work.

1. *Cardiac Recovery Ward.* In the cardiac recovery ward, there are eight rooms, one patient per room, one highly skilled nurse per patient. Backup support is provided by readily available house staff (residents and interns) and attending physicians on call. All rooms are equipped with multiple machines. Machines are for sustaining life (IVs, respirators), for monitoring (TV screen and recording of cardiac functioning), for comfort care and prevention (mobile mattress, cooling machine for mattress), for therapy (postoperative blood purifier), and so on. There are ample supplies of medications on the ward as well as various kinds of supplies for immediate use. A bioengineer calibrates machines each day and is on call for emergencies. There is regular servicing of machines both in-house and by machine company representatives. Extra equipment is stockpiled in case a machine breaks down.

The major function of work on this ward is to get the patients through the critical three to four post-op days, keeping their potentially hazardous trajectories on course. The trajectory phasing has miniphases to which the nurses are sensitively cued. Patients are mostly unconscious, and so patient reactions to the work and their participation in it are absent. Also biographical work, taking into account their life histories and concerns, is at a minimum for the staff. Kin are scarcely in evidence except at short visiting hours, so their participation in patient care is also minimal at this phase of the trajectory.

Comfort care is important but subordinate to survival tasks. Psychological care is also subordinate but somewhat visible in and around the more medical tasks. The nurse does a great deal of machine monitoring, too, making certain that the machines are working correctly, that connections are secure, and so on. Body monitoring is done with the monitoring machines, but a major part of body monitoring is done by the nurses through their own observations and perceptions.

> I watched nurse T. working today for about an hour with a patient who was only four hours post-op. In general the work was mixed. She changed the blood transfusion bag. She milked it down, and took out an air bubble. Later she changed it again. Later got the bottle part filled through mechanical motion. She drew blood and immediately put back new blood into the tube. She milked the urine tube once. She took a temperature. She put a drug injection into the tube leading to the patient's neck. She added potassium solution to the nonautomated IV. But all the while she had in focus, though not necessarily glancing directly at, the TV, which registered EKG and blood pressure readings. Once she punched the computer button to get the fifteen-minute readout on cardiac functioning. And once she milked the infection-purifier tube leading from the patient's belly. And periodically she marked down both readings and some of what she had done. Once the patient stirred as she was touching his arm: she said quite nicely then that she was about to give him an injection that would relax him. He indicated that he heard. Another time she noticed him stirring and switched off the light above his head, saying to him, "that's better, isn't it?" At one point she decided that his blood pressure was not dropping rapidly enough and told the resident, suggesting they should do something; he hesitated, she kept nudging, until he went into action; said he did not like the drug she had suggested. So he named another with which she was not familiar. He brought in a medical reference book, consulted it, neither knew whether the drug involved an injection or an IV, but then he discovered it has a ten-minute action, "so it can't be an IV." She got the drug, injected it. The resident gazed at the TV

> screen for about five minutes, then announced to the nurse, "its working." Meanwhile, she had been doing her series of tasks again around and with the patient.

Notable in the nurse's work is that there are clusters of tasks, done perhaps in flexible sequence but repeated serially every half hour or so. And depending on the miniphase and the nurse's judgments, her work can be slowed or speeded up. The intervals between the series of task sequences are important since they allow her to confer with the charge nurse and with the house staff and to get some relief from the otherwise continuous intense work.

During these postsurgical phases, the staff's most salient work with these patients is that of clinical safety. The intense monitoring of the patient's condition during each miniphase of the trajectory, the almost continuous focus on the TV screen, and the constant alertness to any difficulty with the respiratory machine, which is breathing for the patient, all speak volumes about the centrality of clinical safety tasks (see chap. 4).

In doing these tasks, the nurse or physician is implicitly as much focused on trajectory considerations as with the more obvious work itself. Albeit at particular moments a specific task may absorb attention, the patient's location on a hazardous trajectory is never quite forgotten. Unlike an X ray or an EKG technician, who may see a patient only once and who probably is not much concerned with trajectory considerations but only with the immediate tasks at hand, the cardiac recovery unit personnel are involved in a work situation wherein tasks and trajectory considerations are fused. To quote one nurse: "You are thinking about a lot of things, making sure they all come out right and on time." "Things" means tasks, and "time" means trajectory miniphase.

2. *Catheterization Laboratory*. Catheterization of the heart, a highly complex diagnostic procedure, seeks detailed information about cardiac damage. In the catheterization laboratory there is a massing of resources: equipment, medications, skilled personnel, and the like. Equipment includes an electronic monitor, a computer, an X-ray camper with control machines, video monitors, tape recorders, a power dye injector, machines to measure cardiac output, machinery for processing the film from the monitoring equipment, and so on. Supplies for all this machinery are kept nearby and are purchased by the department itself; the technicians share the responsibility of keeping the shelves stocked. The physicians employ a wide range of skills during the catheterization. The technicians have a year's training and

additional training on the job; their work requires close attention, ears and eyes attuned to the constant beeping of the monitors and the EKG images on the oscilloscope. Their work is tense, stressful. Besides running the equipment, adjusting it, and constantly calibrating it, they also prepare the catheterization room and prepare the patients, recording on clipboards during the procedure the time of each injection or drug dose, its amount, and so on. They also assist the physicians during the procedure. They develop film that has recorded the patients' responses on a monitoring machine. For all the staff, there is a high risk from scattered radiation, so all are conscientious about proper protection. There is also maximal attention to keeping everything sterile since the risks of the catheterization to the patient are very high. Speed of procedure is important because of the risk factor and, of course, so is accuracy.

Utilitization of the total set of procedures differs, depending on the patient's condition. Decisions are made individually for each patient. If a patient appears to be having difficulty, one or more of the multiple tests may be eliminated. During the sequence of complicated, risky procedures, the patient does much work: lying still, holding breath, not coughing, coughing on instruction to eject dye from the heart. The patient's composure work (see chap. 6) may be considerable; for instance, sometimes a piece of equipment fails to work for a while, and procedures are then delayed. The staff does composure work, too, in an effort to remain calm and project an image of efficiency and trustworthiness. If something goes wrong, they try to keep the patient unaware of that fact.

Here is a bit of interaction exemplifying the division of labor, the patient's part in it, and composure work. The interaction also reflects something of the sequence of tasks.

> They were now doing the angiography, each time telling the patient to take a deep breath and hold, now breathe and cough. (A physician explained to me later that "this is when the patient can go into cardiac arrest; there is only dye in the heart, no blood; momentarily the vessel is occluded." The cough pushes out the dye each time that a picture is taken.) It is necessary to rotate the patient for different shots. . . . The procedure was continuing: X-ray shots controlled by the technician from two big machines, the physician controlling the injections and the timing of the shots. Each time a technician or physician says "breathe and cough." Next they gave the patient nitroglycerin, asking the patient which strength he was used to. Another technician reports "87, stable, pressure looks good."

Another machine is rolled up to measure intracardiac pressure; they give the patient another pill.

A word about the sequence of the tasks: in general there is a rough sequence of things to be done, beginning before the patient is actually in the catheterization room, for example, the physician readying the medical records, the technicians readying the machinery, the ward nurses scheduling the catheterization and perhaps preparing the patient psychologically, the patient doing likewise, the transport personnel taking the patient down for catheterization. During the diagnostic session itself, there is a sequence of tasks, but these are somewhat flexible depending on which tests are done and in what order. Moreover, the staff is prepared for machine breakdown, which does happen sometimes. There are not only delays but some shifting of *task sequencing* and additional clusters of tasks to be performed (see chap. 3).

Unlike the cardiac recovery unit, with its intense focus on survival medical and nursing care, the work here is all in the service of diagnosing precisely the location of cardiac damage. Since risk to the patient of the diagnostic procedures is high, there is quite literally embedded in the medical and technical work the demanding requirement that carrying out those tasks be clinically as safe as possible. We call this latter, *clinical safety work*, and, of course, it involves tasks, too (see chap. 4). Bits and pieces of those tasks can be seen in the description above: the physician's decision to omit certain tests or to delay slightly certain procedures until he is certain of the patient's immediate physiological reactions, the tense attention of physician and technicians to many tasks, reflecting not just their concern for diagnostic accuracy but for upcoming danger, and, of course, the careful monitoring of the patient's physiological condition. The other salient type of work, of course, is composure work—everybody is working very hard to make certain that no breakdown of composure occurs, for that would interfere with the primary diagnostic work (see chap. 6).

As in the post-op work of the preceding case, focus is very much on the immediate tasks, on the work to be done, but again, the patient's trajectory is very much in the foreground of attention. For one thing, the diagnostic focus is on locating precisely the kind of trajectory this patient is on and where he or she is on it; for another, the potential danger of catheterization itself is related to the patient's cardiac condition. So, again, work and trajectory are tightly linked.

3. *Misorganization of a Spinal Scan.* In contrast to the two smoothly functioning and organizationally successful types of activities depicted above, the next situation, which also involves diagnosis, exemplifies faulty organization in sequencing the tasks. The result is a setback in

the patient's trajectory. Previous therapeutic action is at least partly undone, and the patient would have faced even worse consequences except for a supplementary factor in the division of labor: a knowledgeable and aggressive kinsman.

> An eighty-year-old woman had been hospitalized for very severe back pain, eventually relieved by a combination of medication and the use of a cutaneous stimulator. Since she could not be relatively mobile, a diagnostic scan of her spine was ordered. The patient was transported by a gurney to the radiology department. Unfortunately, there was an unanticipated delay because another patient got higher priority since his case was an emergency. Waiting there a full hour, the elderly lady became quite cold and developed severe back pain again. A daughter who had accompanied her to the radiology department finally found an unidentified hospital worker and requested some blankets. Covered with them, the mother, now in considerable pain, was transported back to her bed.
>
> There the nurses rushed into the breech with pain medication and heating pads. Immediately thereafter dinner was served, but the patient being in such pain could not yet eat. Right on the heels of the delivery of the food came the transport man, wheeling his gurney into the room. The daughter asked him to hold off for a while until her mother felt better. When she did, then again covered with blankets, all three (patient, daughter, transport man) made the trip to the waiting scanner. After scanning was finished, the radiologist telephoned the transport department informing them that the patient was now ready to return to her bed. But the department was too busy; there were no transport personnel available. So again the patient was kept waiting. After a few minutes, the daughter pressed the radiologist for action, but the delay continued. Finally a radiological technician was pressed into service, so both she and the daughter pushed a gurney—mother lying atop it—back to the patient's bed. Once there, the lady said, "And I was feeling so comfortable—now I'm back where I started."

Thus, the mistiming of tasks (transporting the patient to the scanner and the delay in scanning her) and the failure to anticipate the necessity for another vital task (keeping the patient warm) resulted in untoward consequences for the therapy, which was already relatively succcessful (relieving her intense pain). The sequence of expected tasks took longer than anticipated. New tasks were not foreseen, and so the requisite organization for doing them was lacking. Work by kin filled in that organization, preventing still worse damage to the patient. This *kin work* was concerned not only with clinical safety, but, of course, directly with comfort care and at least implicitly with psychological care. The hospital personnel were only concerned with diagnosis and with what we call *body work* (moving the body to the machine and back in this case), except for the brief flurry of nurses' activity when the patient returned the first time to the ward very much in pain.

Notable in this case also is an organizational phenomenon that is always potentially present: namely, that patients are in competition for available resources. The clinical error in allowing the lady to become cold and her pain to increase again was due not only to failure to foresee a possible delay at the radiology department but also to her being "bumped" to lower priority by another patient's emergency. Resources are always finite, and this kind of patient competition can be annoying (being made to wait) or destructive (as in this woman's case) or sometimes even fatal (nurse's failure to answer a buzzer call by a patient). Competition for finite resources certainly does not often result in fatality but can result in contingencies which affect, whether in small or large degree, the shape of a trajectory.

4. *The Organization and Misorganization of Comfort Work.* In the case of Mr. Einshtein described at the beginning of this chapter, there were four trajectories involving heart, lungs, anemia, and back pain. A couple of days before entering the hospital, Einshtein had a barium X ray in an attempt to locate the source of his blood loss. The night he entered the hospital, he was given a milk of magnesia tablet to prevent possible bowel constriction. The following evening no tablet was given, whether by design or forgetfulness. The next morning, the patient awoke with constriction and much pain and could not manage to pass any stool. He defined this situation as needing immediate attention and asked the nurse assigned him to give him an enema. The nurses were all very busy that morning with a number of new and critically ill patients, and so no enema was forthcoming. No enema was forthcoming because the nurses did not hear his request; that is, they defined the operational contingency differently. The head nurse, when later summoned by him, spoke of a stool softener but ignored his reply that he needed quick action. Finally he asked for the intern, who listened, said she would be back in twenty minutes, and vanished, not to reappear until the next morning, not from malevolence or avoidance, but because she too was busy, unusually so since she was covering three wards instead of her usual single one. Meanwhile Einshtein was metaphorically climbing the walls of his room. Finally, about four hours after his original request, he convinced the head nurse that an enema was needed, but there was another hour's delay while this little-used equip-

ment was brought up from another department. Moments after the enema, Einshtein's pain vanished.

Commentary on this case can be brief, in light of commentaries on the preceding cases. Here the patient's work was essential to getting relief (comfort work) from pain caused by misjudgment in handling the anemia trajectory. The delay in getting the enema was due to four conditions. First, there was a difference in the definition of the nature of the contingency. Second, the nurses and intern were hardly cognizant of the anemia condition (Einshtein was identified as a cardiac case). Third, there was intense patient competition for personnel's time, energy, and attention. And fourth, *comfort work* (for this patient) had very low priority. After all, the staff had been, and was still, working to insure proper monitoring of his blood pressure and pulse and proper scheduling of his medications and various lung treatments; they never were particularly concerned with any comfort care during his two weeks' stay. It was not that they were callous; other work, related to two hazardous trajectories, took total precedence over any concern with discomfort or comfort. They never skipped a beat in getting the necessary tasks done on time or in sequence, and the organization was there to see that those things were done well. The patient had no quarrel with any of that, but only resented his "battle-of-the-bowel." (See chap. 5 for comfort work.)

Concluding Remarks

In closing this chapter, we shall underline a few points already alluded to. First, and in relation especially to the cases just discussed, it is noteworthy that trajectory work may require or involve some among several different kinds of work. As later chapters will clarify further, they include: comfort work, clinical safety work, machine work, composure, biographical, and other kinds of psychological work (subtypes of what will be termed "sentimental work")—plus the work of coordinating (articulating) all of the many tasks involved in the total arc of work. These may have higher or lower priority, depending on the trajectory and its phasing.

Second, trajectory work of whatever species involves the organization of resources. This is why trajectories cannot be conceptualized as pertaining only to the physiological course of an illness or involving only medical, nursing, and other technical tasks. Even the construction of an effective intensive care nursery or intensive care unit for adults, for instance, can involve the work of an imaginative or at least competent architect who can, to quote the comments of one of them, design an "appropriate spatial environment" for the personnel's work. As the discussion in this chapter should have made clear, the organization of resources is a matter that involves both a multiplicity of resources and a complexity of organization for their utilization.

A third point touched on but not especially emphasized so far is that work on trajectories can have significant consequences for the various participants. True, some trajectories are relatively uneventful, so that the experiential and biographical consequences are minimal, especially for the personnel. But even with routine trajectories, there can be consequences for some persons since work relationships are directly related to the illness trajectory with which they are all involved. When trajectories of any kind become problematic, however, then the impact on working relationships can be visibly great, whether deleterious or beneficial. And in some instances, the impact on staff members is more lasting, having consequences for their immediate or long-term self-regard. The concept of trajectory is especially useful in thinking about the experiential and identity impact of work in hospitals because it brings out the *evolving* character of that work and work relationships over the course of the entire case.

3

Machine Work

In this chapter, the central focus in on *machine work* done in the service of trajectory managing and shaping. Not incidentally, our discussion will include the relationship of machine work to the technical aspects of medical and nursing work, as well as to others mentioned in the preceding chapter: comfort, psychological, clinical safety. We begin with machine work primarily because it is easily visualized and because many areas of the hospital are being equipped with machines manned by personnel working with or around that equipment and, in conjunction with the equipment, using drugs, surgery, and other procedures—a trend that necessarily will continue.

General Considerations

In the first chapter, we touched on a few features pertaining to medical technology and its wider consequences for hospitals as organizations, for their personnel, for the relationships among various types of personnel, and in the most general sense for health care itself. To provide further background for examining machine work, especially for those who are unfamiliar with hospitals, we begin with a few additional remarks about the disposition of machines in the hospitals, the training of personnel to use those machines, and further remarks about the machines themselves.

A walk around a relatively large or medically advanced hospital will quickly reveal which sections of the building rely most on machinery. Some sections, departments, and wards are machine-rich while others are relatively machine-sparse. Diagnostic sections are full of equipment and people working with it: for instance, if there is a clinical laboratory, virtually all of its testing will utilize a large number of machines. Radiological departments include varieties of X-ray machines and nowadays perhaps a scanner or two. The hospital may have a department with echogram equipment. Cardiological diagnosis depends heavily on electrocardiograms (EKGs), equipment used in catheterization, treadmill equipment, and perhaps machinery for the nuclear tracing of cardiac damage. Among the clinical wards most heavily equipped are the surgical, including surgical theaters, the recovery rooms, and the post surgical units, and a ward where damaged kidneys are dialyzed. Even small hospitals nowadays have intensive care units with machines, and in the typical ICUs of large hospitals the medical and nursing care are directly associated with the multiplicity of machines found on these units. If there is a cardiac care unit, then equipment for monitoring will be much in evidence. If there is an intensive care nursery, the array of equipment is likely to dazzle even knowledgeable spectators who look in on it. On medical wards, the patients may be less often hooked up to, or worked on with machines, but in those wards we may see various types of respirator equipment in use, notice automated intravenous (IV) equipment standing at bedsides, and both see and hear the digestive tracts of patients being suctioned by the appropriate equipment. These medical wards send patients to other parts of the hospital for therapy and for monitoring the progress or deterioration of their conditions, and they also have machines brought into the rooms for use with patients who are relatively immobile. A specialized ward for those acutely ill with cancer will not have much machinery in evidence, but X-raying is done at the bedside or patients may be taken down to the radiology department for diagnostic tests as well as for radiation therapy.

What is the training for working with this equipment? In general the picture is as follows: Medical schools scarcely emphasize working with the machinery, except for some training in interpreting the results of a few machines, for example, X-ray films and EKG printouts. (Interviews with a sample of medical students at our own university suggested that they had machinery very little in focus, except in interpretation, being much concentrated on other features of the clinical scene: knowledge, procedures, surgery, drugs. Our thanks to Robert Broadhead for this data.)

When young physicians move along to their internships and specialized residencies, then, of course, they learn how to interpret a variety of products of machines (EKGs, cardiac monitoring screens) and in some specialties, like radiology and anesthesiology, machine operation itself as well as interpretation of machine products is at the heart of their learning. While some medical specialities use little or no machinery except for diagnoses done in the radiology department or in the clinical lab, others could scarcely continue without equipment, which the young physicians learn to use or whose products they learn to interpret, or both. Sometimes the physician will rely on technicians, as does a machine-skilled respiratory physician whom we interviewed, but will occasionally do the testing himself or herself as well as interpret the printouts. As for nurses, in collegiate and university programs, the emphasis on machine work is probably not much more extensive than in medical schools, although the students may learn about some facets of machine work in their hours spent on wards where equipment is much in evidence. (In hospital-associated schools, nursing students actually work as floor nurses, encountering whatever machinery is used on the wards.) Unquestionably, however, most of the very extensive machine-oriented skills that nurses possess are learned on the job. To a lesser extent they may learn some features of this work through hospital in-service programs. By contrast, the various technicians who work with specialized equipment (Xray, EKG, respiratory machines), either autonomously or as physicians' helpers, by and large learn their initial skills through training programs offered by state colleges, community colleges, and the like. Of course, they, too, continue to learn additional skills on the job. The nonclinical personnel who work with machines (bioengineers, safety engineers, nuclear technicians) have technical training in varied kinds of specialized programs. It is noteworthy that the medical world is replete with extramural workshops, training conferences, and continuing education programs, some of which bear on working with equipment. In sum, generally it seems safe to say that physicians learn machine work during the advanced years of their training and on the job, whereas nurses learn mainly on the job and specialized technicians learn through training programs and on the job.

The machines themselves, of course, are immensely varied. They include machines utilized for diagnosis, therapy, and monitoring, for relieving discomfort, or as a substitute for an impaired bodily part or system, and frequently they function as life-sustaining machines. There is also communication equipment used for locating key personnel when they are urgently needed. Beeper machines are used all over the hospital along with the paging system and the telephone. Understandably, machines performing those very different functions (for instance, fluoroscopes, cardiac monitors, pacemakers) will look quite different; indeed, different kinds of equipment in the same category (therapy, diagonosis) will also vary in their characteristics and in the kinds of work they entail.

Anyone who has had little experience with hospitals is likely to visualize medical equipment only in terms of diagnostic machinery like the X-ray behemoths (since we have all been X-rayed at one time or another) or scanners (much in the news since they are the most glamorous machines of the decade) or the kinds of machinery used in surgical theaters (seen on TV) or pacemakers (a friend has one) or cardiac monitors (virtually everybody knows someone who has been monitored). But our walk around the hospital will have shown us that the range of machine characteristics is extensive. We will have noticed that some are large, some small; some probably cost more than others; some look old while others are glisteningly new. Here is a partial list of differentiating properties of medical machines, which vary by:

cost
size
skill required to operate
ease of operation
risks involved in operating (to environment, to operator, to patient)
reliability
numbers of operators required
resources required to operate (electricity, oxygen, etc.)
calibration required (frequency, degree)
movability
durability
servicing (amount required, difficulty)
connections, their number and difficulty (to electricity, to other machines, to patient)
used alone or with other machines
attention required when operating
discomfort (to operator, to patient)
old or new model
external to patient's body or internal
common (numbers of) or rare (few)
storability
availability
preparation of the machine (setting up, taking down)
substitutability on breakdown or malfunction (by other machinery)
number of patients on the machine (simultaneously or sequentially)
used with drugs or without
used with nonmachine procedures or not
supplies (degree of perishability, fragility, etc.)
replaceability on breakdown or malfunction
frequency of use (say, per day)
physical effort required to operate
prestigious or ordinary

visibility of working with
visibility of potential error in equipment's operation
old or new
materials worked on (i.e., patients, their fragility especially)
expense of operating

For any given type of equipment, those machine properties can be salient to some degree. For instance, EKG machines are small and easy to move (they move *to* the immobile patient's bedside); each machine is frequently used, servicing many patients; if they break down, they are easily replaced since EKG departments have many machines; they require relatively little skill to operate but their printouts require considerable skill to read. Compare that with the scanner—so costly that the government regulates how many there can be in any given geographic area. Every minute of unused time costs the hospital money, but every minute of employed time can make the hospital money (it can be a "moneymaking" machine despite its initial great cost).

It is easy to imagine, also, how the machine's properties affect work done with and around it. Nuclear tracer equipment requires great care to protect everybody from potential radiation danger and so does the disposal of its wastes. Echogram machines, which bounce sound waves off a patient's heart, require relatively little skill to set up and maintain in good service, but a very high degree of interpretative skill. Automated IV equipment is found virtually everywhere in the hospital: it is easy to move, set up, and take down; it requires an easily learned amount of skill to connect to the patient correctly; it has to be carefully monitored because it may rather easily go awry, but a patient, too, can easily monitor this equipment since when the drip becomes too fast or too slow, that change is easy to see. One further instance: careful and continual calibration for the various equipment used in cardiac catheterization, as touched on in the preceding chapter, is a major activity for minimizing the potential clinical risks to patients and maximizing the accuracy of clinical interpretations. In the pages below, we shall see or sense the dynamic interplay of machine properties and staff or patient work with and around various types of equipment.

Machine work can reasonably be discussed in three general categories. First, there is *machine production*—work insuring that the machines are invented, tried out experimentally, manufactured, sold, bought, and installed. In chapter 1, our discussion touched on the invention processes and on the generally fragmented nature of the manufacturing industry. The purchase of machines involved not only salesmanship but consumers' learning about and knowing about the efficacy of machines and models and convincing funding authorities that the machines were needed. All this represents different clusters of tasks and skills from the machine work an observer sees on the clinical wards and in diagnostic or service departments. It is the latter, represented by the next two categories of machine work, that is the focus of the present chapter.

The second category of work is *machine tending*—work insuring that machines are monitored for various features (safety, efficiency), stored, supplied with parts and necessary materials, disposed of when old or obsolete, and so on. In those regards, medical machines are not very different from automobiles, airplanes, lawn mowers, or washing machines. On the other hand, medical machines are different in some ways; they differ considerably among themselves and are used in a different organizational setting.

A third category of the work pertains to the medical use of machines, that is, their use for *medical production*—their utilization for diagnosis, therapy, or maintenance of life. Those illness-oriented activities include monitoring patients on machines for their clinical safety (as with dialysis procedures), interpreting the machine's information (films, printouts), connecting patients to machines and taking patients off them, telling patients about given machines and the machine work presently to be done, calming patients' anxieties when on machines, coordinating the scheduling of patients with the use of machines, moving equipment to patients or vice versa, weaning patients from life-sustaining machines that are no longer actually required, teaching patients and kin how to operate medical equipment with clinical safety and accuracy after they go home.

These activities are closely linked with types and phases of trajectories. In the strictest sense of the term, they are *all* instances of trajectory work. So, of course, different clinical wards will exhibit different degrees and combinations of those three kinds of machine work and the typical clusters of tasks that constitute each kind of work. Again, medical machines are not so unique that they do not share some of those activities with computers or automobiles, but as the above listing suggests—and as their linkage with illnesses and trajectories necessitates—they certainly do differ in some regards. Moreover, virtually all of this equipment is used on, in, or with the bodies of people, who are reacting either to the machines or their operators, or both, and who are potential machine workers themselves.

Machine Tending

Since various sections of hospitals are increasingly taking on the appearance of a variegated set of machine shops, they are increasingly tied to the relentless requirements of their equipment. This means that, just as there must be a system of supply for autos (parts, oil) and for servicing them, there must be systems—or at least systematic provision—for keeping those machines functioning as efficiently and safely as possible. But because hospitals tend to be decentralized in their plurality of workplaces—which jealously guard their respective degrees of jurisdictional control—the systems of supply, maintenance, and so forth tend to be somewhat independently set up and to function strongly to attain a more centralized control over those systems. (Perhaps government hospitals in the United States come closest to this centralized control.) For instance, in private hospitals the administration, or a representative hospitalwide committee, may be the last court of appeal concerning amounts of money spent on machine purchase or maintenance for various wards or departments, but the latter usually decide on precisely which type or model of machine they need and on when it is obsolete or requires servicing. Those decisions are based on experiential knowledge and inevitably are tied to the type of work done with the machines in relation to varied illnesses. Indeed, the medical and technical specialists know the intimate details of models, necessary supplies, and the companies or personnel that are best at producing, servicing, supplying, and so on—know all this better than outsiders to the ward or department can possibly know.

As with all machinery, medical equipment sets several classes of problems for those who use it. In common parlance, all of these pertain to the maintenance of the equipment, and they include how to get the equipment monitored, serviced, supplied, and operated. The variations associated with meeting each of those problems depends on: (1) the nature of the machines, (2) the medical work done with them, and (3) the organizational contexts within which the medical work takes place.

Monitoring the Equipment

Equipment requires monitoring to make certain it is operating properly. One dimension of "operating properly" is, of course, whether the machine is *safe*, that is, not dangerous to the operators, to the environment itself, or to the patient who is on the machine. Consider the difference between different kinds of machinery used for different kinds of medical work. For instance, a malfunctioning electrocardiograph (EKG) machine may give inaccurate results but is not dangerous to either staff or patient. Malfunctioning equipment that uses nuclear substances can be hazardous for everyone, including bystanders. A malfunctioning respiratory machine that is supposedly breathing for the patient can be lethal for the patient but not at all dangerous for the staff. (We once saw a nurse tear the respiratory mask off a patient only seconds after a power failure had knocked out the machine. During another power failure that lasted only three seconds, a nursing clinical specialist realized that a cardiac patient was gravely endangered because his cardiac rhythms were no longer matched with his cardiac machine; she rushed down the hall, into the ward, and breathlessly turned off the now lethal equipment, undoubtedly saving the patient's life.) In general, malfunctioning medical equipment is likely to be more dangerous for the patient than for the staff, and we shall discuss it in greater length in the next chapter.

Since almost all machines are powered by electricity, the safety work of hospitals begins with installing a backup system to take over in the potentially disastrous event that a power shortage occurs. Of course, if some machines are only temporarily without electricity, there would only be delays in the medical work, but patients on life-sustaining equipment (oxygen ventilators, intra-aortic pumps) or whose lives could be saved in an emergency when the necessary machines were working (heart defibrillators) are in great danger when the electricity fails. Since those crucial high-risk machines are usually massed in certain areas of the hospital (ICUs, the ICN, kidney dialysis unit, surgical units), the greatest alertness is found there during power blackouts. If necessary, the personnel may be able to keep the machines going manually. During one blackout we observed staff members on a dialysis unit located in a clinical building where there was no backup electric power source keep the machines running for a full hour before the electricity came back on. And in another instance, when the power was cut off in a surgical theater and the backup system failed, two heart-lung machines (as reported later to us by a nurse working in the theater) were manually run by three technicians for twenty minutes, a job requiring not only endurance but considerable knowledge and skill concerning both the machines and the patients' physiology.

To maximize the safety of machines, many large hospitals employ safety engineers or, indeed, may have safety departments comprised of several experts who are collectively familiar with different kinds of equipment as well as with dangerous chemicals, fire hazards, and the like. These personnel not only help to enforce government safety regulations but act as consultants and educators to clinical personnel concerning the machinery they utilize. Often the latter simply are not cognizant of the degree of hazard involved in their use of equipment: the potential for electric shock, fire, or explosion, the possibilities for worker or patient radiation overdose, the proper procedures for handling radiation spill, contamination, or disposal. Apparently, sometimes the safety personnel need to be very persuasive, since their policing power in relation to the more powerful medical staff is low. Also to paraphrase one safety engineer, "Unfortunately, a lot of our recommendations for increasing safety mean money, either in terms of materials, changes in space arrangements, or new kinds of job categories." So their safety work consists partly of monitoring the equipment and the staff's procedures and partly of preventing hazardous situations, educating the machine operators, and sometimes attempting to police the more extreme offenders, especially with regard to government regulations. Of course, technicians and nurses who work daily with familiar equipment are trained or learn to monitor it for clinical hazards and often for potential danger to themselves and to the environment.

Another kind of monitoring pertains to the *accuracy* of the information produced by the machines. A term commonly used for this is "calibrating." The hospital's bioengineers may appear daily or periodically on clinical wards, especially the machine-dense ones, to calibrate. As one bioengineer who worked with cardiac equipment said, "The machines are only as good as the person who calibrates them—you can't trust the machines." Calibration error, in fact, may go undetected for some time; one famous medical center which had the most expert of calibrating agents discovered after a number of years that their experts had miscalculated what the calibration should be for a particular type of important machine. And in rural or small town hospitals that have no bioengineers, there may be only an annual or biannual checkup by a visiting engineer, including checkups of monitoring machines. During the intervals, we might suspect the equipment is not recording with the greatest accuracy! Periodic or episodic calibration of medical equipment is much like having your automobile checked by a garage mechanic. Some operators need to calibrate precisely more often or even rather continuously, as in the last chapter we saw physicians and technicians do when working with cardiac catheterization equipment.

Another major monitoring task is, of course, keeping an eye on the machine's *efficiency*. The bioengineers do this kind of checkup work but those who operate the machines daily—the nurses and technicians and for diagnostic machines also the physician specialists—are most likely to recognize when a machine is not working well, is running down, or is soon or immediately in need of service, repair, or replacement.

Servicing

Indeed, the greatest difficulty in managing medical equipment probably is keeping it maintained so that it works at maximum efficiency. On the daily operational level, the personnel are accustomed to tinkering or fiddling with slightly malfunctioning machines (although we have observed scenes when quite fortuitously a young physician will be called on by less knowledgeable or innovative nurses to do the tinkering). One variety of tinkering is fine tuning done by an operator who has a good eye or ear for a specific machine, getting a better performance from that machine than someone less familiar with it might.

But genuine servicing usually needs to be done by nonoperators, experts in servicing or repairing. Some hospitals and hospital departments build into their purchasing contracts provisions for that kind of servicing by the service departments of sales companies. This practice usually is associated with the large companies that manufacture equipment such as X-ray machinery, scanners, and EKG machines. Clinical and diagnostic departments, however, often have special preferences for the specific servicing companies they believe have special competence in the maintenance of their particular types or models of equipment and may even avoid official administrative channels to use them. Large hospitals may have service departments with personnel on call for emergency breakdowns or quick repairs. (Proper repair, as we all know from experiences with automobiles, is crucial since a poor servicing agent can commit a repair error, thus making the equipment even less efficient.) In large hospitals, the service department may pick up defective machinery routinely but may also be so inundated with work that the equipment, as one nurse said, "disappears for weeks." One tactic for minimizing the need for repairs is to maintain an oversupply of machines so that none is used too frequently or for too long a period of time. And when the breakdown of a machine without the prospect of quick or immediate repair actually threatens a patient's condition or life, then backup equipment will be on hand for that crisis.

The problem of servicing and repairing in machine-dense clinical wards can be rendered very difficult by at least six frequently encountered conditions. First, much of the medical machinery produced today seems not to be very well constructed or checked through careful quality control measures or is so complex as to be very delicate and so breaks down or is frequently in need of at least minor repairs. Second, unlike drugs, which are carefully tested under controlled experimental conditions before market distribution, medical machines are essentially tested for efficiency, durability, safety, and the like only during the first months and years after their sale. Third, there is a strong desire among hospital personnel, especially physicians, to have the latest and presumably the most effective models in this fast-moving equipment market. Fourth, because of cost considerations some hospitals do not replace equipment very often. Thus, there is the ironic situation that teaching hospitals, which are on the forefront of medical knowledge, specialization, and patient care, sometimes have older machines and older models than do large community hospitals, which trail in introducing all of that medical technology. Fifth, there may not be a well-organized maintenance or preventive program, the servicing being largely a matter of crisis management or, as an ICU head nurse remarked, "haphazard." (She added that the physicians were little involved with the machines on her ward, other than interpreting their information, and that therefore it was the nurses who paid attention to maintenance and service—even coming up with detailed data about machine breakdowns and their consequences, which were necessary to convince the hospital administrators that certain of the ICU's machinery was obsolescent and needed replacement.) Sixth, only the mass-produced equipment such as scanners and X-ray machines are likely to be sold in conjunction with assured company servicing since only they can afford regional offices, density of servicing personnel, and quick service. Most medical equipment, as noted earlier, is not mass-produced and the manufacturing companies are quite small. In short, there is a high level of technology produced but an organization lagging far behind in its service, repair, and maintenance, both in the industry itself and in the hospitals. Most manufacturers have no incentive and possess insufficient resources to provide efficient servicing. Most hospitals do not have the resources (including requisite financing) to support effective servicing even if they recognize its need.

The consequences of poor service, especially when combined with old equipment, are that the operators of the machines are much frustrated. This is especially true of nurses. Indeed, while most of the literature on nurses' psychological stress ignores that due to machine inefficiency, some of their stress is surely due to that. Thus, one ICU nurse figured she spent two hours of every night on machine maintenance problems or in locating a substitute machine for one that was malfunctioning. And on an ICU observed by us, nurses frequently hunted around to find someone who had worked on a specific malfunctioning machine: "Have you worked with this machine? With this model?"

Nurses may also do considerable minor repairing, keeping screw drivers, wrenches, and other tools on the ward for ready use. (They do Scotch tape repairing, too, as did one nurse wih an EKG machine whose gears were so worn that they jammed the readout tapes; to correct this, she put tape over the gears.) During the change-of-shift sessions, they may inform each other about how to fix equipment. Old timers share with nurses new to the ward information about the idiosyncracies of specific machines, which parts are likely to break down, how to replace a broken part with one from another machine, and how to fiddle with the machines when necessary. Nurses also work out informal systems of matching more efficient and reliable machines with relatively high-risk patients; once the patient gets past that trajectory phase or is relatively stabilized, he or she is shifted to an older, less efficient machine. Nurses may also work out standing arrangements for borrowing equipment like an EKG machine from another ward when one breaks down.

Maintenance problems are added to by a fair amount of machine "abuse," a term used by service personnel when referring with denigration by a hopeless shrug to the unnecessary repairs engendered by operator ignorance, negligence, carelessness, or indifference as well as anger at the machines or anger over other matters that gets taken out on the machines as handy and uncomplaining victims. But, of course, the equipment gets moved around a great deal, sometimes in great haste, and space may be very cramped so that machines get bumped against one another and against walls. Moreover, too many people may be using the machine or using it too frequently. These conditions do not really constitute machine abuse, but merely additional circumstances that wear the machines down more quickly. Nevertheless, there is enough abuse so that equipment salesmen may make a point of emphasizing the durability of their particular machines and how well they can take abuse. Portable machinery, understandably, is more likely to go awry or lose its fine tuning, either because of the sheer fact of being moved or moved carelessly. Ward personnel may try to limit any lending of their machines in order to minimize potential abuse.

In any event, one can empathize with the electronics engineer who told us that the ideal solution for abuse and for lack of staff skill was to automate the machines completely, with multiple machine connections within one enclosing frame. While there are technological and cost reasons for such multiple-linked machines, this engineer's ideal can only be fantasy as far as most medical equipment is concerned. On the other hand, the maintenance people may sometimes be correct in believing that when operating personnel report to them that a machine has gone wrong, it is really a "user problem." Or as one said, "people who work on the innards have respect, people who don't just want results."

In short, maintenance and service of medical machinery entails at least three different systems. First, there is not much organizational structure in the medical equipment industry itself for servicing machines. Second, there is an increasing if still inadequate organizational structure building up in large hospitals for that service and maintenance. Third, there is much informal structure which is ever functioning but not very apparent (except, perhaps, to researchers!). The last system, and its related operator tactics, are so implicit and organizationally nonaccountable that the personnel cannot really tell us accurately what portion of their time and effort is spent on servicing, repairing, and maintaining—except often "It's a lot!" Getting this work done successfully is frequently dependent on fortuitous circumstances and on intimate acquaintanceship with specific machines. In fact, between particular personnel and specific machines there gets built up an interactional history—much as between the reader and his or her potentially ailing toaster or vacuum cleaner—a history that is snapped when there is staff turnover, reducing thereby the effectiveness of that aspect of the informal system for machine maintenance. This informal system is an organizational cost that is neither easily quantified nor explicitly recognized by the hospital's administrators at any level.

Supplying and Storing

The daily struggle to keep machines running efficiently or running at all requires that machine parts be available to those who operate them. This leads to preventive hoarding of parts, which are stockpiled—"just in case." Indeed, entire machines may be stockpiled in anticipation of their use. Hospital corridors are full of extra machines kept on the ready, and hospital closets are used as storage and even hiding places for collections of spare parts as well as for backup equipment. (In one hospital at which we did our research, spare parts and other supplies were warehoused some miles away because of a shortage of storage space in the hospital, but since this usually meant a delay of some days in obtaining requisite parts, the personnel often circumvented this system by covert stockpiling.) It is not only the personnel of clinical wards who do this storing in closets and down the corridors but also others like those who work in transport and respiratory departments.

Departments also borrow machines and machine parts from each other. These may be returned in bad shape or not returned at all, which leads to bad feelings and sometimes refusal to loan again. Borrowing can be hazardous, too, because the requesting personnel are not necessarily aware of the condition of the equipment borrowed—a source of horror stories following later discovery of their defective state. One condition that reduces the possibility of borrowing spare parts is that departments may have purchased the same type of machinery from different companies (leading one nurse to comment that she wished her hospital would standardize purchases to make things easier for her own ward).

What is true for machine parts is also true for the supplies without which the medical equipment might function ineffectively or not at all. One class of such supplies consists of the varied drugs used in combination with different machines. A second consists of materials used in the information recording process: paper for printouts, film, tapes. A third pertains to the connections between the machine and the patient: tubing, catheters, and so on. If any of these supplies are unavailable, then the equipment may be as effectively grounded as an airplane without fuel, And like fuel, these supplies are consumable. Contemporary hospitals are remarkable for the rate at which they use up such supplies; this is understandable for the drugs and paper and film but just as true for the third class of supplies, because the generalized concern about infection and the requirement for sterile objects leads to a throwaway rate that is, to the uninitiated, quite astonishing. So a major task, and potential problem, for the operators of medical machinery is to insure that requisite supplies are quickly available. Ordinarily those materials are stored on the ward or in the department, and they, too, are stockpiled, whether the administrators are aware of that or not. In short, for the personnel, concerned and busy with the daily trajectory work, the problem of supplies is virtually synonymous with "flow"—that is, with continuity of supplies. Stockpiling and borrowing are simply contingency tactics for handling that basic and often harassing problem.

Setting Up and Taking Down

The preceding discussions have touched on features of the next class of problem: the actual operation of the machines. One such operation is that some machines have to be readied in order to be used and taken down after use. Those tasks may require putting in or taking out the requisite supplies (drugs, film) and call for differing amounts of time and skill. Machines used for blood circulation have to be cleaned after use and that may be a fairly arduous job. (A nurse who uses such equipment pointed out that while "that machine over there" was probably a better machine, "this one" required much less time to set up and to clean, and so the first one was no longer used very much.) Setting up may also include positioning the machine in relation to the patient, and vice versa. We are all familiar with those particular machine tasks from having been X-rayed and with the fact that ineffective positioning means further positioning work in order to get better machine results, which is a bother to everyone. Positioning may also require medical work out of concern for clinical safety, as well as additional work pertaining to comfort and composure.

Medical Production Work

A few machines used in the hospital are *not* used with bodies, for example, equipment in the clinical lab that utilizes only body products such as blood and urine. Most machines are body-related, that is, they are used with, on, or in patients whose bodies must be brought into some conjunction with the machines. Thus, there will be transporting either of bodies to machines or vice versa; there will be connecting of machines to body parts and disconnecting, too. There will be simultaneous or sequential monitoring of machines and bodies and of the interaction of machines with bodies. In short, the machinery used with bodies involves complicating aspects that machines not used with bodies do not have. It also calls forth explicitly or implicitly more types of work than those that pertain purely to the tending of machines or to the physiology of the patients' bodies.

Transporting Machines or Bodies

In modern hospitals, then, a considerable amount of machine work involves bringing the patient to the machine or the machine to the patient (or in industrial terminology, bringing together the machine and the material on which it will work). As touched on in the introductory chapter, the traffic of machines going to bodies and bodies being brought to machines is astonishing, and in large hospitals the distances traversed may be considerable. Every sizable hospital has a transport department with its requisite wheelchairs and gurneys as well as movable equipment. The piling up both of those objects in the corridors and of patients being transported in and out of the clinical wards and diagnostic departments is a striking though familiar sight to hospital regulars.

This transporting work intersects with other kinds of trajectory work. For instance, patients often grow irritable at the interminable waiting for X rays and other diagnostic work. Often they are parked en masse in the corridor outside the department while the transport person dashes off to the next job. This means work for the technicians and nurses who must deal with complaints, irritability, and anxiety, as well as with the machine procedures themselves. (On a pediatric ward for children with cancer, the nurses spend much time "picking up the pieces," that is, doing composure work with the children after they have been subjected to frequent diagnostic or therapeutic procedures, done by strangers at the radiology and chemotherapy departments.) After transport, too, the staff must frequently deal with matters of clinical safety engendered by the trip or the waiting (as illustrated by the case of the elderly lady with back pain described in chap. 2). We have observed nurses making the decision to accompany a high-risk patient on the gurney trip, especially when the patient is hooked up to an IV, not quite trusting the transport people, who are often regarded as mere vehicle pushers. As for transporting neonatal infants to surgery or the heart catheterization laboratory, special transport incubators equipped with their own battery power are used, with special oxygen equipment. Such transporting requires a special team involving a respiratory therapist, a person who monitors the infant, a person who pushes the equipment, and possibly a physician.

Patients have to be prepared for transport, both physically (comfort work) and psychologically. Moreover, all transport, whether of patients or machinery, has to be scheduled, and the burden of that often complicated task falls on the head nurses who nowadays spend much time on making such arrangements (this is part of their articulation work; see chap. 7). On busy days, the scheduling problems for her, for the transport service, and for people at the machine site itself, can be horrendous.

Transport personnel have similar scheduling problems, of course. They also have problems with choosing the speediest or least difficult routes to and from the wards. Some routes are impossible because of stairs or because a corridor is crowded with protruding lockers, while other routes are avoided because the corridor floors are in bad condition or because an elevator en route always has a pile up of traffic or is full of passengers. These problems may be somewhat less dismaying in newer hospitals if they have been properly planned, but the continual increase of machine and body traffic to and from numerous machine sites insures that they will not disappear altogether.

The transport personnel also have storage difficulties, for their equipment sometimes gets lost or borrowed, and delays in transport occur, with consequent irritability all around. It is worth emphasizing, however, that despite all this transporting around the hospital, in the machine-dense clinical wards a great deal of equipment is actually in the rooms or kept on the ward itself. So while there is some internal moving of equipment, it represents only a minor chore for the ward personnel on these particular wards.

Connecting Work

Every machine used with patients, as briefly noted earlier, requires connection with the patient—a different task from body or machine positioning. Connecting machines and patients is a major category of machine work involving considerable time and effort by technicians, nurses, and sometimes physicians. The connections required vary greatly from machine to machine. They vary somewhat according to the patient's trajectory phase and the condition of the receiving part of the body:

- — inside or outside the body
- — temporary or long lasting
- — fragile or durable
- — routine or potentially dangerous
- — discomforting, painful, or distasteful to the patient
- — solo connection or many simultaneously
- — highly visible or not
- — correctability of errors or not

Such properties, of course, affect the connecting work itself. Routine connections may often be done quickly and require relatively little skill. Potentially dangerous ones require much care, considerable skill, and sometimes more than one connecting agent. Connections made inside the body will be done by physicians, highly trained, one hopes, and the monitoring of those connections will be frequent, as with pacemakers, endotracheal catheters, or aortic pumps. Potentially painful connections may require informing the patient beforehand, reassuring during the actual work, and comforting the patient afterward if there was anxiety or actual pain. To the properties of the connections, we should add what has already been alluded to, namely, the properties—actual or perceived—of the connecting agents. Are they competent or incompetent, careful or careless, strangers to the patient or familiar, and so on? Connecting work sometimes brings on a battlefront atmosphere between nervous connectors and watchful or accusing patients. This type of work can necessitate considerable work of other kinds, especially comfort and composure work, which may, of course, take more time, effort, and skill than making the connections themselves.

It is important also to recognize that the patients' properties affect the connecting work, not only their temperaments, moods, mental states, whether they are sentient or not, familiar with the procedures, and the like, but also their body properties. These latter include, first, the condition of the body part to which the connection is made, such as poor or used up veins or infection at the site. There are many variations in the condition of a receiving site as well. There are also numerous such sites: limbs, ears, eyes, skin surface, veins and arteries, organs, body cavities, body orifices, spinal canal, and so on. Second, there is the phase of the illness, since with very sick and high-risk patients connections may need to be accomplished more carefully, skillfully, and speedily, as well as monitored more frequently and with more alertness. Alternative machines can be used, too, depending on the graveness of the patient's condition, for instance, a respiratory face mask with a rebreathing bag for carbon dioxide. Equipment such as a pneumonia machine is only used during the acute phase of an illness, but an asthma machine is used extensively during an acute phase and intermittently thereafter. With certain kinds of trajectories, at given phases, a patient may be connected to more than one machine. Thus, in the recovery room, he or she may be hooked up to numerous machines: respiratory, urinary, cardiac-monitoring, automatic IV, and so on. This connecting work is done in quick sequence and, of course, is carefully monitored thereafter for slippage or malfunction.

Different connecting tasks also involve different divisions of labor. Many connections can be accomplished by only one staff member, but some require several personnel either for the connecting itself or for accompanying tasks. For instance, a mother or nurse may be doing the psychological or comfort work with a child or holding a child still while the physician connects the machine. Or in a cardiac catheterization lab, the division of labor can be quite complex: while the sequential connections are being made inside the patient's body by one or two physicians, another monitors the video screen and a nurse or technician reassures the patient, who is also probably doing composure work on himself or herself, as well as the work of remaining absolutely still so the catheterization connections can be made safely and efficiently.

The work of monitoring the connections, once they have been made, varies: some need scarcely any attention and some frequent and careful attention. Patients may play an important role in this monitoring. For instance, a patient may point out the inadvertent disconnection of an EKG connection. On dialysis units, the patients during their long sessions on the equipment keep an eye not only on their own but often on their neighbor's machines, noting the malfunction of machines and their connections. During Mr. Einshtein's hospitalization (see chap. 2), the day after the IV had been removed from the connecting shunt into his arm, his wife noticed a possible infection in his arm around the shunt, called this to the attention of the nurse, who then quickly removed the shunt. Such events occur with fair frequency whenever malfunctioning connections can be seen by patients. They and their kinsmen, then, will either fix a connection or call staff's attention to the problem. Intravenous machines are monitored regularly, sometimes anxiously, by patients and their relatives. Experienced or overanxious patients may also, during the staff's connecting work or just afterward, point to inadquately or incompetently made connections. Moreover, unless a patient is completely immobilized by his or her condition, there is always the possibility of the connection becoming loosened or disconnected. So, for both staff and patient, connecting work is inherent in the use of much of the equipment.

Finally, there are complex interrelationships among several sets of conditions, namely, (1) the trajectory phase itself, (2) the properties of connections, of connectors, and of their division of labor, (3) the properties of the machines, (4) the machines' impact on the body, (5) the site at which the machine work is done, and (6) ultimately the organization of the hospital itself. A few concrete examples should suffice to illustrate some of those complicated relationships. Thus, ICUs are organized around acute states of illness where immediacy of machine action is required, and machines are multiple, requiring great skill and resources to make body connections, to operate, monitor, and maintain. In the X-ray department, the size of the machine, the potential danger both to patient and staff, the skill required, all mean that the usual pattern is of a flow of body traffic to the department. If the patient is too sick, portable X-ray equipment may be brought to the bedside. If a patient is very sick but the body connections are complex or dangerous and require specialized X-ray machines, then personnel from the patient's ward or other departments will converge on the radiology department to help with the work. In the cardiac catheterization department, as we have seen, the catheterization procedures require that the patient be transported there because of the multiple machines, the connections made inside the body, the constant monitoring of both the machines and the body because of high potential clinical danger. For EKG machines, the body connections are easy to make and are outside the body; it requires minimal skill to run the machine, and the machine is easily portable, so machine and technician come to the patient's bedside. When making inside body connections is combined with very specialized skills and considerable resources for monitoring machine and body (as with kidney dialysis), then the surgical theater will be the site for making connections (the shunt), while the ward will be the site for the remainder of the work. When an internal body connection is very temporary, the clinical danger is negligible, and the resources required are few, the connection can be made at the bedside, as with a gastric connection for suction. But if the connection requires specialized skill, yet does not require much in the way of time or other resources, then a skilled connecting agent will come to the bedside, as when an arterial line connection is made with an esophageal varices tube.

Before ending this section on connection work, which is a highly visible feature of body-related machines, we should add that there are various consequences of carrying out that work inadequately. There is a potential clinical danger, even of death, to the patient. There can be interference with other work while the defective connections are being made all over again. There can be "fallout," such as patients' annoyance, frustration, mistrust, accusations of incompetence, anxiety, fear, even panic, and corresponding reactions among the staff. Hence, it is important to make good connections in the first place, as well as to recognize and rectify quickly any errors or inadequacies in the original connection. This and the monitoring involved are together an important part of staff work in the more technologized sections of the hospital.

Monitoring Machined Medical Work

Since medical machines are used on and with bodies, their monitoring is not at all limited to concern with their mechanical functioning. In fact, "monitoring" is a term much heard in today's hospital, but, given the various contexts in which personnel use it, a thoughtful listener can be confused about exactly what it refers to. Attempting to avoid the analytic tangle inherent in their use of the term, we begin this section by noting the various types of monitoring involved in highly skilled work done with high-risk premature infants. On entering an advanced ICN, what strikes an observer is the array of glass boxes (isolettes), each with its enclosed tiny child, over which a nurse is hovering or with which she is working. The isolette insures a carefully regulated protective environment without which the infant could not survive. In addition, the observer is likely to be dazzled by the number of wires and tubes attached to the isolette or the baby itself.

Now if we ask what kinds of monitoring are going on, the answer typically must take into account the following, aside from any monitoring of the mechanical functioning of the equipment itself. There will be a conspicuous machine attached to the infant by leads and pads, which monitors various dimensions of cardiac functioning (tachycardia, brachycardia, systolic pressure, and heart rhythms) and respiratory functioning (low rate, high rate, inspirate rate). The machine is busily doing its monitoring and reassuring the nurse through continuous beeping noises, but ringing an alarm if something goes awry with the infant. It also has dials with digital readings, giving information which the nurse monitors. So she is monitoring the machine's signals by ear and its readings by eye. The isolette's internal temperature is registered on a gauge, which the nurse adjusts in response to the infant's temperature. She does this every 1–3 hours, depending on the relative stability of the infant's condition. She reports the isolette's temperature on a chart next to her recording of the infant's temperature, so that later scanning will reveal at what external temperature the baby does best. She is monitoring both the machine's information and the child's temperature, recording all that information, and acting in accordance with her interpretations of information. Attached by a small electrode to the infant's skin is likely to be a transcutaneous oxygen monitor recording the amount of oxygen in the blood. This equipment yields computer printouts, which the nurse reads and records; here, too, she is monitoring the machine's information. There may also be a continuous positive air pressure (CPAP) machine, which has a hose like that of an ordinary vacuum cleaner, an inflatable rubber bag, an adjustable meter attached to a wall outlet, and a stream of oxygen, and is operated by hydraulic pressure. Again the nurse is monitoring the equipment and its relation to physiological functioning as well as the information given by the meter. In addition, there may be apparatuses which, strictly speaking, are not machines but which require monitoring nevertheless, especially with regard to their therapeutic impact. One is a "bili light," used to prevent jaundice; it is plugged into a wall socket. Another is a hyperalimentation tube insered in the infant's jugular vein, through which flow nourishment and drugs. There may also be an umbilical line into its umbilical artery from which blood can be drawn so that the blood gases can be measured. Of course, not all of the equipment will be used with every child or even during every miniphase of its trajectory.

A fourth type of monitoring is the close and almost continuous attention paid to signs yielded by the infant's body and behavior: movement, skin color, temperature, respiratory rate, and the like—this reading being done by sight, hearing, and touch. If the baby is taken out of the isolette for a necessary procedure, then various other nurses, physicians, even a respiratory therapist may converge, most doing monitoring of one kind or another. A fifth type of monitoring might be termed "second order," exemplified by the physician or head nurse who listens to or reads the nurses' reports of *their* monitoring; the nurses' monitoring is closer in to the machine and body functioning, while second-order monitoring is more distant, being laid on top of the other. Of course, the physician or head nurse may wish to double-check the infant and its attached equipment, using his or her own senses and judgment. This latter is a type of monitoring usually called "supervision" or "using your own eyes." Just to keep the empirical record straight, not all monitoring may be of equal importance, for that depends on trajectory phase and the infant's immediate condition; hence decisions are being made about how frequently to monitor what, with what degree of alertness, and so on.

Of course, trajectory work done without machines involves the monitoring of bodily and behavioral signs, as well as the impact on physiological systems of drugs and other medical interventions. The addition of one or more machines only increase the monitoring and usually makes it somewhat more complex. It is a moot point whether most machines make for less work or more work than before they were invented: our impressions—and the next pages will support them—are that the monitoring has become generally more complicated even though it has provided some short cuts, mainly through the mechanized information.

All of this monitoring, including that by or with machines, is designed to keep the staff abreast of one or more things: let us call them "dimensions." First, there is the monitoring of trajectory stabilization or change, whether negatively or positively, and how much change has occurred. An important aspect of that is "present condition," meaning precise location on the trajectory. Second, if the negative changes are drastic, then clinical safety is at stake and that is being monitored, especailly for high-risk trajectories or during dangerous phases. Third, there may be monitoring along at least two other dimensions, neither strictly medical although each may greatly affect the medical course. One pertains to the patient's comfort (for instance, does the machine cause undue discomfort) and another to the patient's "psychology" as affected by the machines and their operations. In fact, each of those dimensions may take precedence over strictly medical monitoring during some moments or even entire days of the patient's hospitalization.

Different trajectories call for different totalities (or arcs) of work, including monitoring work, the implicated tasks varying according to phase of the trajectory. Therefore, depending on trajectory and phase, different machinery will be utilized, whether for therapeutic or monitoring purposes. What makes the staff's work both variable and potentially further complicated are the many properities of the machine-body monitoring. A listing will immediately suggest why this is so. These properties include:

- frequency of monitoring
- duration of monitoring
- intensity of monitoring
- number of items (including body and body systems) being monitored
- number of dimensions being monitored
- clarity or ambiguity of signs being monitored
- degree of discrimination required in sign interpretation
- number and kinds of sense modalities involved in monitoring
- sequential or simultaneous monitoring of the signs

To make this discussion a bit less abstract, let us visualize the monitoring done in ICNs and in CCUs (cardiac care units). The former, as already noted, involves almost continuous attention, high alertness, multiple body systems, hosts of items, and probably often ambiguous signs, high discrimination of signs (since the infant is so fragile and the physiological changes often so minute), often virtually simultaneous monitoring, and the use of most senses. Life is rarely if ever dull in the ICN! By contrast, in a CCU the nurses may complain of boredom. All day long, monitoring TV screens record the heart rhythms, which in turn must be monitored by the nurses. A nurse may keep her eye either on the machine located at the bedside or on another located at the nursing station. Though each patient may be in great potential danger, the work entailed in watching just a few monitored items is not difficult, for only if a patient is thought to be in a hazardous condition are the monitoring tasks likely to be challenging. Otherwise the nurse's focus on the monitoring screen need not be intense, though her observation of body signs, reflecting especially cardiac and respiratory functioning, may be both intense and frequent, involving sight, sound, and touch as well. The nurse may also be monitoring through her checking of pulse and blood pressure. However, as the patient moves further from his or her heart attack and seems to be improving, the intensity and frequency of such monitoring will decrease depending on the nurse's wariness, concern, and experience, as well as on the competition for her attention by other patients with more dangerous conditions.

Again, think of dialysis, which involves only one machine (it has alarms but no information-giving printouts); it and the patient must be closely monitored early in the dialysis session, but not so frequently between then and the period of disconnecting the patient from the machine. The comfort dimension is also likely to be monitored (if only by the patient!) along with the patient's psychological state, especially if he or she is new to the dialysis procedure or is in a difficult trajectory phase. The nurse in the ICN need not monitor an infant's comfort nor its psychological reactions to treatment, but the CCU nurse may have to monitor patients' stress, composure, and other psychological matters because those can profoundly and negatively affect cardiac functioning, whereas discomfort caused by the monitoring machinery is an irrelevant issue, though, of course, she must be monitoring for other discomforts engendered by drugs, bed, or malfunctioning physiology. Comfort or psychological work is also monitored (one degree removed) for its impact on further physiological condition.

Another source of variability in the monitoring will be the agent, adding thereby to the variability engendered by the diverse trajectories, phases, drugs, procedures, and machines. Those who do the monitoring may be variously skilled, experienced, concerned, attentive, alert, and so on. In turn, the accuracy of their monitoring can be affected by resources on hand (efficiency of the machinery, lighting, time available, numbers of monitoring agents, number of patients being monitored). Another source of variability in monitoring has already been alluded to, namely, the salience of items, body systems, or dimensions which are perceived as requiring the monitoring. That perception is affected by various conditions including the nurse's experience, her conviction that the physician's orders are on target, the impairment of a sense modality, whether she is tired or full of energy, and her ideological convictions (comfort care is deemed essential, or psychological nursing is an important ingredient of excellent clinical nursing). All those conditions will affect the accuracy of monitoring—indeed, whether it is done at all.

An important aspect of this work is the proportion of attention given to machine-related monitoring compared with human monitoring. Some personnel complain that there is now undue reliance placed by both physicians and nurses on the monitoring of machined information, to the detriment of careful observations of body and behavioral signs. Nurses admit that when they are first learning to handle and monitor machines or new models of equipment, they tend to focus less on what used to be the essence of "real nursing," that is, making observations about patients and their bodies. It is not unknown for patients to worsen and even die because attention was solely on a machine's malfunctioning and monitoring. On the other hand, such a machine can give false information that either lulls or unwittingly alerts the personnel, as when its alarm sounds, either because the equipment is malfunctioning or because the patient has unwittingly set off the alarm by moving too quickly or too far.

Paying attention to alarms—whether they are balky or actually performing correctly—constitutes a fair proportion of the nurse's monitoring work, which is sometimes complicated by the noise of alarms going off on machines other than the ones which she is attending and by the constant beeping of some of them or by their emitting other noises. Personnel are prone to turn off the alarms sometimes just to get relief, trusting to their own eyes, ears, and hands. (Or they tune out psychologically, placing their attention elsewhere, yet tuning in subliminally so as to be alert if their particular machine sounds an alarm.) Nevertheless, alarms are vitally important since their action is based on precategorized limits; like alarm clocks, they go off when their limits are reached, except that the number of parameters involved may be many more than the "no more time" that shatters our sleep.

Monitoring work must be learned. The reading of body and behavioral signs is taught to nurses and technicians during their respective schooling, but undoubtedly they learn more while working on the job. They also learn about machinery as related to bodies mainly while working, learning through their own experiences and teaching by the older hands. Usually, the teaching is quite informal, personnel of different professional categories teaching and learning from each other.

For nurses especially, learning to monitor can hardly be done apart from working on the wards, since after several years they are likely to encounter numerous types of machines, either by working on different wards or because of the continual introduction of new machines. Clinical physicians, however, because they are typically specialists, work directly with many fewer types of machines in their lifetime. Their monitoring work is primarily interpretative, and much of it is of the second-order variety, which they learn mainly while they are residents although they improve with years of additional clinical experience.

One other actor in the monitoring system, the patient, should not be overlooked. Machinewise patients, familiar with equipment from their repeated hospitalizations, need not be taught monitoring chores and usually require no urging to do them. They know the machines and they also know the vagaries of their own bodies better than anyone, and that combination can make them valuable partners in the monitoring work. But that combination also makes them impatient or critical of staff members' monitoring work when they perceive it as incompetent or negligent (we saw instances of this in the chap. 2). By contrast, patients new to their disease or to particular equipment may require persuasion to engage in some measure of monitoring, by staff who wish thereby either to share the work or increase the clinical safety. Nurses will evaluate patients in accordance with their probable trustworthiness to learn and to do this monitoring. Those who are deemed too sick, unintelligent, or unmotivated to monitor themselves are likely to be placed in rooms closer to the nursing stations. Teaching patients to monitor themselves is usually done on the wing rather than through formal instruction. Of course, some kinds of monitoring, like reading cardiac waves, which dance across the screen, require too much medical sophistication for most patients to monitor even if they had the requisite energy and motivation.

Patients will also monitor each other (as already noted in our discussion of dialysis sessions), especially their roommates, but alert patients will refrain from doing this work for a variety of reasons: it is not their business, or they have taken a dislike to their roommate, or they do not trust their own judgments. Some nurses are loath to share rooms with anyone when they are hospitalized because the floor nurses are likely to expect them to keep an eye on roommates when they would prefer to avoid that work. (See chap. 8, on patient work, for further discussion of these issues.)

The most explicit teaching of patients understandably occurs a few days or hours before they go home with equipment which they must learn to operate and monitor (they must also learn to monitor its impact on their bodies). Survival machinery, like dialysis equipment, calls forth the strongest and most formal of training programs for the patients and their kin. Nevertheless, the teaching of patients about to be released is still at a relatively rudimentary stage, and since many patients live in rural areas with a low density of informed professionals or technicians or live quite far from hospitals, the followup on the effectiveness of their training is minimal.

To return to the personnel's work: an immense amount of transmission of information yielded by their monitoring is characteristic of any section in the hospital where monitoring goes on. The transmission takes the form of verbal or written reports, or both. In addition, printouts and film can be personally delivered or sent to the responsible interpretive agent, sometimes along with the notes of the person who did the bedside or laboratory monitoring. Nurses will also be found putting directly into their recorded notes the machine's recordings. Side by side there may be the machine's information, the nurses' recorded monitoring of machine information, her own observations of body signs, and her written comments on all that. Transmission of information laterally and upward is, then, a major industry engaged in by nurses, technicians, residents, and attending physicians, and, for the machines themselves, additionally by bioengineers, safety personnel, and various other calibrators, maintainers, and regulators of equipment. (Readers of this book may be amused to know that some years ago, when its senior author first began to do research in hospitals, he was much relieved to find the personnel so much absorbed in their own recording, for that allowed him to write observational notes at the nursing station without calling undue attention to himself; but he did not then understand that the staff writing had so much to do with the multiple forms of monitoring.)

All this transmitting of monitoring information is, ideally, in the service of allowing the physicians to make informed interpretations bearing on patients' trajectories: location, movement, and relationship with past medical interventions. Future courses of medical action—options perceived and chosen—depend primarily on those interpretations, pyramided atop the information gathered by technicians, nurses, residents, and the personnel of specialized labs. At the bedside operational level, transmission of monitoring information, as from nurse to head nurse or to a resident or attending physician, may result in decisions bearing immediately on a patient's safety, comfort, or anxiety. It is analytically useful to make a distinction between these two levels of information transmittal: they correspond to the distinction made earlier between option decisions made quickly on the floor and those made upstairs by the physician or physicians who are the main shapers of a patient's trajectory. Inaccuracies or blunders in monitoring can run the gamut in their consequences, from immediate fatality to throwing the physician's calculations quite off the most effective course of action. Therefore, good monitoring is the very bedrock of high-order interpretations and trajectory decisions. (See chap. 10 for further discussion of information work.)

For those who do the operational monitoring, there are consequences, too, perhaps principally boredom, excitement, and stress. We have already alluded to the ennui associated with repetitive and unchallenging kinds of monitoring, especially when trajectories are stabilized and patients are no longer in much danger. By contrast, monitoring is challenging and rewarding under a variety of conditions: when the worker is first learning how to monitor or is learning about a new machine; when the trajectory phase is at high risk and so the monitoring is vital; when the monitoring indicates that a worsening trajectory is reversing itself and the monitoring is indicating good news or has contributed to it; when the monitoring itself challenges craft or professional abilities (including those associated with ideologies that emphasize the importance of monitoring, as with comfort or psychological dimensions or as with the physician's joy in his "sixth sense," composed in part of craft and in part of ideologically based satisfaction); and when monitoring tasks are varied because the trajectories worked on are varied, hence the monitoring agent is somewhat in the situation of an orchestral musician confronted by contemporary music—difficult but interesting—rather than playing the same old music.

Finally, monitoring can result in varying degrees of stress for those who do the monitoring. Quite aside from engendering boredom, monitoring tasks can be emotionally wearying, physically tiring, hard on energies and nerves, sometimes resulting in stressful staff disputes over evaluations or interpretations of monitoring work, and over the long run can contribute to staff burnout. Nurses, especially those who choose to work in machine-dense and high-speed wards on high-risk patients, surely are constantly under stress, not only because of the general nature of their work but specifically because of the large proportion of monitoring tasks entailed in that work, so essential on these wards for the fate of patients.

But whether boring, exciting, or stressful, monitoring in the service of trajectory work is a vey large and important aspect of all medical production work. Increasingly, visibly, and dramatically, nowadays monitoring involves body-related machines.

Multiple Biographies and Machine Work

Except for the opening pages of this chapter, our discussion of machine work has ignored its historical and processual features. Working with and around equipment is sufficiently complicated and absorbing a topic to keep the analytic observer busy just outlining the types of work that is done daily in the hospital. Analytic discussion, however, should not stop with that rather cross-sectional, temporally flat, picture of daily though persistent activity patterns. So, linking back to the first two chapters we need to add the following.

There are multiple biographies, to use this term loosely, which are profoundly affecting machine tasks, so that these tasks are continually on the brink of change (Weiner et al. 1979; also see chap. 9). As noted earlier, machine (and other) technology is rapidly evolving. With each introduction of new equipment (or drug or procedure) into the market, something new has been added which will soon affect the specific tasks performed by hospital personnel. That technology is both the product of progressively evolving medical knowledge and specialization, but in turn furthers the latter. One important outcome is the production of profoundly new kinds of trajectories—shortened, lengthened, with different and novel phases and miniphases—meaning not merely the courses of illness but the tasks and organization of work implicated in those trajectories' change.

All these influences wash over and through (although at differing rates and depths) the various clinical wards. There we find machines, older and newer, each with its own history or biography of use in the general market as well as its history of consumer use and experience. The state of the art of various medical specialities is also a visible presence. It affects in the first place which types of machines (drugs, procedures) are on the ward and in the second place which kinds of illnesses, and at what stage, predominate on a particular ward. Moreover, each ward has its own biography, deeply implicated with the technological, medical specialization and trajectory biographies. Add to that the biographies (and the fairly constant turnover of personnel on highly technologized wards helps to make the point) of individual workers each of whom, of course, has experiential and personal histories pertaining to the work at hand.

A major conclusion that can be drawn from all these considerations is that the tasks carried out around and with equipment do *not* change with glacial slowness! They may change slowly on some types of ward, but certainly not where technology and medical specialization and forms of illness and ward organization are interacting furiously. Yet, if the range and kinds of tasks change with visible speed ("after two years away from the ICU, I could not just go in there cold"), nevertheless, it should not be assumed that the *types of work* change so quickly. Reflection on the divisions of this chapter will suggest that the basic issues attending machine work, with bodies, with persons, are fairly persistent. How those issues present themselves and how they are struggled with together yield the daily drama. Those issues are not immutable but they are certainly endemic to the carrying out of trajectory work, today and in the foreseeable future. In the next chapters, we shall focus on various types of work, all of which are much affected and intertwined with machine work. The first will be clinical safety work, in one sense the central work of the hospital staff.

4

Safety Work

Because the raison d'être of hospitals is to give medical care, a substantial proportion of their personnel inevitably are involved with issues of *clinical safety*. We use this term to indicate an important distinction between the safety of patients and the safety of personnel or the environment in which they work. It may be that hospitals are unique insofar as clients' physical safety is at the heart of the work in which personnel engage.

At the ward level, of course, the immediate aim is to manage and shape hazardous courses of illness so that patients are saved or made safer from the contingencies of their illness. Diagnostic services are essentially organized to locate the source of and degree of danger from an illness, and treatment units are organized to reverse or compensate for the damage done by illness. Contemporary intensive care units are organized to care for patients who are in maximum danger from illness. As the patient's condition becomes less dangerous, he or she is moved to intermediate units and later, if need be, to rehabilitation units. At each of those work sites, varying kinds and degrees of potential hazard are anticipated and resources are organized to cope with them.

An earlier version of this material appeared as "Chronic Illness, Medical Technology, and Clinical Safety in the Hospital," in *Research in the Sociology of Health Care*, vol. 4, edited by J. Roth (Greenwich, Conn.: JAI Press, 1984).

This blocking, slowing up, or reversing of hazard deriving from patients' illnesses is, after all, the core of illness work. But adding to that physiologically derived core are risks engendered by medical interventions (surgical, procedural, pharmacological, mechanical), which can threaten the safety of patients, whether their illnesses are similarly threatening or not. In the days when infectious and parasitic diseases were prevalent, hazard from the diseases themselves was very great, given the relative ineffectiveness of medical knowledge and skill in altering the course of disease. Medical intervention then was minimal and sometimes risky, though not startlingly so. The situation today is drastically different. Many of the chronic illnesses for which people are hospitalized do not immediately threaten their lives. Nevertheless, some are threatened immediately, or soon, unless there is skilled medical intervention. Ironically, that very intervention can be exceedingly hazardous either to life itself or at least to bodily functions. Hence, physicians are engaged in balancing whether to intervene, and how and how much, against whether to allow a disease to run its unimpeded natural course. For purposes of clarity, we are going to refer to the hazards of medical intervention as "risk," reserving the term "danger" for those arising from the illness itself and from various contingencies arising to threaten the clinical safety of the patients.

Chronic Illness, Technology, and Hospital Organization as Sources of Hazard

As noted in chapter 2, trajectories have been extended and new phases of trajectories have evolved, along with multiple trajectories, which have impact on each other. One implication of all this is that there are many unknowns in terms of the illness dangers *and* the risks of the associated trajectory work done on those illnesses. In short, one major source of safety work—whether actually threatening to life or not—done on and around patients is the problematic character of many of the chronic illnesses. For physicians and assisting personnel, the uncertainties of disease courses can scarcely be separated from the other trajectory work. (For example, the extended life of a person suffering from cancer is threatened both by the properties of the disease itself and from old or new chemotherapeutic drugs used to control the disease.)

Turning now to the intervention side of the equation, one can easily grasp some of the risks of, say, open-heart or brain surgery or even some of those attending diagnostic procedures. Numerous types of therapy can also be potentially hazardous—whether procedural or pharmacological, whether or not they utilize machines—and especially hazardous for particular trajectories or their phases. While many procedures and drugs are relatively standardized, others are quite experimental. Even the standard ones can have a negative impact on particular patients whose idiosyncratic physiological reactions may be unknown.

An example of potential risk in using a fairly conventional procedure is the Swan-Ganz catheter, which is used to monitor hemodynamic dangers accurately. Quite aside from the careful monitoring for safety that must be done during the procedure itself, there are some twelve possible problems involving hazard, for which there are twenty-six possible causes and an equally long list of actions intended to rectify things that have gone wrong or errors that have been committed. Of course, the number of tasks designed to minimize the risk during the procedure itself is astonishing.

While this is a riskier procedure and piece of equipment than many others, it is safe generally to characterize medical intervention as being much more of an art than a science. A great deal of it is relatively unexplored and untested, if often courageously carried out. As much to the point is that the work associated with medical intervention may contribute to its risk. All kinds of contingencies can arise from staff's mistakes or from malfunctioning equipment. The wrong drug dosages can be ordered or given. Diagnostic errors can be made in the clinical lab, or results reported for one patient that were actually those of another. Machines can become disconnected and nobody notices. (Apropos of that particular machine function: a colleague of ours was connected to a stomach pump, but during his second night the pump was accidentally disconnected from its electrical outlet, and until the patient awoke in the morning that disconnection went unnoted. The same pump was disconnected temporarily the next day by a careless EKG technician who had come to work on the patient's roommate.) Virtually every step of medical procedure and intervention, then, is dogged by the possibility of contingency and error, and hence risk to the patient, all of which require alertness and skill in preventive, monitoring, and rectifying action, that is, in what can be conveniently termed "safety work."

Potentially increasing both danger (illness-derived) and risk (intervention-derived) are various contingencies that arise from a third source: the hospital's organization. Discussion of a few organizational conditions bearing on hazard and safety will underscore the potency of that source. Perhaps the first condition, as noted in chapter 1, is that hospitals are generally quite decentralized in terms of their ward functioning and work. That decentralization has several implications for the safety of the patients. Centralized control over safety features, even environmental hazards bearing on patient as well as staff safety, tends to be weak. Recollect that a safety department—if indeed the hospital has one—tends to persuade or negotiate with ward personnel, rather than to order, command, and challenge. Safety personnel supply the wards with regulations and guidelines derived from federal, state, or city governments or from the hospital administration. But a combination of relative ward autonomy and safety department weakness in authority and resources means that only a few regulations and guidelines can be monitored.

Safety personnel are not likely to be confident about strictly clinical safety issues unless they are directly affected by safety features falling within their own realm of competence. Thus, the field researcher discussed a recent electrical blowout throughout the hospital with one environmental safety functionary:

> He had been discussing, with the dialysis staff, emergency plans for evacuating patients in case of disaster. When he found out it takes an hour to unhook the patients, he hit the ceiling. He kept mentioning during the interview twenty minutes for evacuation, like it was a magic number—the usual time required to get people out. He has been pushing the physician, he said, to come up with a plan so that patients can be unhooked as quickly as possible without dangering them.

But when asked about the unhooking of patients in intensive care areas:

> He didn't answer except by bringing up the dialysis unit, though he did state he was in no position to make medical judgments about how to evacuate a patient hooked up with the machinery. He gave me the safety plan for the hospital. Reading it, I find that instructions are made to O.R., patient units, X-ray, lab, etc., but missing are the critical care areas. Not a one is mentioned.

The delicate balance between clinical and environmental hazard is illustrated by the safety personnel's need to monitor the hospital's generators, which take over in case the city's electrical circuits fail. This means that they must alert ward personnel to exactly when the generator system will be monitored, so that any patient plugged into a life-sustaining machine . . . ! On some older ICUs, in fact, not all wall outlets may have been connected to the generator systems, so the ward's monitoring must proceed in tandem with the generator monitoring. Thus, the latter monitoring can heap potential clinical risk on top of ongoing clinical risk—just as careless machine servicing or incorrect calibrating of machines can add to risk to patients.

Hence, it is apparent that the interplay between wards and safety specialists can be important, possibly crucial for clinical as well as environmental safety, and can involve different relationships between the various wards and various types of safety specialists. For instance, on machine-dense sites, new personnel must be oriented toward the dos and don'ts of electrical hazards—don't touch the cardiac monitor and the patient at the same time, and so on. Experienced ward personnel do the teaching, but originally the guidelines came to the ward from the safety specialist.

There are certainly many governmental regulations (e.g., when patients have radium implants, the beds must be 10 feet apart, but if beds are closer, there must be walls between beds) that must be adhered to closely. On all wards, of course, the pharmaceutical regulations are followed unless personnel are careless. Yet the country over, surgical procedures are largely unregulated, let alone supervised, by either government functionaries or hospital administrators, although peer review boards may look at suspect surgical work and records. But, for the most, the surgical ward's control over safety features is internal.

Government regulations run far behind most ward practice and are much less stringent for machines than for drugs. The ward personnel are relatively on their own. Besides, they will bend and adapt both government and hospital guidelines or regulations in what seem sensible ways in order to accomplish the ward's work.

In intensive care units, of course, the equipment is calibrated and monitored regularly and frequently if the particular hospital has the necessary resources. The relative autonomy of hospital wards does not necessarily make for increased risk to patients, but it is a factor in safety *and* hazard.

Another feature associated with decentralization is that each ward is autonomous only to the degree that it is independent of the resources and services of other departments—and it never is. Insofar as a ward's personnel must depend on or deal with the external hospital world, that, too, enters into safety and hazard. (A patient admitted to the emergency room in great pain was suspected immediately of having either a cardiac or digestive condition. While she was waiting for the requisite diagnostic tests, food trays were brought and the patient was asked if she wanted breakfast. Unthinkingly and without being noticed by the nurses, she ate a light breakfast because her pain had already subsided. Immediately she began to have intense pain, for eventually she would be diagnosed as having a digestive problem.)

Patients transported to diagnostic sites can be at risk if visits are not properly prepared for and supervised; lab tests can be disastrously erroneous; patients can be served the wrong food, and so on. If all such interdepartmental connections work badly, clinical hazard is increased; if they work well, the patient benefits.

A third important feature of hospitals pertains to problems of adequate staffing. Maximum clinical safety requires skilled or at least competent personnel in sufficient numbers and good physical shape to operate safely. Even the most affluent hospitals encounter difficulties with one or more of those problems. The reluctance of a great many well-trained nurses to work in hospitals is a recognized phenomenon today. The increased numbers of nurses being placed temporarily in hospitals through registry services means that many either will not be competent to handle the ward's characteristic illnesses and equipment or will not be familiar enough with ward practice to function with maximum safety to patients. (There have been aberrant cases reported, too, where such temporary—or not so temporary—personnel have deliberately killed patients; the point is that supervision of their activities may be slight or ineffective.) Many, if not most, nursing administrators resort to shifting their nurses around to make up for daily shortages on wards, and these "float nurses" may not be as skilled at work in one ward as another. Intensive care unit nurses complain, too, that they can be understaffed because one or two personnel have been shifted temporarily in order to help out elsewhere. When wards are unexpectedly overflowing with patients, some patients may be bumped to another ward where personnel are not so familiar with their diseases or with accompanying equipment or they are moved too quickly from the ICU to a medical or surgical ward, to their hazard. Nurses aside, the various technicians who visit the wards or receive patients at machine sites may not be well trained, highly motivated, or adequately supervised. The same can be said about physicians. (And in teaching hospitals, interns and residents need to learn the ward's trajectories and routines, before they can contribute to maximum clinical safety. "I just get tired of having to teach the young doctors" is a frequent complaint among nurses everywhere.) Even when personnel are highly skilled, motivated, and present in sufficient numbers, their efficiency may be impaired by overwork, tiredness, even boredom derived from the work, not because of individual peculiarities or capacities, but because of ineffective ward or hospital organization. All of that contributes to increasing the hazards to a ward's clients. Added to the issue of adequate staffing is another striking feature of hospitals: they operate for twenty-four hours and seven days a week. Evening or night shifts may be understaffed or staffed with less competent, or even incompetent, personnel. Backup services decrease in the evening and virtually vanish at night, except in the intensive care units.

We are, of course, referring to relatively affluent hospitals. Many are not. In these, the extraordinary number of organizational resources that bear on clinical safety and risk are minimal or missing. If really sick persons are sent to those hospitals, their safety is quite threatened. On the face of it, patients are safer in those hospitals which are better serviced and practice the best and most advanced medicine. The qualification to the phrase "on the face of it" is that patients in those hospitals are often sicker, or they would not be there. The very complexity of treatments given as well as the complexity of their coordinated organization affect the level of hazard. In short, all three sources (chronic illness, medical technology, and hospital organization) have a profound impact on clinical safety.

Machine and Machine-Body Safety

We have already touched on hazards associated with various elements of medical technology (machine, pharmaceutical, surgery, procedures). In this section, our focus will be directed at some special risks to patients associated with equipment used in diagnosis and treatment and how those risks are potentially minimized, monitored, assessed, and corrected.

As noted in the previous chapter, a striking visible feature of acute-care hospitals is their vast amount of equipment. To a considerable degree, clinical safety, then, depends on properly functioning equipment and appropriate work by competent or skilled workers at many levels. Each of the properties of machines also has relevance to clinical safety, as, for example, size. A large machine may decrease the personnel's work space in an already tight unit, thereby affecting efficiency and work flow. Storage may be a problem; equipment may be stored in an area not usual for it and may create delays in delivery of the machine to the crucial site. New machinery often requires extensive orientation of staff to its safe use, or the learning of new skills, or it may necessitate the incorporation of new personnel onto the ward. More often than not a period of time is required to "get the bugs out" of a new machine or model, work out details of the division of labor, and determine the machine's reliability. Machines placed permanently in the body (e.g., pacemakers) call for both machine safety and the patient's physical safety. When the patient goes home, there must be training for safety work there, plus the development of organizational mechanisms so that both machine and patient can be monitored.

When equipment is invented, it must be tried experimentally, manufactured, sold, and installed. Later it must be monitored for efficiency and safety. From those varieties of work which are involved in producing, using, and servicing machinery, we can sense the great variety of safety jobs engaged in by many different types of persons, and the dense organizational arrangements—both inside and outside the hospital—upon which machine functioning and associated clinical safety rest.

Machine Production Safety

Machine production safety is concerned with safety when innovating, manufacturing, selling, purchasing, installing, and preparing the proper environment (space, lighting, electric wiring, etc.); it involves complex relationships not only within hospital departments and services, but also between them and manufacturers and government safety regulation agencies. During the innovation process, physicians and allied professionals together with engineers attempt to perfect the machine for safety as well as efficiency. There is an ongoing exchange between the manufacturer's representatives and health professionals in order to improve efficiency and safety, an important exchange because only through actual use of the machinery are most clinical inadequacies and safety hazards discovered. It is impossible to anticipate all the clinical conditions and contingencies that might affect a machine's efficiency and safety. Not infrequently users make improvements that are incorporated into the later machine production. For example, the number of alarms for signaling impending danger may be insufficient in clinical situations, and so a hospital engineer may then devise and add new alarms. This improvement may later be adopted by the producers. Or a machine may be proven safe in test situations and meet safety regulations, but unexpected situations in the hospital may affect its safety. For example, the amount of insulation needed to protect the machine's functioning from outside electrical magnetic interference may be quite inadequate for shielding it from interference when used in a hospital located near a transmission power station.

When safety hazards are discovered, a complex communication must then be set up among producers, safety regulation agencies, hospitals, and other users. Also communications must be set up within the hospital, not only concerning specific hazards and how to rectify them, but also for recalling defective machinery and parts. Safety communication is not confined to equipment but also includes hazardous bio-materials, drugs, and chemicals—as witnessed by the innumerable safety bulletins circulated in larger hospitals.

Since most machines are powered by electricity, safety work begins with proper electrical wiring, and a backup system to generate electricity to take over when a power failure or shortage occurs. Along with this there are requirements about training and drilling health professionals and other hospital personnel for emergency action and for minimizing or preventing clinical hazards should the power fail.

Considering the many different properties of machines that pertain to safety, the purchase of machinery necessitates consultation among many hospital personnel and with technical experts. Even when machines are proved safe in test situations and through long usage and are produced by a reputable manufacturer, there may be manufacturing defects: ground wires disconnected, cords broken, and plugs improperly installed. Maximizing safety then requires that an engineer test and evaluate newly purchased machines for defects even before their use.

Machine-Tending Safety

Just as machine production safety calls for complex relationships among producers and hospitals and between repairers and suppliers within and outside the hospital, the same is true for machine-tending safety (which includes monitoring, servicing, and repairing of machines, as well as machine supply and storing and disposing of equipment when old or obsolete). Developing adequate institutional arrangements to assure machine-tending safety is fraught with difficulties because of the great numbers, diversity of types and models of the machinery produced by many companies, along with the rapid diffusion of this equipment. The diversity—constantly changing—produces a lag in the organizational resources and arrangements required to cope with the safety tasks within both hospitals and the equipment industry.

Hospital administrators' attempts to maximize safety by centralizing control over aspects of machine-tending safety encounter difficulties. First, each medical specialty service tends to think its safety concerns are unique, a belief based on experiential knowledge gathered through working with given machines in relation to various illnesses. Often the personnel feel they know better the intimate details of models, necessary supplies, and the companies that are best at producing and servicing them than outsiders to the ward or department can. For example, at one hospital where we observed, efforts were made by the administration to standardize cardiovascular monitors for all the intensive care units, since it was reasoned that this would assure better servicing and repairing. Consensus among the ICU staffs could not, however, be reached since each unit felt its clinical needs were unique and could not be met by using a single company's product. And since some producers compete for markets, their models are eventually improved. Hospital staffs did not want to be saddled with one company's product should more safe and efficient models be obtainable from another company. Moreover, each department had different equipment priorities: some, for instance, having newer generations of cardiovascular monitors already, would prefer expending their resources in purchasing other equipment.

A second consideration is this: although many hospitals now employ safety engineers, bioengineers, and technicians to service and repair machines, these resources are rarely sufficient because of the constant introduction of new technology to the wards. Its rapid absorption is hastened in part by hospital personnel, especially physicians, because of their desire to have the latest and presumably the most effective model that appears in this fast-moving equipment market. (Even small-town hospitals may do this; we interviewed on hospital administrator who was, happily, about to attract a specialist through purchase of a second-hand scanner!) Moreover, hospitals compete to attract physicians and patients by possessing the latest technology. At the same time, while new technology rapidly makes equipment obsolete, cost considerations may prevent replacement of those particular machines whose malfunctioning may be potentially hazardous and parts necessary to repair machinery may not be available through the manufacturer because of the age of particular models.

Machine-Body Safety

The machine-body interface for maximizing safety is extremely complex, for it involves safety in setting up the machine, connecting the patient to the machine, monitoring both the machine and body systems, while interpreting the interaction of the machine and machine products (printouts, films, body products, etc.), drugs, and other therapies. For each of those kinds of tasks there are potential hazards, including those produced by error. There is always a chance, in fact, that error can occur. The machine, machine product, drugs, and other therapies present particular problems for assessing, preventing, monitoring, minimizing, and rectifying clinical hazards. Those are maximized when multiple body systems are involved and when linked with the use of multiple machines and multiple therapies as is the case with many problematic trajectories. The interaction of danger sources places a heavy burden on the personnel concerning their decisions on which of the many hazards are to be risked. Such decisions are difficult purely from a clinical standpoint but become more so when the risks taken also involve potentially negative impacts on the patient's identity, on the legal security of the staff, and on the costs of reducing anticipated risks. Moreover, the risking must take into account available resources, not only for the individual patient but for groups of patients. (For example, in the ICU that was saddled with old machinery, the staff attempted to match their resources with the danger profile of the patient. While the patient was in a high risk condition he or she was cared for on the more efficient equipment, but once past that condition was shifted to older and less efficient equipment. Risk decisions were difficult there when the machine risk could not be taken because of a danger profile or when there was an overfllow of patients.)

We should add that the interaction of various sources of danger presents problems in assessing, monitoring, preventing, minimizing, and rectifying clinical dangers. For example, a machine readout indicates changes toward a more dangerous physical condition. Assessment then involves determining if the altered printout is due to a malfunction of the machine, the body connection, drugs, actual worsening of the body, or combinations of those various sources.

Controlling the Trajectory

Controlling trajectories for an outcome as successful as possible and with minimum harm from intervention requires that health professionals, particularly physicians, have some notion of what the trajectory shape will be, some imagery of the trajectory phases, the kinds and degrees of dangers and risks in each phase, the therapeutic actions required to keep the trajectory satisfactorily under control, the resources and skills required, and the anticipated contingencies that might cause problems for successful trajectory management.

Complexities of Diagnoses

As a consequence of advances made in diagnostic technology, the diagnostic process has become more rapid, efficient, and reliable, particularly for the more recognizable diseases. Yet there is much variation in the diagnostic approaches to various illnesses. They may vary from very reliable to very questionable, be easy or difficult to carry out, require a minimum or maximum of skilled resources, and vary in degrees of potential risk to the patient. Depending on the illness and characteristics of the means of diagnosis, the physician must contend with different kinds of problematic issues, for example, whether to subject the patient to a potentially dangerous diagnostic procedure or to wait and see how the illness develops symptomatically.

In spite of the array of diagnostic approaches available today, the diagnostic search may encounter many problems, especially in estimating the reliability of diagnostic means. As noted earlier, physicians need to be careful in assessing reliability since clinical laboratories and X-ray centers can vary in the quality of their work; a great deal of experience may be necessary to make judgments, which ultimately affect the patient's safety. Yet physicians are increasingly at the mercy of the work of clinical laboratory personnel and other diagnostic technicians whose reliability may not be easy to judge. (Recollect the statement by the wary oncologist in chap. 2.) Errors may arise not only from misinterpretation but from machine error, too, since some machines have to be calibrated carefully and frequently or the test results they produce may be inaccurate.

Complexities of Therapeutic Management

The complexity of organization for therapeutic action, including its import for clinical hazard, derives not only from the problematic character of many trajectories but from the number and range of tasks involved in the therapeutic action, plus the organization of tasks involved in controlling the illness course. If an illness is well understood, standard operating procedure can readily control it, but even relatively expectable ones can develop unanticipated complexities around organizational issues: delays in treatments, errors in treatments, and the like. It is important, therefore, to underline the point that error and failure can occur during the completion of any task. Clinical safety then requires not only purely medical and technical tasks, but the organizational underpinning necessary to carry out the tasks successfully.

Ordinarily, physicians do not concern themselves with the operational details of task accomplishment (see chap. 7). The supervision and articulation of the various tasks usually fall within the provinces of the nurses and technicians. While the latter focus only on the immediate tasks of, say, taking an X ray or drawing blood, being unconcerned with the more general course of the illness, physicians and nurses focus at least implicitly on trajectory considerations as well as on the trajectory work itself. At a particular moment, specific tasks may absorb them, but the patient's location on a hazardous course is never forgotten. An added complexity is that patients are not, after all, inanimate objects, so their reactions affect not only the trajectory phases but the tasks that are necessary to make the trajectory management successful and less hazardous. Loss of patient's composure, wounded sensibilities, uncalled for discomforts—all these may add to the risks of medical interventions.

The tasks done during the various phases and miniphases of a trajectory vary in their properties; these include the degree and kinds of potential risks and the degree to which errors can be rectified. In different trajectory phases and work sites there will be different patterns of work, depending on the properties of tasks and the associated safety concerns. For example, in a heart catheterization done for proper diagnosis of potential cardiac damage, there is a massing of many complicated pieces of equipment and skilled personnel to carry out the procedure and prevent or minimize the many potential risks. There is a carefully arranged division of labor among the personnel, also an exquisite simultaneity and sequencing of tasks. Patient participation is very important in this sequencing. Maximizing clinical safety, as well as minimizing threats to the patient's identity and composure, are both integral to the overall task structure. In contrast, during the immediate postoperative phase, within the recovery room, the task structure is primarily organized around returning the patient to proper physiological functioning following the surgical trauma and the effects of the anestheisa. Much of the work involves monitoring the physiological functioning. Impact on the patient's identity is of minimum concern here. Indeed, patients are often unconscious or nearly unconscious. Clinical safety is at the forefront.

Task Structure and Safety

Anticipated dangers associated with clinical actions must be operationalized into an organized task structure. For each task, varying degrees of complexity are entailed. Among the salient properties relevant to maximizing the safety of a given task (minimizing its risk to the patient) are: (1) the diversity of resources required; (2) the diversity of tasks done by various personnel and a patient and the risks associated with the tasks; (3) the flexibility of the temporal ordering of tasks, both simultaneously and sequentially, as well as speed of action; and (4) the rectifiability of the temporal ordering of tasks and of malfunctioning technology, error, or other unexpected contingencies. In addition, the task structure often calls for a great amount of assessing, preventing, minimizing, monitoring, and rectifying of potential dangers, which are done by many different (and even different kinds) of personnel.

To illustrate those points, here is a vignette observed in a cardiac intensive care unit:

Mr. C., a patient in his late seventies, with serious congestive heart failure, has been the center of attention all morning. He is considered the most seriously ill patient on the unit, so he is placed in the bed unit directly facing the nursing station. The nurses described the patient as being irritable and anxious throughout the night.

The physicians had made a decision to insert a Swans-Ganz catheter to monitor the hemodynamic system more accurately. The nurses were anxious that the procedure be done soon because two new patients were scheduled for admission. However, the resident physician doing the procedure was not immediately available, being tied up in teaching rounds on the unit. Twice during the teaching rounds, a nurse approached the physician to "get the show on the road" because of the impending admission of the new patients.

Since the work pace was slow because other patients were less seriously ill and stabilized, the slow work pace was used as an opportunity to provide "learning experiences" for a novice nurse. The novice was assigned to this task, assisted by several seasoned nurses to tutor and help her.

The novice gathered and brought the necessary equipment, machinery and supplies to the bedside, following the instructions in the procedure manual. A "crash cart" (cart with all the necessary equipment required in case of an emergency) was also brought to the bedside. One of the seasoned nuses assisted the novice in working on the Swans-Ganz set up (which has some 11 tubings connected to various parts of the equipment and to the patient), pointing out the various steps in doing this task, dos and don'ts, and potential errors. Another nurse calibrated the monitoring machine that would be connected. This machine is a very specialized monitor, custom made to meet certain research requirements. Earlier, the head nurse stated that because of the specialized nature of the monitor there were only a few nurses who could finely tune the machine.

The resident came to put in the catheter. He explained to the patient that he would be putting down a tube through a neck vein as explained earlier in the morning. He informed the patient that it was necessary to lie flat during the procedure even though this might make breathing more difficult. The doctor rolled down the head of the bed while the nurse helped to position the patient. The doctor and nurses donned masks.

The seasoned nurse in a nice manner informed the physician that there were two sets of sterile gloves, one to disinfect the skin and the other to insert the catheter. Earlier in the morning this nurse had informed me that she had insisted on a more elaborate, operating room-like set up in these types of procedures. Prior to her coming on the unit there was less strict asceptic technique. Previous records showed a number of infections, but since instituting stricter techniques, the infection rates had noticeably decreased.

While the doctor was preparing himself and readying the equipment, another nurse came with another piece of equipment, a connection for the central monitor in the nursing station. The nurse helping the novice pointed out the proper connections, how they can be identified by the numbers of prongs and color coding.

The doctor prepared the skin where the needle was to be inserted, but before doing this, informed the patient that he would be cleaning the skin, and the solution used would be cold; he asked the patient to be still and to keep his hands out of the way. This completed, the doctor prepared to set up a sterile area. He informed the patient that he would be covering his face with a sterile towel. Throughout all this, the novice nurse helped the doctor while the seasoned nurse whispered the next steps and the equipment to be readied.

Shortly after the doctor had readied the patient, another doctor arrived to help. At the same time, another doctor, dressed in street clothes, stood at the unit doorway. The three exchanged information about the laboratory findings. The older doctor asked what they expected in the pressure readings from putting down the catheter, given the patient's current condition. The resident speculated.

Before the experienced physician got into the sterile gown, he surveyed the situation and immediately removed the pillow under the patient's head. The nurse immediately caught the error and brought a rolled bath towel to place under the patient's neck. The physician explained to the less experienced why this position is preferred. Physician asked the patient if he is "all right."

The less experienced physician anesthetized the vein cutdown area, assisted by the novice nurse. Before injecting the anesthesia, the doctor told the patient he will anesthetize the area and so some pricks will be felt. The seasoned nurse moved over and held the patient's hand. The physician oversaw the less experienced doctor doing the procedure, making suggestions about how to move the needle to get better results. This was interspersed with telling the patient he is doing very well, or asking how he feels. Meanwhile, the novice nurse responded to the doctors' requests for equipment and watched the EKG readouts.

The doctors showed the less seasoned doctor how to locate the vein and the best way to make the incision. The doctor warned the patient he will feel pressure, but no pain. One physician acted as an assistant to the less seasoned physician, giving low-voiced instructions. The procedure progressed nicely and relaxedly, even to the point where the less experienced physician was asking many related technical questions about cardiac management. While this was going on, the nurse remained with the patient, from time to time patting him, uncovering the towel from his face, observing him and informing him that "everything is fine"; also glancing at the monitor readouts.

The physician interrupted the resident's conversation, stating the catheter had better be put in right away because there was a danger of blood clots if they dallied. The seasoned doctor quickly prepared the catheter and took over the procedure, pushing in the catheter. The nurse immediately moved to the special monitor machine, making adjustments to the machine, writing on the paper readouts, and instructed the novice nurse to prepare the various connections. Everybody looked at the monitor readouts. The doctor asked the other physician to pull out the catheter "a tad" because he thought the catheter position needed adjustment. Evrybody watched the oscilloscope for a period. The seasoned doctor informed the less seasoned one that everything went well and complimented the patient for being a good patient. The doctors exchanged technical information, with the seasoned doctor informing the less informed one that the suturing task would be left to him. The nurses helped the patient get comfortable and cleaned up the mess. The nurse discussed various critical points of patient observation and care with the novice.

This not uncommon scene in the cardiac intensive care unit indicates the complexity of clinical safety. It illustrates the varieties of bundles of tasks involving several personnel which must be done sequentially and simultaneously—organized, in other words, into a task structure that bears directly on safety. First, the nurses assessed the potentially dangerous procedure in terms of the overall anticipated work on the unit, because procedural safety requires time and personnel. Aftes surveying the unit's overall level of hazard, time was used to train a novice so that she would become a safe nurse. A seasoned nurse was assigned to help the novice, as well as to do the catheterization tasks. In essence, the nursing staff was building safety resources. In preparing the necessary equipment, machinery, and supplies, backup was also made available for possible dangers should anything go awry.

The physician doing the procedure engaged in interactions with the patient to assure that the latter would not be a source of hazard, especially through untoward movement or loss of composure. The nurse prevented the physician from breaking the aseptic rules, and this was done very nicely so that his identity would not be threatened. In general, with each minitask that might endanger the patient, the physician preceded it by interacting with the patient.

Personnel took into account the risk potential of the task's phases: the seasoned physician taking over the task when the risk was at its highest (putting in the catheter). Likewise, the nurse took over tasks that required great skill, especially tasks involved with the special monitoring machine. The experienced personnel engaged in much monitoring and preventing of risks which might be incurred through the actions of less experienced personnel. When the physicians were engaged in tasks that required much concentration, the nurses engaged in much composure work with the patient to minimize the potentially hazardous impact of any loss of composure.

The field note quotation also shows some consequences occurring when structural conditions are altered. As can be seen, the consequences would have been quite different if: (1) the number of seriously ill patients was very high; (2) there was a shortage of experienced nursing staff; (3) the latter did not take the less experienced personnel's identity and composure into account; (4) the experienced nursing staff did not take the patient's identity and composure into account; (5) the tasks were out of sequence; (6) skills were not matched with the high-risk phases of the tasks; (7) unexpected breakdowns of equipment occurred; or (8) there were changes in the patient's physical condition during the carrying out of this procedure. Different combinations of these conditions will, of course, have different consequences for clinical safety.

The safety requirements needed here are quite different from, say, a cardiac resuscitation task structure (where the patient is in grave physical danger, and the tasks may have potential physical risk for the one being resuscitated) or with a procedure for manipulating a cardiac catheter in order to connect a patient to an intra-aortic balloon pump. These call for a special space and teams of skilled personnel working on different parts of the patient's body simultaneously and sequentially.

Generally, to manage the risks more efficiently, efforts are made to group patients who have similar trajectories and similar danger profiles all on the same ward. This enables a routinizing and patterning of the overall safety-task structure, with the likelinood that fewer major task readjustments and reorganizations need to be made when a patient's danger profile changes. Hence, there is a strong drive for each specialty and subspecialty to have its own special unit if the hospital's space and funds permit. However, many problems are posed because of the increase in problematic trajectories, and finite resources do not permit an exact matching of resources to the danger profiles. There is also the reality that task safety rests on a complicated and easily upset organizational underpinning.

Safety Measures and Routines

What other safety measures and routines do wards possess for minimizing danger and risk to their patients? Besides adequate staffing, good interdepartmental relations, frequent calibrating and monitoring of equipment, stockpiling of equipment, and the like, wards engage in standard safety measures. They have emergency fire drills, electrical short circuit drills, cardiac massage, and defibrillation practice. There are organizational arrangements that minimize the risk of giving the wrong drugs or the wrong dosages. There is the teaching and coaching of less experienced personnel. Staff will study various safety guidelines and regulations, memorizing them.

In ICUs, especially, the staff members try to anticipate potential hazard by routinizing certain tasks, such as checking out alarm systems and other machinery features at the beginning of their work sessions. They change tubing on respiratory equipment daily to reduce the risk of infection. The nurses develop protocols of nursing care wherein hazards, actions, and resources are identified. These protocols become part of standard operating procedure. The development of these protocols and procedure manuals takes time, because a great deal of discussion is required and the input of many persons (nurses and others) may be involved. However, their revision is required for maximum clinical safety because of the rapid development of new knowledge, the introduction of new technology, and the constant appearance of new organizational contingencies. Resource building on the ICUs through the upgrading of knowledge and skills and the use of backup staff is striking. Among nurses, the amount of informal teaching is not always apparent to the casual observer. Nurses continually apprise each other of new information. Periods of slack in the work often are used to refresh infrequently used skills, to upgrade protocols and procedure manuals, to teach novices who are unfamiliar with risky procedures, and so on. Because slack periods are essential for resource building, resentment against nursing administrators on these units runs high if a nurse is transferred to an intermediate unit because her service is not deemed nearly as essential to the ICU as to some understaffed ward.

The ICUs are perhaps a bit exceptional since their patients are among the sickest and their medical interventions are the most extensive, but such safety measures and routines are characteristically diffused over all the wards and are followed more or less closely depending on the competence and concern of their respective personnel and the resources at their command. One additional condition that bears on those standard modes of maximizing clinical safety is that an experienced staff develops what might be termed "local knowledge." They learn the idiosyncracies of specific pieces of equipment. They learn which drugs to be particularly wary of or alert to, given the illnesses prevalent in their ward. They learn the physiological peculiarities, too, of particular patients, especially when these are repeaters to the ward (and people with certain chronic illnesses tend to be repeaters). They learn, too, modes of dealing with the hazard-producing contingencies of other departments and their personnel. That local knowledge possessed by ward staff and shared among them and their knowledge of protocols, procedures, guidelines, and regulations, all contribute to the maximization of clinical safety. Any structural condition or contingency that decreases those two kinds of knowledge thereby increases the chances of clinical hazard. Given the variability of those contingencies and conditions for hospitals around the country and for their wards, obviously some are safer places for patients than others.

Assessing and Monitoring Clinical Hazard

Accurate, efficient, and intelligent assessment and monitoring of hazards (associated with the illness course itself and with its clinical management) are the bedrocks of clinical safety. Since assessing and monitoring often occur simultaneously, they are frequently used as synonymous terms by health workers. Their close interrelatedness stems in part from each requiring criteria of safety limits, interpretative skills, and the use of senses (seeing, hearing, touching, smelling) plus various kinds of measures (lab reports, machine readouts). Though closely related, assessing and monitoring can be considered for analytic purposes as distinct activities.

Assessing is concerned with estimating and evaluating the graveness, controllability, and rectifiability of risks and dangers. In turn, these are associated with the medical interventions, with the illness itself, and with various expected or unexpected contingencies which have appeared, and weighing those risks and dangers so as to judge courses of action effectively for preventing, controlling, and rectifying. Assessment implies assigning priorities to hazards and often implies a higher level of cognitive process than occurs in monitoring.

A central aspect of monitoring is the tracking of specific items and indicators that are defined as potentially hazardous because of their frequency, rate, change, or duration. An interpretative process is also involved here, but the main emphasis is on preventing potential dangers and risks before they get out of hand. More often than not, the totality of tracked items and indicators, rather than single ones, is used in making assessments. Moreover, effective assessment rests on effective and accurate monitoring but, in turn, effective and accurate monitoring depends on equally effective assessment. Consequently, a continual interplay of both processes occurs throughout the entire trajectory, and together they constitute a large portion of the total trajectory work.

A central issue in accurate assessing and monitoring is the reliability of criteria for determining safety limits. There is great variation in the criteria used in establishing safety limits for kinds and sources of hazard. Here are a few properties of these criteria:

- the degree of clarity-ambiguity of signs, indicators, and measures used
- the degree of skill and experience required to obtain the signs, indicators, and measures
- the degree of skill and experience required to interpret the signs, indicators, and measures
- the number of signs, indicators, and measures involved
- the frequency of signs, indicators, and measures
- the numbers of workers involved and the degree of cooperation required among them
- the degree to which the patient's cooperation and interaction are crucial
- the degree to which the sequencing of various criteria is crucial

The use of much of the medical technology is fraught with uncertainty, and when this is combined with chronic illness—where many body systems are involved and affect each other—then the interaction of multiple interventions makes it very difficult to establish reliable criteria for safety limits. More often than not, the weighing and balancing pertain to making judgments about which of the hazards are more or less worse. Moreover, finding the cause of some identified hazard may be very difficult and often requires the expertise of several specialists. (See the case of Mrs. Price in chap. 2.) The complexity of balancing and weighing is heightened because various actors may be weighing and balancing quite different matters. Moreover, they may not be fully aware of each other's assessments. Also the concerns over weighing and balancing can alter over time for each, and there may be varying degrees of awareness of one another's weighing and balancing.

On the ward, each type and level of staff will vary in the scope and level of assessing and monitoring that is permitted, or at least generally engaged in. These jurisdictional boundaries are determined by training, education, and legal code. The fact that many persons and levels are involved necessitates that team members seek assistance from appropriate persons or groups when a safety limit exceeds their respective jurisdictions. (For instance, an LVN may go to an RN or the RN to the head nurse.) However, there is much overlap between the assessing and monitoring of safety limits because the sources of potential risk and danger are many and they interact. This overlap necessitates further communication among multiple levels and groups of workers as they attempt to make accurate assessments. Moreover, because of the overlapping, staff engage in assessing and monitoring each other for reliability and competence, Interactional difficulties arise around matters such as: (1) stepping beyond one's jurisdiction; (2) not taking responsibility for hazards thought to lie within one's jurisdiction; (3) forcing assessment and monitoring responsibilities on lower-level workers, which others or they believe to be beyond their proper scope and level of competence or responsibility; and (4) discounting of the assessments made by different levels of workers.

Though there are commonly agreed upon, or legally mandated, safety jurisdictions for each level of hospital worker, the overlap of jurisdiction poses problems. There is a tendency for different kinds of personnel to set different priorities without having an awareness of the total trajectory. They may assign differing importance to different indicators, signs, and measures in terms of the degree of reliability and creditability. Therefore, they may miss crucial indicators seen by other personnel. Physicians, for instance, tend to rely heavily on various types of laboratory tests to make assessments, whereas nurses depend more on patients' bodily and emotional responses.

These differences in work responsibility also result in different solutions to problems. For example, nurses are largely responsible for preparing, hooking up, and monitoring the machines that are connected to patients. Thus dangers arising from machine malfunction are often of greater concern to nurses. (In one situation that we observed, the nurses were much concerned with the potential dangers from old cardiovascular monitoring machines, which, of course, greatly increased the monitoring and rectifying work associated with them. The physicians were sympathetic to the nurses but were not sufficiently concerned to force the hospital administration to correct this situation.) The differences in the focus of monitoring and assessment, then, have consequences for the ward's work organization, staff interaction, and staff morale.

Some varieties of the varied monitoring system and assessing can be seen in the accompanying chart. The extent of divergent views, and the degree of agreement or disagreement, among health workers, patients, and family can be identified on such a chart. All that is necessary is to use letters for type of worker, and numbers for the particular staff member, thus: for physicians, D^1, D^2, D^n; for nurses, N^1, N^2, N^n; for technicians, T^1, T^2, T^n; for kin, K^1, K^2, K^n; for the patient, P^1, P^2, P^n. Then match and D, N, T, K, or P against others on this chart:

	Potential Sources of Hazard				
Hazard Dimensions	Patient as a Body System	Patient as a Person	Diagnostic, Palliative, or Therapeutic Measures	Personnel	Environment
Graveness					
High					
Low					
Specificity					
Known					
Unknown					
Predictability					
High					
Low					
Duration					
Long					
Short					
Controllability					
Difficult					
Easy					
Rectifiability					
Difficult					
Easy					

Monitoring and Mismonitoring

Bodily and psychological reactions to the illness and to the various interventions are monitored in order to: (1) provide a basis for the assessment of current trajectory status; (2) be alerted that something has gone wrong or is going wrong; (3) be alerted to the effectiveness or ineffectiveness of various therapies; (4) recognize discomfort and pain suffered by the patient; and (5) note the side effects of the various interventions. Much of this, of course, has direct or indirect bearing on assessments of clinical safety and hazard.

Numerous items then must be monitored, and they vary widely in their properties. A partial list would include:

- the degree of predictability of their occurrence
- the degree of ambiguity or clarity
- the skills and experience required to discriminate altered signs
- the degree to which the patient's cooperation and communication are involved
- the number of instrumentalities (senses, machine products, lab findings, etc.) involved
- the skills and experience required to interpret signs
- the salience of signs

These properties are taken into account when setting priorities for the monitoring of various items and incorporating them into a task structure. Thus, because of their salience certain items are monitored at very frequent intervals, while others occur periodically and so allow more flexible monitoring. Some items, of course, are routinely monitored.

The transmission of monitored information becomes a major activity for the health personnel. It takes the form of oral or written reports and recording on charts—or both—of observed patient reactions, printouts, lab monitoring, etc. Transmission occurs both laterally and hierarchically: it is engaged in by everyone—nurses, technicians, residents, attending and staff physicians, bioengineers, safety personnel, and various maintainers or regulators of equipment. For both short- and long-term trajectory management the transmission of information concerning the specification of the trajectory, a patient's trajectory status, the movement of the trajectory, and so on, is a necessity. Inaccuracies and blunders in monitoring can have many untoward consequences including those affecting clinical safety *and* fatality. For instance, noting the exact time of a cardiac arrest is crucial, since the time limit for rescuing a patient is very narrow. (See chap. 13 for information work.)

As mentioned earlier, mismonitoring can flow from an incorrect initial assessment (such as mislocating the patient's status). This is so particularly when the intensity of monitoring is decreased because a patient appears to have improved. Only later will the full-blown clinical consequences of that misjudgment be recognized. Related to this is the mistaken setting of priorities. Still other mismonitoring is due to a malfunction in the machine itself, to a mishap in the machine-body connection, to incorrect calibration, to a monitoring agent's inexperience, either with the particular type of trajectory or with the technology being applied, to a shortage of adequately skilled personnel; or to an inadequate support system for maintaining the technology. A large number of very ill patients can also bring about a decreased intensity of monitoring of the less ill. And, of course, when a monitoring agent is tired or preoccupied, there are additional sources of mismonitoring. A less obvious condition is that when the monitoring is highly routinized the work becomes boring, it requires much effort to stay alert (as when on a cardiac critical unit all the patients seem quite stabilized).

Hazard Sources and Assessment

A final word about assessment in relation to accurate and efficient monitoring of indicators, which in turn are related to potential sources of hazard. These include: drugs, machines, procedures, personnel, environment, ward organization, patient as body, patient as person. A change in one of these sources will have different effects on others. When multiple drugs, procedures, and machines are used with a patient, the number of monitoring and assessing items increases. Levels of interpretation, then, are related to the scope and depth of assessing and the degree of discrimination and knowledge required for accurate assessment. In reality, however, the assessment process is three dimensional, since multiple assessments are occurring simultaneously.

In short, assessment involves estimating *how* the change in one source will alter another, *why* it is altered, *how to determine* the change, and *when* a change is hazardous, as well as *how to alter* the danger, *who* the appropriate agent to do that is, and *when to alter* it. This process is continual—and sometimes virtually continuous.

We can also see that for maximum clinical safety, especially in relation to the more complicated trajectories, an immense amount of information must flow, a multiplicity of kinds and levels of assessment must be reviewed and scanned, and the articulation of various levels of work is required (see chap. 7). Misassessment can result from not knowing how a change in one source affects others, or how this is manifested in body symptoms and signs or other measures; or from focusing on the wrong indicators or not taking enough indicators into account, or misreading and misinterpreting the indicators; as well as by not knowing safety limits. The conditions for misassessment are quite similar then to those discussed under monitoring for dangers and risks.

Patients' Monitoring, Assessing, and Rectifying of Clinical Hazards

Just as health workers are busily engaged in monitoring, assessing, and occasionally rectifying clinical danger and risk, so are the patients themselves and often their families. (See chap. 8 for patients' work in general.) The patients' monitoring and assessing is quite intense since it is their bodies and selves that are endangered. Their watchful eyes are not simply on potential dangers and risks as such, but also on the possible negative consequences of either staff's or their own mismonitoring and misassessing. They make their appraisals about themselves and others in highly charged situations. Their judgments may be very different from the personnel's. What may appear to be a major risk or danger to them may be trivial to the staff. Structurally, too, the context within which patients must indicate their fears, anxieties, judgments, and even discoveries (they do indeed discover dangerous errors) makes expression of them additionally difficult. First, patients are part of the hospital's division of labor (see below), but not formally so, and often only implicitly or in scarcely recognized ways. Second, when indicating to staff judgments of actual or potential hazard, they not infrequently operate from weakness in any accomplishing, persuading, or negotiating that they deem necessary; that is, they experience difficulties in legitimating their work.

Division of Labor, Implicit and Explicit

In the actual division of labor during the monitoring and assessing, varying degrees and types of cooperation may be required of a patient. For the staff to make accurate assessments, a patient may have to engage in important collaborative actions: for instance, accurately supplying information about bodily and emotional reactions to the illness and to various medical interventions, or complying with various diagnostic tests or in doing various therapies. When patients cannot collaborate because of the severity of their illness or are unable to talk, are confused, hard of hearing, and so forth, then families and other appropriate resources may be substituted. Thus, in pediatric units, parents are important agents for assessing and monitoring. Patients also supplement the staff's monitoring and assessing by apprising them of something being "not quite right" or "going wrong"—new or altered bodily signs and discomforts, altered machine sounds, or a disconnected tube. Supplementary action can be essential for instituting measures to prevent or reverse a potential risk. How well a patient performs these actions depends on whether the patient and kin understand both the degree of danger or risk and the degree to which participation in the work is deemed necessary by the staff. Also important are the degree of patients' medical sophistication and other capabilities.

However, because mutual participation and responsibility remain for the most part implicitly understood rather than explicitly stated, much monitoring and assessing is done independently. It is also often invisible to each person and unshared. Those invisible and unshared actions guide each person's managing of danger and risk, so that when the judgments differ, either in items or their dimensions or in priorities, then management action may be at cross purposes and is apt to be mutually misconstrued. Thus, it becomes the basis for interactional difficulties which arise between the respective parties. However, to make explicit the monitoring and assessing which the staff judges as appropriate for a given patient is not without its problems for the staff. Patients vary widely in their experiences with illness and in personal experiences, medical sophistication, and willingness to accept responsibilities. Judgments must be made about a patient's competence to take on the requisite tasks.

There is also the question of timing. This may call for varying degrees of interactional skill by the personnel, so that potential hazards can be made explicit to patients and families without their being unduly alarmed by the information. Then, of course, many illnesses and medical interventions can be so uncertain in outcome that the attendant risks cannot be specifically predicted to the patients. A great deal of biographical information about illness and medical experience is required from a patient before the staff can reasonably make the patient's responsibilities clear. This informational work is becoming especially important with the increase in chronic illness, since patients now are having long and complicated illnesses with their associated experiences. So this work calls for much interactional skill on the part of staff members, but also much time spent with the ill—time often not available on a busy ward. Thus, a considerable amount of patients' monitoring and assessing goes unnoticed by the personnel, unless directly brought to their attention or called for explicitly by the need to have patients "cooperate" in therapeutic and diagnostic actions.

Mutual Assessment of Risk Potential

Since both patient and staff can be a source of danger and risk, both play a silent game of assessing each other's potential as a source of those hazards—whether the other is competent, alert, reliable, and trustworthy. The cues and signs utilized by each may be accurate but also can be quite off the mark. For instance, a patient who has a reputation as a "crock" or a "whiner" will experience extreme difficulty in getting the personnel to accept the reliability of his or her assessments concerning the seriousness of, say, a bodily reaction. A tricky silent game is played wherein both parties size up each other, as well as present themselves in such a manner that they are accepted as reliable, competent, and believable. Patients' conversations with each other and with kin are replete with judgments of staff competence: "Boy, nurse so-and-so sure knows her stuff." "You got to watch Miss Jones." "I feel worse today because I don't think she knows how to do the treatment." Patients and families are constantly engaged in consulting about and comparing observations concerning the competences of various personnel.

More often than not, patients are at a disadvantage because they have neither the experience nor medical knowledge—and often recognize that—to make accurate judgments about hazard. However, some become quite expert. For example, kidney dialysis patients, because of their treatment sessions each week, become expert not only in assessing staff competence but in monitoring both the treatment and their bodies while on dialysis.

A patient's focus on assessment, as well as on monitoring, is often based on very personal experiences with illness, health personnel, and hospitals which often are not known to the staff. These experiences color the patient's priorities, making some hazardous items quite important, though others may be actually of equal or more importance medically. For example, one patient had gotten an infection at the intravenous puncture site during his previous hospitalization, so he assessed and closely monitored the personnel who were now doing that procedure—whether they washed their hands, and so on. He even refused to have anyone he judged as clumsy and physically untidy carry out the procedure. The staff, in turn, thought of this patient as "being a bit fussy" and "a little on the paranoid side."

Patient-Staff Differences in Criteria

A central problem in getting a better matching of patients' and staff's assessment of hazard is that generally they apply different criteria. Health professionals tend to rely on technical medical measures, whereas patients rely on bodily reactions and sensations, mainly pains and other discomforts. Pain and discomfort are highly subjective matters, and many discomforts are highly ambiguous. (See chap. 5 for discussion of discomfort). This poses particular problems of assessment for both the patient and the staff, since this difference in assessing discomforts may be relevant to the more crucial assessing of clinical safety.

Important for our discussion is that in daily life one's discomforts tend to be kept private. There is a tendency not to burden others with them. Even when discomforts are directly related to illness, people attempt to normalize or hide them when in social situations. This normalizing (as well as avoiding placement of burdens on others) is drastically altered when someone becomes hospitalized. First of all, the medical orientation of the hospital staff encourages the viewing of discomforts as symptoms of disease. Assessment of symptoms is important for proper diagnosis, treatment, and location of the current illness status, as well as for monitoring reactions to therapy. However, because discomforts are ambiguous—stemming partly from the many sources which may not be directly related to the patient's illness—he or she may have a problem of deciding which discomforts are important enough to make public. At the same time, because the discomforts are no longer mundane but possibly life threatening, this tends to encourage patients to dwell on and exaggerate bodily discomforts.

Moreover, specifying the source and sometimes even the nature of a discomfort can be extremely difficult for the patient. If he or she suffers a headache, is that because of a missed breakfast or a diagnostic test, or is it the tenseness and anxiety engendered by waiting for an impending test result, or is it from a newly administered drug? Not infrequently, the personnel are also caught up in those same ambiguities.

Interactionally, the reporting of discomforts can be tricky for patients. They might be viewed as making a "mountain out of a mole hill" and so be made to feel foolish. Then there are implicit norms about proper behavior of patients, concerning their styles of reporting and requesting relief. Ordinary rules of politeness govern how someone should ask for relief: not too demanding, nasty, or with screaming and shouting. There are also norms pertaining to enduring and tolerating discomforts, and how the latter should be expressed. Thus, the patient should tolerate an uncomfortable procedure because it is necessary for getting well. Indeed, the problems that a patient has in figuring out the implicit rules of reporting discomfort and for requesting relief are great, as evidenced by the amount of patient-to-patient and patient-to-kin checking out and prompting of each other. "Don't you think you ought to report this to the nurses?" "Do you think I ought to tell the doctor?" "I think you have put up with this long enough." For the patient to dwell constantly on bodily discomforts and to express them (or sometimes to underexpress them) may have grave interactional consequences. Overexpressing may result in patients' being labeled "hypochondriac" or "overanxious," while underexpression may bring labels like "macho" or "a denier." Discrepancies between patient and staff judgments, including the staff's discounting of the patient's assessments, may have drastic consequences not merely for their interaction, but, of course, for clinical safety.

It is important to understand that patients use these bodily reactions to assess the trajectory locations, such as whether they are out of danger or not. When their perceptions of bodily reaction and discomfort do not match the medical criteria used by the staff, then interactional conflict may arise, endangering future trajectories. Staff may discount patients' expressions of discomfort, or patients may discount the staff's assessments. These differences in assessment have consequences for how patients cooperate in the treatment process. Thus, patients may engage in risky activities because they feel better or refuse to engage in activities because "I'm not over the danger." (This is a particular problem when patients engage in self-assessment and monitoring while at home. Drugs and treatments may be discontinued or monitoring of bodies may be discontinued because one feels better.) On the other hand, staff's discounting of the bodily indicators as reported by patients may have serious consequences. Horror stories abound about the serious dangers of being neglected because of staff's heavy reliance on objective, measurable medical approaches.

In the highly technologized hospital, many pains and discomforts experienced by patients are technologically and/or staff-inflicted (see chap. 5). Patients must suffer various painful and discomforting procedures and tolerate uncomfortable tubes in various body orifices. Patients often use the discomfort and pain-inflicting potential of the staff to assess their overall clinical competence. Thus, when the latter do not make explicit the unfortunately necessary pain and discomfort, patients may assess the staff as incompetent and negligent (Fagerhaugh and Strauss, 1977). Although they may be fully aware that some pain and discomfort must be tolerated in the service of getting well, the suffering that they must withstand may be well beyond their tolerance for discomfort, not to mention their ability to maintain composure. In other words, a patient assesses pain and discomfort not only for relevance to the illness trajectory, but in terms of personal composure. When a necessary pain or discomfort exceeds the composure limit, a patient may pull out a tube or refuse further painful treatments. Of course, other balancing factors may enter into the decision to cooperate in the treatment—such as tolerating terrible discomfort and pain just to live a bit longer. Patients' communications about their pains and discomforts may constitute both assessments of perceived dangers, but also request for relief. Thus, those communications can be fraught with ambiguity or carry double messages. All of that adds to interactional difficulties between patients and personnel, which in turn can negatively affect the safety work of both.

5

Comfort Work

Weaving in and out but always on the margins of the discussion in previous chapters have been references to comfort work. This type of work is familiar to us all, since so many illnesses are associated with aches, pains, nausea, and other physical discomforts. That is true whether the sick person is at home seeking to minimize and relieve those discomforts or in the hospital. Failure to do comfort work to the satisfaction of patients when they are hospitalized is a major source of their anger and frustration—leading often to bitter complaints and accusations of incompetence or negligence. Patients endure the perceived or actual incompetence and negligence because they are powerless to change the situation and because they believe, at least minimally, in the potential effectiveness of contemporary health care. Older people sometimes remember that before the days of penicillin, the physicians' armamentarium was relatively ineffective even though they may have offered plenty of tender love and care. And some segments of the health occupations, especially nursing, are much concerned with rectifying the more depersonalized aspects of hospital care. However, combined as complaints about comfort care often are with others about the more psychological aspects of care (see chap. 6 on sentimental work), the patients' criticism has led to a veritable outpouring of publications about the dehumanization of health care.

In general, we ourselves are inclined to lay the blame for whatever inadequacies of comfort work may occur primarily on the staff's usual "technical medical-nursing care first, comfort care second" focus, along with the technological and organizational features of medical and nursing work which are emphasized throughout all of this book. Of course, there is also incompetence, negligence, callousness, even, alas, instances of brutality in hospital care. But the weakness lies in the minimal accountability of staff for comfort work, as compared with the more technical features of their work.

What is important to grasp is that the hospital setting and the trajectory work done there, together, complicate the comfort work almost beyond belief as compared with comfort work done during the pre–chronic illness era. Giving tender loving care (the centerpiece of traditional nursing identity) has so many novel features that it warrants being awarded the status of genuinely new "news." The questions for the analyst, then, pertain first of all to how a triad of structural changes have affected the context and nature of today's comfort work. These changes have occurred in medical specializations and their associated technologies, in the chronic illness trajectories, and in the hospital's organization in tandem with the first two changes. Other important questions are: What *is* comfort work? What types of such work are there? Specifically, how is the comfort work done and by whom? What happens if it is not done or is perceived as done incompetently? And how does the work differ in accordance with various trajectories or phases of trajectories?

Structural Changes Affecting Comfort Work

The overwhelming prevalence of patients bedded down with chronic illness in the hospital means there is a great deal of illness-related discomfort that requires handling by the staff, and inevitably by the patients, too. Of course, there were discomforts aplenty associated with infectious and parasitic disease before the antibiotic era, but chronic diseases bring discomforts dramatically to the fore. Each illness has its characteristic pattern of symptomatology, and many of the symptoms represent some degree of episodic or persistent discomfort to the sick person.

Running down a list of symptoms, one can see this quickly. Lessened mobility often means aching bones, discomfort when sitting down or getting up, and painful movement when moving around. Lessened energy brings physically uncomfortable moments associated with the sudden need to fall out of conversation from sheer weariness, or the exhaustion of making it up the stairs or opening heavy doors, even of just moving around. If lungs are affected, as in emphysema, the ill person hurts when coughing or even when moving. People with injuries to or deterioration of the spine have backaches and pains.

Arthritics suffer from numerous discomforts associated with doing domestic chores, with aching hands and limbs. Persons with ulcerative colitis have immense colonic discomfort. Cardiacs may experience frequent periods of dizziness. Other illnesses bring persistent itching, thirst and what not.

Furthermore, the changed nature of trajectories (stretched out, new phases) may involve various kinds and degrees of discomfort. For instance, many people with Parkinson's disease now enjoy additional years of life because of effective drugs but may need to endure discomforts associated with the pharmacological side effects as well as with physical deterioration itself. Moreover, since many chronic illnesses bring about other systemic disturbances or affect unrelated illnesses, the discomforts that afflict the sick person can be varied and feed into each other. And unlike short-term infectious diseases such as pneumonia or measles, chronic illness is likely to be associated with long periods, even as long as life itself, of uncomfortable living. Not that discomfort is always at peak intensity, but the discomfort is apt to be intermittent, repetitive, sometimes persistent even if not so intense as to be completely immobilizing or debilitating.

Specializing and Technology

Quite aside from the contingencies of disease itself, the contemporary explosion of medical specialization with its attendant therapeutic intervention contributes to the discomforts of ill persons and complicates their comfort care. In the hospital especially, during the acute phases of an illness, the interventions can, of course, be diverse and intrusive. As we have seen, patients must be transported to and from machine sites, their bodies positioned in relation to the machines, their stomachs suctioned, their arms punctured for IV connections or for drawing blood. Machines aside, there are numerous procedures that also give degrees of discomfort, both during and after the staff's procedural actions. As for medications, however necessary and effective they may be, they can also result in digestive disturbance, dizziness, headaches, or any number of discomforts. The essential point here—essential but easily missed—is that medical interventions can and often do *inflict* discomfort. That is so even when the personnel are competent and careful; when they are not, the chances of inflicting discomfort are greatly magnified.

For the management of many trajectories, the medications, procedures, or machine work deemed necessary are well-nigh continuous over the course of hospitalization (and often afterward), engendering discomforts that may feed into each other, raising the pitch of discomfort geometrically progression. This may sometimes stretch over many days or weeks of hospitalization. If the patient develops multiple trajectories (as Mrs. Price did; see chap. 2), then the discomforts visibly mount. Since many a patient already has multiple trajectories—whether visible to the staff or not—medical interventions in the service of the main line of trajectory work may add to the discomfort which has its source in any ongoing illness.

In their giving of comfort care, that is, in doing comfort work, the personnel now have at their command a number of technological modes and technical devices. Given the health professionals' penchant for adopting the latest technology available, it is not at all surprising that comfort work is also being technologized, no longer relying simply on empathy and common sense or on words and gestures related to staff's recognizing the physiological grounds for a patient's discomfort.

Evolution of the hospital bed exemplifies the mechanizing of this work at a relatively simple level. In the past, the changing of an immobilized patient's body position in bed was managed manually. After the bed became electrified, patients themselves might shift their own positions merely by pushing buttons. Although the mechanized bed allows them to do this portion of the necessary comfort work, the bed also contributes to the nurse's neglect of proper body positioning, with the consequence that patients may develop still other discomforts. For example, a common sight on the wards is that of patients scrunched up in bed, sitting on the small of the back. This can result in backaches and even in painful infections of the lung because of incomplete lung expansion.

Many other procedures utilized for therapeutic purposes as well as for managing discomfort, such as cold and hot applications, have become mechanized. For example, cool sponge baths given to lower fever and relieve temperature discomfort have been replaced by hypothermo machines. Those machines are also used for their heat. These and similar machines come in many types and models. Also, the do-it-yourself devices for comfort that were invented on the spot by nurses have been increasingly taken over by medical supply companies. New kinds of equipment and devices to relieve discomfort are constantly being introduced, as illustrated by the "briefs on new equipment" published in the medical and nursing journals. While these new pieces of equipment are extremely helpful for doing comfort work, they call for the kind of elaborate organization of supply and maintenance discussed in chapter 3.

Drugs, too, are increasingly utilized in discomfort relief. A vast array of drugs designed to relieve various discomforts is now available to the physicians who order them and the nurses who administer them.

And at home, of course, the patients rely heavily on them, too. Some drugs are highly effective but many have untoward side effects, so that constant upgrading of knowledge and attention is required to monitor the patients' physiological reactions. When someone has many discomforts, then several drugs may be used simultaneously. This, in turn, can pose additional problems, as when a drug used to control one discomfort reacts unfavorably with another. Or when several drugs are used, which one or what combination is responsible for the appearance of yet another new discomfort? Problems of drug incompatibility are further exacerbated because of increasing numbers of patients with multiple chronic disorders. In the larger medical centers, pharmacists have become important in carrying out therapeutic work and comfort work because of their knowledge of drug impact and of the range of pharmacological options now available.

There has also been development in what might be termed soft technology for doing comfort work, technology based on knowledge drawn from both the biophysical and social sciences. This technology pertains to appropriate ways of interacting with and taking care of patients and their bodies so as to increase physical comfort and to give encouragement to patients in their own management of discomfort. The simple, commonsensical way is, for example, to hold the patient's hand, saying things like, "You're doing fine; hold on for just a bit longer," thus assisting the patient to endure discomforts. But new physiologically based knowledge underlies more technical modes of such comfort work. From the social sciences, too, various techniques have diffused into the hospital. Thus, there are psychological approaches (both one-to-one and group) deriving from Skinnerian operant conditioning (including biofeedback methods, which use machines), from the Rogerian tradition (reflective techniques), from Rankian, Jungian, and Reichian traditions, and so on. Various teaching philosophies also influence comfort work: for example, concepts of self-care and independence versus dependence. Thus, current ideology leads some nurses to encourage patients toward independence and self-care, doing their own comfort work. On the other hand, the various strands of the alternative health care movement, which in part represent reactions to medical technology, also have an impact on comfort care. These approaches are very diverse—yoga, transcendental meditation, herbs, folk medicine, acupuncture, diet—each having some potential for diffusion into hospital practice.

While it is safe to say that traditional (hard) technological approaches predominate in hospitalized comfort work, yet the numerous alternative approaches pose the likelihood that patients and personnel will hold potentially clashing views about what techniques are most appropriate and for what kind of discomfort. Among the staff itself, psychosocially oriented nurses may conflict with more physiologically oriented nurses who put their trust in drugs as a major method for relief of discomfort. Nurses and physicians may disagree among themselves about the appropriate medication options. Patients who believe in alternative health techniques may not be able to legitimate their wishes for the use of such nontraditional methods.

Hospital Organization

In addition to the changes in technology, medical interventions, and the chronic illness trajectories themselves, the characteristic organization of today's hospital also contributes to making comfort work a complex issue. A reiteration of only a few of the hospital's standard features should quickly suggest why. The institution is organized principally to give acute care, meaning an intense focus by the personnel around strictly medical aspects of diagnosis and therapy. This, combined with the general hustle and bustle of work life and the great concern with clinical safety, means that comfort will take primacy only under such—and not so frequent—conditions as touched on later in this chapter.

The various technicians who move in and out of patients' rooms are very much focused on their technical tasks and very little trained in the niceties or the physiological technicalities of comfort care. They have little knowledge of any given patient's current discomforts, unless told by the patient, and may have little understanding of how to minimize their own unwitting or inevitable infliction of discomfort. Nurses are still being educated at schools that emphasize comfort as well as more strictly physiological care, but the organization of ward work tends to pull them all toward the latter kind of care and toward the numerous mundane activities that help to keep the ward functioning as an organization. New patients must be examined and bedded down, while old ones are readied for going home. Supplies must be checked and double-checked, taken out, kept flowing. Physicians' orders must be filled and carried out. Housekeeping chores must be done. Shortages of nursing staff mean that nurses must often cover for each other. Difficult patients and kinsmen must be managed. Clinical emergencies take precedence over everything. And all the multitudes of tasks attending machine work need to be done. In general, also, the flow of information to nurses from physicians and from head nurses concerns work couched in medical and procedural terms that bears relatively little on patients' discomforts—except for their relief by medications when discomforts are seen as affecting the disease course itself or are highly visible and perhaps complained about by the patients themselves. Comfort tasks tend to be scheduled as routines, thus making the staff's total work easier: hence, there is a time to bathe, to pass out fresh drinking water, to look in on patients. However, the intensity of the therapeutically oriented work schedule often competes even with the comfort routines. In short, all these organizational features of the hospital tend to draw staff's attention away from engaging in the work of preventing, minimizing, or relieving discomfort. Unless discomfort is perceived either as affecting the course of illness or flowing directly from the illness (high temperature, dizziness) or the therapeutic maneuvers designed to manage it.

The work flow of departments other than the clinical wards also tends to complicate as well as minimize greatly the amount and effectiveness of comfort work, which generally fares badly in the competition for staff's time and attention. For example, when X-raying a patient, obtaining a clear picture has priority, while patient comfort is entirely secondary if thought of at all. The daily scheduling of radiological tasks is more efficient, too, if patients come through in an even flow; so it is not unusual to find them queued up on wheelchairs and gurneys, experiencing varying degrees and kinds of discomfort while awaiting their turns. A day of scheduling for radiological work can result in the sick person's own comfort schedule going awry: he or she may miss two meals in a row and as a consequence develop a headache or may be thirsty for an unreasonable amount of time because no interfering liquids were allowed so that a test could be made, or may experience a delay in receiving a medication designed to relieve an ongoing discomfort. After the patient returns to the ward, its personnel are then faced with having to cope with his or her normal reactions to such frustrating situations, as well as having to help alleviate the discomforts thus engendered or magnified.

Inadequacies in goods and services required from supporting departments also enormously complicate the comfort work of ward personnel. A patient, for instance, may require frequent changes of bed linen because of excessive sweating or inability to control bowels or may require a certain drug or comfort-abetting device. Yet there may be a shortage of necessary supplies on the ward or an exasperating delay in receiving them from elsewhere. It is not unusual for a nurse to be heard explaining that a drug or device or piece of equipment has been ordered, "but we have to wait until it comes." It is equally common to hear a patient say something like, "What the hell does it take to get a pill for my headache?" Or "Why don't you have that damn equipment right here? Why do you have to send for it?" Additionally, all the problems of machine maintenance, repair, and supply touched on in chapter 3, affect the timing, amount, and effectiveness of comfort work. Any inefficiency or delay in that work inevitably affects comfort work adversely.

Discomforts: At Home and in the Hospital

Discomforts cover a wide range of body conditions and sensations. Uncomfortable sensations include tingling, itching, soreness, pressure and fullness, coldness, hotness, stiffness, dirtiness, thirst. Uncomfortable physical states include weakness, dizziness, flatulence, constipation. These discomforts are, of course, a part of ordinary living, being associated with routine body functions—eating, sleeping, defecating, bathing—as well as with the daily activities of working, walking, sitting, interacting.

Outside the hospital, one's own body and its occasional or persistent discomforts tend to be private matters. People take care not to expose certain parts of their bodies in public, while personal caring for bodies is usually done in private. Social conventions prevent our talking about intimate "private parts" too openly, and such activities as passing gas or scratching oneself vigorously are frowned upon when done in public. Nor does one dwell on body discomforts or burden others with their details. In short, people usually maintain some semblance of normal health, even when suffering much discomfort; the sick tend to play down or hide their uncomfortable symptoms.

Everyday normalizing and managing of discomforts becomes drastically altered when someone is hospitalized. First of all, as already noted, the medical orientation of personnel encourages viewing discomfort as symptomatic of disease. Symptom assessment is important for proper diagnosis and treatment and for periodically locating the illness status, as well as for monitoring physiological reactions to therapeutic measures. But because discomforts tend to be ambiguous—stemming in part from their many possible sources which may or may not be directly related to disease or therapy—the patients themselves may experience difficulty in deciding which discomforts are important enough to tell the personnel about. Over time, because of the personnel's questioning and through their responses to expressions of discomfort, patients may learn which discomforts are significant to report and for which ones they can successfully or at least reasonably request relief.

Second, in the hospital a patient's body becomes much more open to public scrutiny, shared territory for all kinds of personnel who lay claims to its examination and manipulation. When carrying out their various trajectory tasks, nurses, physicians, technicians, and other health workers manipulate and expose the body, inserting instruments, needles, tubes into it. The state of the body is so openly discussed among the staff that even visitors and other patients may overhear the talk.

Routine matters of hygiene involving actual or potential discomfort for the patient are done under conditions strange for him or her and with unfamiliar equipment. Sometimes minimal information is given about how to go about these tasks: a basin of water is plunked down with, "OK, get started on your bath." Moreover, some tasks are difficult, such as cleansing oneself after using a bedpan, but as this is a very private matter, patients do not ordinarily request staff assistance.

Third, hospitalized patients are required to cede management of their discomforts to others. When acutely ill, in general one readily relinquishes this responsibility. However, chronically ill persons have had much experience and done much experimentation in managing their own discomforts. Often they have tried many different types of drugs and know which are more or less effective, how much to take, when, and what the potential side effects may be. They have learned which body positions "work best" and which to avoid "like poison." They know a great deal about pacing themselves and about which foods not to eat. So in many respects they are much more knowledgeable than any staff member can possibly be about managing their characteristic discomforts—however little they may know about managing other discomforts that result from medical interventions done at the hospital. Additionally, since many suffer from two or more chronic illnesses, they, rather than the staff, are likely to be concerned with minimizing or alleviating discomforts associated with all except the primary illness, upon which the personnel are focused almost exclusively.

Fourth, besides all the discomforts inflicted by the personnel while doing diagnostic and therapeutic tasks, patients' discomforts can be heightened by the hospital environment: it can be noisy, untidy, poorly ventilated, too hot or too cold, and full of unpleasant odors. A fifth consideration is that the mundane quality of most discomforts tends to render invisible much of the comfort work engaged in by patients—or conversely, the necessity for staff sometimes to do comfort work which goes unrecognized. For example, before a procedure begins, a sick person may prop a pillow because of "a touch of arthritis," or position his or her body in a specific way so as to "avoid having my back go out." If patients do not inform them, the personnel do not necessarily notice such actions; or if so, regard them as unrelated to comfort care. A counterpart of this blindness is that similar actions carried out by personnel, especially the nurses, may be invisible to or misinterpreted by patients. Comfort work often requires considerable knowledge about physiological functions, much skill, technique, and art; even meeting hygienic needs can be important in its therapeutic implications. Yet the patient may regard this work or assistance as nontechnical, ordinary, or just being nice or helpful. Even close monitoring and assessing of discomfort-relieving procedures and medications can be quite invisible qua work. Hence, the oft heard criticism, "The only thing nurses do is pass out pills," shows little awareness that monitoring and assessing may accompany this seemingly menial task.

In sum, management of discomfort at home and in the hospital cannot but be enormously different. That is so even when patients rely to lesser or greater extent on their own tried and true or now desperately experimental methods. Everything in the hospital—organization, technology, work routines, staff orientations, the physical setting itself—compounds both the relative simplicity of comfort work done at home and the relative autonomy of sick persons (and kin) in doing their own comfort work. The contrast between home and hospital is epitomized by the remark of a long-time user of aspirin: "They even take away your aspirin, but don't pay attention when you ring the bell."

Awareness of and Agreement about Dimensions of Discomfort

Adding further to the complexity of comfort work in hospitals is the awareness of, and agreement or disagreement over, various dimensions of discomfort. The dimensions include duration, graveness, specificity of cause, predictability, preventability, controllability, and rectifiability of any discomfort. Each dimension, of course, constitutes a continuum running from high to low, short to long, ambiguous to clear-cut, and so on.

In some illnesses, both the numbers and kinds of discomfort and their associated dimensions may not present particular problems insofar as they are easily recognized, easily agreed upon, and measures for handling the discomforts are relatively effective. Standard surgery without undue complications thereafter is an instance of a trajectory characterized by those features. However, as noted earlier, problematic trajectories have markedly increased; hence the nonrecognition of and the disagreement over each and every dimension of a discomfort is a potential hazard to effective comfort work, as well as to harmonious relationships between staff and patient and among the staff itself.

In more specific terms, various participants in the trajectory dramas may misunderstand each other's readings of discomfort dimensions, not recognizing that others have placed different interpretations on or given different weights to whether a discomfort—if it is noticed at all—is important or unimportant, critically grave or not, ambiguous or unambiguous as to cause, will quickly pass or be persistent, is generally relievable or not, and so on. Even if each party recognizes how the other is reading the situation, misunderstanding not really being at issue, the disagreement still may result in impatience, irritability, frustration, anger, or downright fury. Consequently, rhetoric may flow easily and action reminiscent of the battlefield is not uncommon.

Discomfort Vignettes

The management of discomforts engendered by the contingencies of the illness itself, the medical interventions, or the hospital environment involves potentially eight different kinds of comfort tasks. These are: (1) preparing the patient for discomfort, (2) assessing discomfort, (3) preventing discomfort, (4) minimizing discomfort, (5) relieving discomfort, (6) legitimating discomfort, (7) enduring discomfort, and (8) reporting discomfort. The last three are the patients' job, though he or she may also engage in the others. Before scrutinizing what these tasks entail, we shall present several vignettes taken from field notes to illustrate some of their features in relation to other kinds of work and to phases of trajectories.

Mrs. Hofnagel's Travail

Mrs. Hofnagel was operated on for an anal fissure; she was given a spinal block, sent to the recovery room for an hour, then back to her room.

> For the next day or two she had some anal discomfort, but was readily given relieving medication upon request. However, one nurse the second day "struck me as really mean, implying 'you're a coward because you can't wait' " for the medication. "She said something also about how I was handling the packing when I was peeing and I had to point out that I was trying to keep myself clean."

1. Discomfort and slight pain following this operation are anticipated by the physician, so he writes orders for *relieving* medication including on patient's request.

2. But one nurse has a different philosophy of pain *relief* and perceives the patient as lacking proper *endurance*. She *assesses* the degree of discomfort differently than the patient, the latter having no effective means of *legitimating* the degree of her discomfort.

3. The patient is engaged in *preventing* potential discomfort from an unclean packing, an action which the nurse misinterprets.

> Two days after the operation, Mrs. Hofnagel experienced her first bowel movement. She had not been *prepared* by the staff for the potentially great pain that might attend this activity. There was an aide in attendance, called by the patient who had been told that the first bowel movement might make her feel faint. The aide filled the bathtub with water while the patient began to defecate. "It was like passing splintered glass! I was so shocked. You expect you'll be uncomfortable but . . . And I had had no previous experience with this, so did not know what to expect." The aide helped her off the toilet and put her into the tub, afterward helping her back to bed. A nurse then gave her clean packing and more medication.

1. This shows failure to *prepare* the patient for great discomfort.
2. Assisted by the aide, the patient gets *relief* by sitting in hot water.
3. Afterward, the nurse engages in *preventing* or *minimizing* more discomfort through medication.

> Mrs. Hofnagel's reaction to the episode on the toilet? "Horror! And scared about next time. When the physician came, I yelled at him: 'You didn't tell me! What if the aide hadn't been there?' " The physician, whom she liked very much, only laughed. "He was pleased that I went, that I was functioning with no problems. He regarded all this like a minor cosmetic job—but up the anus."

1. A negligence accusation is lodged by the patient, who remarked that (*a*) no one *prepared her* for the discomfort; (*b*) there might have been nobody there to help *relieve* her.
2. The physician's focus is on the successful phase of the trajectory management, to the exclusion of any comfort work except his previous *orders for medication on request.* The physician sent her home—though she was frightened of future bowel episodes—with instruction to fill her bathtub in case of a repetition of the "splintered glass," and to sit in the hot water occasionally between bowel movements.
3. This also shows *minimizing or preventing* of future discomfort.

Mr. Einshtein's Enema

Recollect that in chapter 2, we referred to Einshtein's discomforting episode, which he later referred to as his "battle of the bowel." We repeat it briefly here in order to use it for a different purpose.

> Two days before he entered the hospital with a severe cardiac attack, he had a barium enema with an X-ray, done to

> check a possible source of anemia. The first night in the hospital, a nurse gave him a milk of magnesia pill to prevent possible bowel blockage and attendant discomfort. The second night, however, though he had not yet moved his bowels, he was given no medication. The next morning, at about seven he felt like defecating but was impacted—and really hurt—so believed he needed an enema. He told the nurse that two or three times, when she came to take blood pressure readings, and finally asked for the head nurse, repeating that he was in much discomfort. The personnel were very busy that morning, so scarcely heard his relatively mild expressions of discomfort or his requests that they relieve it. The head nurse spoke of a bowel softener, but the patient insisted—the second time around—but again to no avail that he needed relief "right away!" An intern supported the head nurse's judgment about a bowel softener, although the patient repeated his own firm belief. About one o'clock his discomfort was so extreme that he called for the head nurse and insisted flatly on an enema: the nurse acceded but said, "in a while," because the necessary equipment had to be brought from a servicing department. In about an hour, the enema finally was administered. It yielded immediate relief: the discomfort vanished entirely.

1. The staff failed to *prevent* the discomfort, though it might have been anticipated.

2. The patient failed to *legitimate* the extent of discomfort and the need for its relatively immediate *relief*, for the staff *assessed* differently the extent and importance of the discomfort. They judged this in some part by either misreading or misinterpreting his *expression* of his discomfort.

3. The patient chose not to *endure* any longer, now *expressing* himself vividly and strongly, so managed to get *relief* for his discomfort.

A Child's Unavailing Expression

An infant girl, about a year and a half old, was being treated for a badly bleeding wound on her thigh by one nurse, assisted by another who mainly held the child down with a steady hand.

> The child cried incessantly, reaching frequent crescendos. When treatment of the wound was finished, the second nurse washed the child's whole body starting with the groin and vaginal area, making no sentimental gestures of any kind. (The entire episode took about fifteen minutes.)

1. There was inflicted pain and other discomfort, but no *preparation* of the infant through nonverbal gestures or words of reassurance.

2. Personnel are intent on main task of treating wound and minimizing chances of infection. Perhaps they make some attempt to *minimize* inflicted pain when treating wound through technical skill, but there are no apparent attempts to do so when washing the infant.

3. Since child is so young, there are no accusations against her for not *enduring* her discomfort or for mode of *expressing* it.

Comfort Work in the Recovery Room

In chapter 2, a portion of a field note was reproduced: it described sequential tasks carried out by a nurse at the bedside of a patient just back from a cardiac operation. We repeat those few lines, to illustrate how the comfort tasks are done and how they fit into the sequence of the tasks necessary for the patient's survival.

> The nurse changed the blood transfusion bag. She milked it down, and took out an air bubble. Later she changed it again. Later got the bottle part filled through mechanical motion. She drew blood and immediately put back new blood into the tube. She milked the urine tube once. She took a temperature. She put a drug injection into the nonautomated IV. But all the while she had in focus, though not necessarily glancing directly at, the TV which registered EKG and blood pressure readings. Once she punched the computer button to get the fifteen-minute readout on cardiac functioning. And once she milked the infection-purifier tube leading from the patient's belly. And periodically she marked down both the readings and some of what she had done. Once the patient stirred as she was touching his arm: she said quite nicely then that she was about to give him an injection which would relax him. He indicated he heard. Another time she noticed him stirring and switched off the light above his head, saying "that's better, isn't it?"

1. Patient was injected to *minimize* or *prevent* expected discomfort. It should be added that the temperature of the bed was controlled by a machine, used both the *minimize* potential discomfort and in the service of the trajectory itself.

2. Switching off light to *relieve* discomfort was done in response to *assessment* of the patient's expression of discomfort.

3. Patient is nonsentient so there is no need to *endure* or further *express* his discomfort—and certainly no need to *legitimate* because *expected* or "reasonable" given phase of trajectory.

We shall next discuss in detail the complexities of comfort work—and what happens when there is disagreement about it—as well as the specific organizational conditions for doing or not doing this work. We use data bearing on pain. What is true of "pain management" is simply a more evident instance of what transpires with nausea, dizziness, digestive discomfort, and other instances of discomfort. (This material is taken from Fagerhaugh and Strauss 1977, pp. 61–69, 86–97, 116–22.) The discussion will cover routine surgical trajectories and their associated pains, back pain, which at least in degree tends to be difficult for patients to legitimate, and the inflicted pain of medical procedures.

Pain and Routine Surgical Trajectories

Routine surgical trajectories can be characterized as predictable, involving few risks, unambiguous, and of short duration. Barring complications, the recovery courses and their accompanying pains are predictable and nonproblematic. Both the hospitalization and the pain courses are anticipated to be short. . . . Staff anticipates that pain will be relatively high for 24 to 72 hours postoperatively and will then quickly taper off.

There is a relatively high degree of specificity as to the causes of physiological . . . pain and discomfort. So patients generally need not legitimate the presence of pain. . . . Because of the physiological bases of pain, specific drugs and specific nursing and medical measures are utilized to relieve pain. Of equal importance . . . are the prevention of complications and the returning of the patient to physiological equilibrium, both of which may unavoidably require inflicted pains and discomforts. . . . Usually patients are aware that severe pain will last a few days, but that all pain will eventually end.

The Staff's Pain Work

The pain tasks of the staff include assessment, prevention, minimization, and relief. The approaches to these pain tasks may be physiological, pharmaceutical, or psychological. The tasks are an integral part of the overall work done to accomplish a successful surgical outcome. The division of labor involved is the usual one in medical organizations. The surgeon and the anesthesiologist determine the preoperative drugs, treatments, and anesthesia for a successful and painless surgery. The surgeon prescribes the drugs and treatments appropriate for relieving postsurgical pain and discomfort. The professional nurses administer the drugs and treatments and assess, observe, record, and communicate the patient's pains and responses to the various pain-relieving approaches. When the approaches do not control the pains, or when new pains and discomforts develop, the nurses consult personnel such as head nurse, medical house staff, or surgeon, for appropriate action. Auxiliary nursing personnel are accountable to the professional nurses, to whom they report the patient's pain and responses to the pain-relieving approaches.

Preoperatively, the staff attempts to minimize the degree of anticipated postsurgical pain by relieving the patient's apprehension about the impending surgery and pain. This is accomplished by talking with the patient about pain tolerance and anxieties concerning the surgery. The necessary preoperative procedures are explained, as are the surgical course, the accompanying pains, and the measures available for relief. The staff explains painful but necessary procedures which require patient cooperation and tolerance in order to avoid complications. In nursing vernacular this stream of information is called "preoperative patient teaching." Its purposes are not only to relieve patient apprehension and thereby reduce pain perception but also to assure a cooperative patient for a successful surgery.

For the first 24 to 72 postoperative hours, the staff . . . members monitor vital signs, maintain fluid and electrolyte balance, prevent complications, and do other treatments specific to the surgery. Together, the treatments require a multitude of tasks, some involving no pain (taking blood pressure), others giving some discomfort (intravenous infusions, irrigations, or dressing changes). Circulatory, respiratory, and other complications associated with bodily immobilization must be minimized at the cost of "patient-induced pain" caused by deep breathing, moving around in bed, and early ambulation. Achieving patient cooperation is vital.

Incisional pain will probably be high for the first 24 to 72 hours postoperatively. . . . The nurses' tasks include assessing the pain and giving the [relieving] drugs at appropriate intervals. When the dosage or frequency of administration of drugs does not "hold" the pain, then the surgeon or house staff is notified about changing the drug order. The pacing of drugs must be sufficient to control the worst pains [and discomforts], but it must not cause sleepiness or drowsiness when cooperation with treatment is necessary.

There are many additional pain-minimization tasks such as splinting the incision when the patient coughs, vomits, or changes body position. A variety of discomforts can be anticipated: dry mouth, headache, urinary and bowel retention, irritations from tubes placed in various body orifices, sore throat from an endotracheal tube used for the anesthetic. For each . . . there are appropriate discomfort-minimization measures. Reassuring and encouraging the patient are, of course, related pain-minimization tasks, . . .

Usually by the third or fourth postoperative day, the patient is expected to be "over the hump" and is encouraged to be more physically active, take foods by mouth, and be more self-sufficient. As pain decreases, less potent drugs are used.

Patient Pain Tasks

When the patient accepts the decision to have surgery, an implicit contract is made with the staff. . . . the physician is responsible for as successful a surgery as possible and as comfortable a hospital stay as possible. The patient is to cooperate with the physician and other health personnel for this common goal. . . . two of the patient's pain tasks are to apprise the personnel of existing pain and to give appropriate information (where, when, and the character of the pain) as requested. Using this information the staff assesses the pain and takes appropriate action. The patient also must keep pain expression within reasonable limits by avoiding prolonged loud crying and moaning. . . . One of the patient's major tasks is to cooperate with and endure painful but necessary procedures. . . . Noncooperation can unnerve the staff members and affect their technical performance.

Ward Work and Pain Accountability

Considering, then, the properties of routine, low-risk surgical trajectories (predictable, unambiguous, short duration, and finite) and the specificity of approaches to pain prevention, minimization, and relief, we can assume that much of pain management is nonproblematic—as perceived by the staff. We can also assume that when the surgical trajectory is routine, there are well-developed, well-organized approaches for managing pain. There is a discrepancy, however, between what is possible and what is neglected in effective pain relief. This discrepancy can be understood only when viewed from the combined impact of (1) the work demands of the clinical setting, (2) the institutional accountability surrounding pain management, and (3) the complexity of patient-staff and staff-staff pain interactions.

Surgical units are usually very busy places, with innumerable and complex tasks requiring much skill, frequently involving a considerable use of machinery. Compared with medical units there is a constant flow of new patients, and the rate of patient turnover is quite rapid. There is a mixture of routine and complex problematic cases which require more or less of the staff's attention. When emergencies occur or when there is a shortage of staff or when there are several critically ill or problematic surgical cases, attention is naturally focused on the critical or problematic patients at the expense of the routine, low-risk surgical patients who are recovering on schedule.

When we asked nurses what kinds of preliminary information were routinely given to patients about surgery and pain, the answer invariably was, "It depends. . . ." It depended, in fact, largely upon the amount of competing ward work and the number of patients admitted to the unit. . . .

The consequences of work pressures and the high priority accorded medical and procedural matters relegated informational exchange and the psychological preparation of patients to a catch-as-catch-can basis, determined by individual inclinations and the pain management philosophies of the nurses or the competing work priorities on the ward. . . .

Relief versus Minimization: Reliance on Drugs

There is also a lack of pain minimization through nursing-comfort measures. Paradoxically, this dual neglect is due partly to the very properties of routine, low-risk surgery. Because the causes of pain are unambiguous and of short duration, there is high reliance on manipulating either the frequency or the dosage of drugs in order to relieve pain. . . .

Thus, when patients complain of pain, the nurse's immediate response is to check when last a shot was given and whether the drug can be administered again within the limits of prescribed frequency. The reliance on drugs for relief is also due to the fact that patients, like nurses, tend to see drugs as the only solution to pain relief. Consequently, patients tend to initiate pain interactions by saying, "I need a pain shot." This reinforces the nurse's stereotypical responses: "Let me check the last time you had a shot";

. . . "You just had a shot an hour ago." These responses also reinforce a patient's perception of drugs as the major means of relief. When asked their reactions to the nurses' stock answers, patients replied: "It made me angry"; "I felt devastated"; "It made me feel stupid"; . . . .

The anticipated short duration of the surgical pain also encourages reliance on drugs. Anxiety or no anxiety, when there is no danger of complications or problems of drug dependency, such as those that might arise with an extended trajectory, the severe pain will last only two to four days at the most. Adding a tranquilizer or increasing the dosage or frequency of medication will control the pain. . . .

Nurses have other measures available to minimize pain and give comfort, such as splinting an incision when the patient has coughed or turned, giving a back rub, positioning, or pacing the drug to minimize the pain in ambulation. But these are volunteered rather than mandated, [because of] the great emphasis on drugs as the relief measure. The exceptions that we observed were in situations such as involved cardiac or respiratory surgery, when coughing was absolutely essential to avoid complications and when the surgery itself caused much coughing with pain. Here the pain minimization measures were "ordered."

Although the patients we queried were critical of both the staff's management of pain and care in general, they were not likely to express disgruntlement or to voice criticism directly to the staff. Several factors contributed to the lack of overt critical expression on the part of patients. Generally knowing that severe pain would be short-lived, the patients were concerned with getting past the acute phase of surgery and back on their feet to resume their former social roles and were, therefore, willing to endure the pain. They were also concerned about staff reprisal should they voice their criticism. Enduring pain and discomfort was also related to their comparisons of themselves with others who were more critically or seriously ill; they considered themselves more fortunate. The relative absence of overt fussing and complaining by patients tended to encourage the staff's assumption that their management of pain was adequate.

Variable Pain Philosophies: Problematic Aspects

What may be routine and nonproblematic to the staff because a patient does not complain may be very problematic for the patient. Patients know they must cooperate in the recovery process, but how they are to behave is not made explicit by the staff. This is due, in part, to the routine nature of certain surgeries which fosters a taken-for-granted attitude, so that the who, what, when, and how of patient-staff informational exchange and interaction are not considered essential. This results in each staff member interacting with the patient in terms of his or her own philosophies about pain. These philosophies may very widely on issues like threshold assessment, pain legitimation, giving of information, kind of control administered to the patient, pain trajectory, and limits of endurance.

The staff usually assumes that drugs can control surgical pain, yet the effectiveness of drug control calls for a complex set of staff-staff and patient-staff interactions. The patient must know the appropriate times and ways to request pain relief, the amount of pain he or she is expected to endure, the rules governing drug administration, etc. Unless the patient has had previous experience in hospitals or has been given explicit cues by the staff, drug transactions can become quite problematic.

The varied philosophies of pain greatly influence transactions involving drugs. Wide variations were noted in the decisional prerogatives of doctors and nurses regarding drug-related tasks. Some nurses thought that giving information to patients about pain medication was solely the responsibility of the surgeon; others thought it was a shared responsibility. Variations were noted concerning how much information should be shared with the patient about anticipated pain and about pain drugs, and who should give this information. When a patient asked about pain drugs, some nurses would respond, "You'll have to ask the doctor." Others freely gave information about the drug, its dosage, and frequency of prescription.

A nurse who believes that patients should be told about anticipated pain may have difficulties with a physician who believes that informing only increases the patient's "anticipatory pain." Variations were noted on the degree to which nurses adhered to the prescribed frequency of dispensing drugs. Variations were also noted on how much pain the patient had to endure before a nurse would consult a physician for changes of the drug order. And physicians varied in the discretionary latitude they allowed nurses in dispensing drugs. . . .

There are also staff variations on the amount of control patients are allowed to have, the willingness to act on patients' suggestions, and the degree of adherence to bureaucratic rules. . . .

The staff may assume that a patient has been given adequate information about his or her responsibilities in the drug transaction, but in fact the information may be far from adequate. Take, for example, a surgeon's assurance to the patient that pain shots will be available every three hours. If three hours have passed, should the patient ask for the next shot or wait for the nurse to act? . . .

Among the consequences of the many unshared, individual pain philosophies is a tendency for patients to become very confused and generally dissatisfied with their care, or to develop distrust of professionals. . . .

In addition to variations among nurses, there are group variations among work shifts on the same ward. The latter depend upon the pain-management philosophies and the degree of accountability demanded by the charge nurse for the given shift, on the numbers of staff assigned to the shift, and on the kinds of competing work demands. . . .

It is noteworthy that when patients complained to the researchers about the ways their pains were mismanaged, they attributed many of the problems to personality defects in the ward personnel, calling them unsympathetic, unkind, mean, and so on. The patients were totally unaware that the personnel were acting on the basis of their individual pain philosophies. Nurses criticized each other on the same basis. We should add that the patients often had *their* own pain philosophies, which they might or might not openly express. . . .

Back Pain and Its Legitimation

Discrepant Perspectives and Their Sources

With low-back pain, the discrepant perspectives of staff and patient pertain basically to staff's actual inability to diagnose accurately. . . . back pain remains exceedingly difficult to diagnose. . . . Diagnostic problems stem partially from the unreliability of clinical findings. Neither X-rays nor myelograms are always conclusive. . . .

The patients studied here were all diagnosed as having disk or vertebral problems. Some conditions clearly had started with an injury; in other cases the etiology was ambiguous and onset gradual. Treatment had included bed rest, traction, ultrasound treatments, bracing, or surgery.

Most of these patients had long medical biographies. Some had returned to the hospital because fusions did not "take"; one had had a period of relief, but the deep-seated remainder of an operated disk was shedding disk matter and there was new pressure on a nerve; some now had new herniated disks. In some cases the back disease had progressed too fast or for too long, and there was permanent damage to nerve roots. Many patients had had suspicions or verifications of previous medical mismanagement and were, therefore, often mistrustful and sometimes angry, still looking for a miracle. Others were hoping for long-term but not necessarily total relief. Many were guarded in their expectations.

Understandably, the staff does not view such patients as highly desirable. Their course of illness is unpredictable, the difficulties in objectively validating their pain and its source cast suspicion on its degree, and the limited relief options available when pain appears intractable lead to the staff's frustration and helplessness. Herein lies the initial discrepancy in perspective—over the issue of etiology.

Staff believes strongly in psychogenic factors as an important source of back pain. Patients, however, while not denying that emotions can intensify the pain, are not willing to accept a totally psychogenic explanation, which would imply that their pain was not "real." Although the staff's different perspective is not explicitly communicated to the patient, it does affect staff's interpretation of patient behavior and the actions taken to deal with it.

A second discrepancy in perspective occurs over the signs of visibility of pain. Even when X-ray or myelogram clearly indicates some pathology, staff is still not always convinced of the degree of pain that patients claim, for a similar abnormality will distress one person but not another. The patient usually does not know of the staff's skepticism regarding visibility. Persons who have had an unsuccessful medical experience or previous legitimation-of-pain problems feel vindicated when the doctor reports that clinical tests show a substantive basis for their pain. It never occurs to them that the staff's doubt has not been totally dispelled. . . .

A third discrepancy in perspective occurs over relief procedures, whose efficacy is often questioned by the staff. In large teaching centers, the personnel on an orthopedic ward rarely see successful back patients. They are more likely to see those who are returning for a second and third operation, and they have no way of knowing whether those who do not come back are simply "living with it," are shopping elsewhere, or are actually cured.

Many of them, therefore, question why patients expose themselves to surgery when there is such a low rate of success and so high a risk. Patients, on the other hand, have often tried all the options—had no permanent relief after traction, for instance, or found the discomfort of a brace outweighed the potential benefit—and now see the risk as worth taking when weighed against the unrelieved pain and the consequent interference with the normal conduct of their lives.

Yet a fourth discrepancy in perspective relates to the endurance of pain. It stems from the failure of patients who, for one reason or another, might have higher degrees of pain tolerance [and so can endure more of it than others might]. . . .

Considering all the circumstances just described, the staff's assessment of pain is obviously not a simple matter. Although they look for signs by which accurate assessment might be made, they observe these signs in interactional situations that affect their perception about the handling of expression and endurance of pain. Patients may be inhibited from natural expression or, in their inability to endure and their zeal to convince, may adopt modes of expression which are unacceptable to staff. This interplay will be examined . . . but first we shall look at the organizational features involved in the assessment of low-back pain.

Assessment: Minimal Information Base

An initial problem is that the assessments are based on minimal information. The patient's record will provide information about why he has been hospitalized, drugs to which he is allergic, his weight and vital signs, and previous hospitalizations. This, however, does not provide a composite picture of the "whole person." Many other important aspects of the patient's biography (for instance, his experience with illness, pain, and medical care), while integral to his perspective, are not generally known to the staff.

Lacking such information, the staff's knowledge of patient biographies is composed of bits and snatches pieced together from incomplete accounts and, therefore, subject to distortion. Furthermore, the communicated information is highly limited and selective, often obtained when the patient is in distress, crying, or begging for relief.

The staff frequently has the most information about patients with poor reputations. Sometimes, when a patient's back disease has been diagnosed on another ward, he may be transferred to the orthopedic ward along with an already damaged reputation. His reputation and biography may then be further distorted [because of] inadequate communication among the day, evening, and night shifts.

Most important, the biographies rarely contain any acknowledgment that, before entering the hospital, the patient has had pain to manage and relationships to deal with or has developed his own coping strategies. Thus, a wide discrepancy occurs between how patients see themselves and how they are seen by the staff.

Interactional Assessment

Assessment, for the most part, is based upon the staff's ability to read the signs—in situ and behavioral, sent out by the patient—a reading that is greatly affected by interactional and experiential variables. Behavior (actually, the patient's pain tasks of expressing and enduring) is read in the light of interactional rules of which the patient may be totally unaware or of which she has inaccurate knowledge or with which she may overtly disagree. Here cooperation over pain work breaks down, and the discrepancy gap between staff and patient widens further.

For example, when asked about their general discounting of degree of pain in back patients, nurses replied, "They make a lot of fuss that everything hurts when they have visitors, but they can get in all kinds of positions the rest of the time. . . ."

Most people with chronic disease have learned to keep pain expression as minimal as possible; they develop strategies for covering up. Covering up . . . is the rejection of the social significance of the handicap. . . . However, people with chronic back pain who have developed this coping strategy may not be aware, now that they are hospitalized, that they must modify their behavior to convince others of the reality of their pain.

Status-Forcing and Limits

There are social conventions for forcing persons into or for making them accept certain positions, however temporary. This process is called status-forcing (Glaser and Strauss 1971). Thus, in addition to deliberate covering up of pain as just described, other persons with low-back problems may be status-forced into keeping their pain expression invisible.

It may be made clear [by families and associates], as one back patient put it, "that they don't want to be around someone who complains all the time." Or others may express disbelief in the pain, especially when they have stakes in the sufferer's remaining active. . . .

As a consequence of such status-forcing, a person with

previous negative experiences in regard to pain endurance enters the hospital with an already "spoiled identity" (Goffman 1963*b*). Such people are no longer coping satisfactorily, according to others' definitions, and will have picked up feelings that they are giving in too easily, not making the best of it—that they are deficient in character or weak-willed. In other words, they begin to view themselves as others view them. They know their pain is real, but their identity is altered and —more important for our purposes—their behavior is altered as well. Consequences run the gamut from stoic teeth-gritters to those who feel driven to employ unacceptable tactics in order to convince.

In the hospital, no one explicitly tells patients of staff policy or of how the staff decides on suitable limits for pain expression. In fact, on wards such as the one we examined, there are differences in these conceptions, both within and between shifts. Patients learn about pain expression from the staff's explicit and implicit cues, cues pertaining to when and how to express pain, as well as to perceptions of pain legitimacy or lack thereof.

Whens and Hows of Pain Expression

People with chronic pain learn not to express their pain constantly, and yet staff members sometimes need an outward manifestation so they can make an accurate assessment. Thus, it is acceptable for the patient to express pain at expected points—ideally, three to four hours after medication—but the rest of the time pain is expected to be endured.

One way that the staff status-forces patients into enduring pain is to place a value on stoicism. The nurse urges: "The doctor says you can have the medication in three hours, but why don't you try to wait awhile?" Or she forces the patient into longer endurance by stretching out the 15-minute promised return. . . .

Staff members signal to patients by facial expression, body posture, or, when pain expression is excessive, by explicit statement, that expressions like loud moaning or whimpering are not acceptable. Or they simply avoid confrontation ("I get busy with bedpans"). Nurses also signal when they dislike the patient's mode of asking for relief—for instance, asking too often, whining, wheedling, or usurping the nurses' authority by phoning the doctor. Observations about the status of the pain are often explicitly stated. "You should (or shouldn't) be having that much pain.". . .

Nurses will admit that they are more sympathetic with

the teeth-gritters than with the overly expressive patients and that they will ask those who are enduring silently, "Wouldn't you like something?" Obviously, however, this tendency does not cover all passive and stoic patients, or there would not be stories such as the one concerning the woman who suddenly demanded to sign herself out because for three days she had not been given any pain medication, although she had a pain order. The nurse who described the transformation of this initially pleasant, placid patient was perplexed: "We didn't know she was in pain; we were waiting for her to ask."

Some patients never pick up the staff's cues; they are not aware that they have exceeded the limits. Sometimes, however, they know the staff's rules but cannot control their pain expression. . . .

To summarize the interactional bases for assessment: The patient is expected to take some *but not too much* responsibility in assessment and to cooperate by asking for relief, *at the right time* and *in the right way*. But this general rule may impede accurate pain assessment of patients who have established a pattern of covering up their pain or who feel status-forced into doing so; those who do not know that it is their responsibility to convince or who are not skilled at convincing; or those who cannot control their expression of pain.

Experiential Assessment

Patients are not the only ones to have biographies; staff members have psychosocial and pain biographies, too. A significant component of assessment is the experiential background of the staff member doing the assessing. Thus, nurses and physiotherapists compare complaining back patients with their own experiences with pain. Comparison may also be based on a pain ideology which has been reinforced by experience. . . .

When staff members are unsure of their assessments, they employ various tactics to test judgment. One tactic is to test for disparities between general behavior and the expression of pain. A nurse who found one patient's mode and frequency of expression unacceptable (the patient always began whimpering one hour after receiving medication) satisfied herself that the expression was disproportionate: "One day I stood outside her door and there was no sound. As soon as my shadow fell across her door, she started to whimper." This patient had employed the wrong strategy; it only proved to the nurse that the pain was really not very great.

Perhaps the best illustration of the influence of discrepant perspectives on assessment is provided by the differing views on distraction. Thus, persons in pain cannot send out pain signals all the time, if only because of the pure exhaustion of constantly focusing on pain. Yet, one can both be distracted and distract himself from pain. Under such circumstances one will feel it less and consequently express it less.

Patients acknowledge this of course. . . . They know, however, that a price is often pain once the distraction is over: an increased awareness of the pain, fatigue, and irritability. Further, they know that when the pain intensifies, nothing distracts them, and then they avoid being with others. To them, the potential of distraction is definitely no criterion for judging the legitimacy of their pain.

In the hospital, there is not only less to distract patients, but also they have an increased anxiety and focus on the pain, a fear of the unknown, and are continually reassessing their condition. (Am I improving? Am I developing a resistance to the medication?) Some personnel do recognize that if distraction were used as a strategy there might be greater endurance of pain. "Maybe if we took the time to talk to patients, they wouldn't need the medication." Others view distractibility as proof, at least with certain patients, that the pain is not as intense as the patient would have them believe. . . .

Inflicted Pain: Accusations of Incompetence or Negligence

It is easy to see that the implicit (sometimes explicit) contract which allows the accomplishment of the primary medical task can be violated, either in actuality or in the opinion of one of the contractual agents. . . .

Since the obligations of the contract are reciprocal, a patient of course can be reprimanded for breaking his side of the bargain. The stage is set, on both sides, for accusations of bad faith or bad conduct. The blaming, as in any political arena, will often be mutual.

From the staff's viewpoint, the patient can be blamed for failing to endure the pain; after all, it is only a byproduct of a task done for the patient's own good. He can also be blamed for failing to control extreme expressions of displeasure and slowing up accomplishment of the primary tasks.

A number of conditions underlie the possibility that the patient will also make accusations. The most general set of conditions is that the patient, like the staff, makes a distinction between necessary and unnecessary pain. The latter, of course, pertains to pain that is an unanticipated byproduct of the primary task, pain that the patient either has not been told about or has been told would not occur. However, unnecessary pain pertains also to necessary pain when the pain is more intense or of longer duration than expected. The inflicter is usually held responsible for all types of unnecessary pain: unanticipated, overly intense, and long-lasting.

As the patient sees it, the unnecessary pain can be caused either by *incompetence* (lack of skill) or *negligence* (carelessness, indifference). The patient may erroneously accuse pain inflicters, believing they have been careless when in fact they are inexperienced or they have made errors involving skill. Or, the patient may think the staff less than competent when in fact there has been some actual negligence displayed. Experienced patients, such as those on extended physiotherapy regimens, are more likely to spot the difference between incompetence and negligence. . . . [Here are] some common organizational reasons for a staff member's actual negligence or incompetence. Concerning incompetence: the main fault usually lies with personnel who either are insufficiently skilled at their techniques or at "working on" particular kinds of patients. That deficiency of skill can stem from insufficient basic training; lack of enough in-service training to keep up with advances in technologies; at the very least inadequate information about types of patients new to the personnel (a newness often caused by such factors as staff rotation).

The organizational conditions fostering negligence are perhaps more complex. To prevent or minimize pain engendered in cardiac patients by postoperative breathing regimens, patients must receive their drugs before doing the breathing, and receive them at exactly the right time. But unfortunately this involves a more complex intermeshing of staff work than is usually accomplished. Hence this kind of pain infliction through organizational negligence seems fairly frequent on CCUs. Other contributory organizational factors include a staff on a tight schedule, or one with a heavy load of medically difficult patients. A staff focused on technical aspects of care to the almost total exclusion of the humanistic aspects is also likely to be negligent in its infliction of pain during the pursuit of its main tasks.

Hospitals and clinics also seem often to proliferate a tendency to discount the patient's opinions on medical and even procedural matters, so that when a staff member and patient do not really know each other, a discounting of the patient's cues or utterances is likely. The patient is even more likely to be disregarded if he has earned a negative reputation on the ward or clinic—a frequent phenomenon, alas, in our health facilities. . . . Quite aside from an actual reputation, however, certain people get additional short shrift, or at least less concern is shown for them, because they are of "low social value": for example, some of the drunks, suicide attempts, victims of knife slashings, "accident cases," and various of the low socioeconomic or "undesirable" ethnic and racial groups who appear regularly at the emergency room of our hospitals.

Now let us return to the differences which a patient's experience might make in accusations of incompetency or negligence. Even without experience with specific procedures, treatments, or regimens, laypersons can sometimes recognize lack of skill in the manner, approach, style or actual words of the pain inflicter. Experience leaves the patient less at the mercy of such negligence. . . .

A patient who time and again goes through the same regimens or procedures can quickly learn to judge the skill of personnel. Essentially, each new potential pain inflicter is on trial. Patients also become better at distinguishing between individual reasons (unpleasant person, doesn't like me) and organizational reasons (overworked, not enough staff) for negligence. Such comparisons go hand in hand with the repeated infliction situation. Also, if a number of patients know they are undergoing the same treatments, as with physical therapy, they will share their evaluative comparisons so that certain staff members, like certain patients, receive reputations. . . .

Patients differ in the manner in which they express themselves to staff when they believe they have suffered from some degree of incompetence or negligence. Sometimes they can be very direct; at other times they choose to remain silent. Conditions eliciting direct comments are fairly obvious: the patient is surprised into angry exclamation, or fears that the same inflicter will return unless somehow reprimanded. Patients may even be quite fearful of potential damage, as well as of the pain itself, and command, as one did to a physical therapist: "Don't touch me again! You obviously don't know what you're doing." Among the reasons for keeping silent: the pain is insufficient to complain about, or is simply overawed by the personnel's authority. Silence can also be a response when the patient fears, sometimes accurately, that there may be reprisals for complaining or blaming. An experienced person

> may recognize the dangers of being defined as a "bad" patient.
>
> Those accusations which patients do level at a staff member are often met by two kinds of counterstatements. The first is based, whether justified or not, on the strategy that the strongest defense is an offense: "You moved!" or "What do you expect with all that racket you've been making?" In other words, the staff member accuses the patient of failing to keep his or her part of the implicit contract.
>
> The second type of defense is to retort that someone has misread the situation; the task is very difficult and a certain amount of pain is inevitable, or what looks like undue and unseemly haste or careless procedure is really nothing of the sort. In short: signs are at best ambiguous, and only the truly experienced (that is, the professional) can read them correctly. Both types of counterstatement can be delivered with a variety of gestural and tonal expression, signifying a range of disapproval running from reluctant countercomplaint through annoyance, anger, fury, disgust, desperation. After all, the main job simply must be done, with or without the patient's cooperation. Understandably, such sets of tactics and countertactics may end in an increasingly vicious spiral of bad feeling, bad temper, and bad health care. . . .

As noted earlier, what is true of pain management is a more institutionally evident instance of what undoubtedly occurs with other kinds of discomfort experienced by patients, as they are subjected both to the intricacies of their own illnesses and to the medical interventions designed to control the illnesses. In the largest sense, then, all trajectory managing involves comfort work. But what specifically, when, by whom, how effectively, how well accepted by the patient the comfort performance is—all that is profoundly affected by the staff's (and patient's) conceptions of the trajectory itself and by the organizational conditions which impinge in such complex ways on the evolution of particular patients' trajectories.

6
Sentimental Work

Our attention now turns to an important, varied, often subtle, and sometimes very complex type of work. It, too, is done in the service of managing and shaping trajectories. Sentimental work, as we term it, is present as an ingredient in *any* kind of work where the object being worked on is alive, sentient, and reacting—present either because it is deemed necessary to get the work done efficiently or because of humanistic consideration. It should have been often glimpsed accompanying the various types of work discussed in the preceding chapters.

In medical situations, a sick person is reacting both to the illness and its symptoms—with anxiety, fear, panic, depression—and to the medical treatments, which can frighten, wound sensibilities, and even threaten self-esteem. Like comfort work, there is nothing especially new about pointing to the existence of sentimental work: the old-fashioned physician's bedside manner and the nurse's "tender loving care" are simply aspects of an earlier era's recognition that there was more to medical and nursing work than its physiological core. But sentimental work done under the changed conditions of chronic illness prevalence plus treatment in today's technologized hospital is something quite different from old-fashioned sentimental work. As will be

An early version of this material appeared as "Gefühlsarbeit. Ein Beitrag zur Arbeits- und Berufssoziologie," *Kölner Zeitschrift für Soziologie und Sozialpsychologie* 32 (1980): 629–51, and a version in approximately the same form as this, "Sentimental Work in the Technologized Hospital," *Sociology of Health and Illness* 4 (1982): 254–78.

seen, too, it is something more than the work of seeing that the patient is made physically comfortable.

Also, to recognize it as a phenomenon is easy; a more difficult task is to answer the following kinds of questions about it:

Are there different kinds of sentimental work?
How is sentimental work carried out?
When and where is it done and when not?
Who does it?
What is its relation to other types of work?
When is it likely to be in focus?
When is it visible,when invisible, and to whom?
What are some of its consequences: for patient, work, staff, and ward?

Sources of Sentimental Work Complexity

Quite like other types of work, sentimental work has been profoundly affected by the same changes in disease prevalence and medical organization. Since those have been detailed earlier and will enter integrally again into the account below, we shall touch only briefly on a few summary points here.

The essential characteristics of chronic illness suggest immediately that these diseases impinge frequently and sometimes harshly on sick persons' situational interactions, on their long-term interpersonal relationships with significant others, on their moods and passing psychological states, on their very identities (Strauss and Glaser 1975). Thus, crippling, deforming, or stigmatizing symptoms are publicly evident and privately depressing. Lessened mobility or energy necessitates the services and goodwill of friends and kin, presenting problems of coping with that dependence. Loss of body's powers—the recognition of and anger at a permanently failed body—presents major crises in the lives of people whose life-styles are profoundly affected and whose identities may be attacked at their very roots—all this quite aside from the impact of an illness known to be hazardous to life or almost certain to bring it to an end soon. It is not as if such problems vanish when an acute phase of the illness is over: they are persistent, often continuous or repetitious, and they can worsen over time. A relatively short period of handholding and expressions of kindliness by kin, friends, and physician will not spirit those problems away. The acute flareup of symptoms or potentially dangerous body deterioration which brings the chronically ill into the hospital does not render them any less sensitive to their existential dilemmas.

Atop all that, in the hospital they encounter situations that can further increase their emotional turmoil. A number of those situations were touched on in previous chapters whenever we mentioned giving, or failing to give, psychological care or doing psychological work, and other such situations can be seen in the descriptive cases where that sort of work was sometimes reflected.

Among the most general sources of sentimental work, however, are the following. First, there is the ever present possibility of *clinical* danger to the patient because of various aspects of the staff's trajectory work, especially when a trajectory is relatively problematic. As we know, various of the diagnostic tests may make a patient anxious and create fright or panic in someone who is encountering them for the first time. Or the medications may produce unpleasant or frightening side effects; their effects may even become defined by a patient as quite out of hand. As for the various machines used for diagnosis, therapy, or life support, they, too, can arouse much anxiety and fright or threaten a patient's poise or self-esteem.

Second, the medical work is usually done by total or relative *strangers* to the patient: they may know little about that person's identity, or his or her medical and social biographies, or attitudes toward illness, bodies, treatments, or themselves. Third, the medical aspects of trajectory work, of course, usually take *priority* over other considerations. Hence, these staff strangers tend to be focused on the main medical jobs rather than on the patient's identity, biography, and attitudes unless those seem especially pertinent to the immediate trajectory tasks. These last two properties (strangers and priority) of trajectory work can together heighten greatly the potential for arousing anger or rage, engendering tension, wounding sensibilities, creating interpretations of insult and so on. During the staff's busy medical work, the patient's inner struggles may go unnoticed or at least not managed to the patient's satisfaction. Personnel may ignore the sick person's attempts to give what seem to him or her quite relevant biographical data. The personnel may also ignore or denigrate a patient's wishes in the matter of making medical choices that he or she deems pertinent either immediately to identity or to posthospital life.

A fourth feature of trajectory work is its *duration*, for it tends to last several days and even weeks, especially when trajectories are highly problematic. Hence, the impingements of trajectory work on patients' moods and identities are more likely to occur than if the hospitalizations were of short duration. Moreover, a lengthy hospitalization may result in a cumulative impact on the patient, so that increasing amounts or different kinds of sentimental work are done—or the patient wishes they would be done—by the staff.

However, trajectory work does not necessarily include sentimental work as defined either by the staff or the hospital itself. That is, sentimental work is not always thought relevant to the work at hand, so that even when it occurs, the staff member is neither held accountable for it nor asked to make the accomplished task visible through verbal or written report. For all that, it does get done and is part of the total trajectory work. Even when done implicitly or on an ad hoc, individualistic basis, its specific appearances, modes, and agents are not accidental but patterned.

Types of Sentimental Work

There are several different types of sentimental work, among which it is analytically useful to distinguish. Although quite possibly there are more, in all, we have observed: (1) interactional work and moral rules, (2) trust work, (3) composure work, (4) biographical work, (5) identity work, (6) awareness context work, and (7) rectification work. It is important, we believe, to give this typology in order to avoid blurring these useful distinctions by the common terms "psychological work" or "working psychologically" with someone and because the typology is necessary in order to specify the different conditions, consequences, tactics, and so on that attend each subtype of sentimental work.

Interactional Work and Moral Rules

At the most elemental interactional level—the level which most of us scarcely note because action there is so implicit—the staff's preoccupation with and focus on purely medical work can often make the patient feel like a veritable inanimate object rather than a human being. At the very least, reactions of being worked on and of depersonalization may be aroused. While knowing that the medical work must proceed, the patient may wish, perhaps unconsciously, that more respect were being paid to himself and to his body and may feel humiliated or depreciated, and, of course, he or she is having to cope with an extraordinary sense of biological and psychological invasion. Some rather basic rules, mostly implicit, of human behavior are being violated, although without staff's intention to do so. (Our thanks to Fritz Schuetze, University of Kassel, for having brought this important phenomenon to our attention.)

For underlying interaction, there are implicit or *taken-for-granted understandings* (or rules or norms or assumptions) that affect behavior, which, if followed, lead each person to regard the other as polite, courteous, considerate, reasonable, pleasant (Garfinkel 1967, Goffman 1963*a*). These and similar synonyms refer to silent contracts about such matters as conversation (listening carefully, not breaking in abruptly on the speaker, not shouting) and about certain actions (not brusque, not brutal, not breaking in on privacy). A physician or staff member who "really" listens when with a patient or who converses informally and with "genuine" interest or who does not move without warning or other human touch will have followed some of the understandings that undergird normally pleasant and nonconflictual interaction. Anyone who shatters those implicit rules or understandings is going to get pronounced or otherwise reacted to as inconsiderate, discourteous, rude, unpleasant, even brutal. A mild instance is that of the woman who reacted to the style of an anesthesiologist during his preoperative visit when he entered her room, sat down on a chair, and did not introduce himself. She asked, "Who are you?" He answered, "I'm your anesthesiologist." Her retort: "Not if I have anything to say about it!" Or more passionately, expressing what many patients doubtless feel when used as subjects for medical demonstrations: "I was in front of a great many students in a big hall and I felt insulted, you know, as a person, neglected as a person." Being treated as a nonperson, without any recognition as a living being, even though nothing brutal is meant by it, *is* insulting to many who encounter that neglectful treatment.

> When my daughter-in-law had that burned retina, they had a parade of thirty doctors come through, and all they told her was that, "You're going to be presented in rounds." That's all. She didn't have any idea of what that meant. So there was this army that walked through, but nobody looked at anything but the eye in the dark. She found it just horrendous, even though it was an emergency.

In addition to the interactional rules there probably are others—more explicit perhaps—that govern work relations as such: for example, the matter of *orienting* the person who is being worked on, one should not surprise a patient unpleasantly, even for a required task, but rather prepare him or her first for what may hurt or perhaps even offend. An elderly farmer was being examined by an intern who, in feeling the abdomen, pushed hard against the patient's liver. The old man suddenly shouted, loudly enough to be heard down the hall, "Hey, what do you think you're doing!"

Explaining is almost like orienting but pertains not so much to what one is going to do as to the nature of the options, decisions, or overall arc of work. Here is a worst-case scenario where explaining was not done, or was not perceived as done:

> A woman in her twenties had been in a severe car accident and spent nearly a year on a neurological ward with several operations done on her brain there. She was very upset because no one had done any explaining about the effects of the lesions and because the whole thrust of the care seemed to be toward surgical interventions. Between operations, she said that they provided almost no care, either of an explanatory nature or for orienting her to her surroundings. For instance, she lost her sense of taste (common for the injury she had) but had never been told that was a direct result of the location of the injury. (Our thanks to Leigh Star of the University of California, San Francisco, Department of Social and Behavioral Sciences, for this account, taken from a field note.)

In trajectory work, there is a fair amount of explaining by staff to patients, much of it not in the nature of teaching or going into depth about what is about to be done, or what has been done, unless the patient presses for further explanations. Our point in referring to the phenomenon of explaining here, however, is to emphasize that this is not necessarily just instrumental work but can be done for composure, identity, and other sentimental-work reasons.

A close cousin to orienting and explaining is *pacing*. Here is an instance (which also brings out the building of trust—a type of work discussed more fully later):

> A physician persuades a wary child to sit on a stool, saying: "This won't hurt." The doctor takes out cotton from nose and asks: "That didn't hurt, did it?" The child nods agreement. The M.D. wants to wipe the bloody nose with cotton, but the child makes a defensive gesture. The M.D. says: "It's soft" and puts a piece in the child's palm. The child holds the cotton, feeling it while M.D. wipes the nose and probes a bit with another piece of cotton.

Pacing is a central rule—in fact, a tactic—used by the nurses debriding of patients in a burn unit described elsewhere by us (Fagerhaugh and Strauss 1977). Physical rehabilitation therapists tend also to be quite careful in their pacing, as they work with patients on often painful exercises. Not only do they take note of capacities for enduring pain and managing sometimes limited energies, but the therapists will allow or prompt negotiation permitting patients' greater control over the pacing of this joint rehabilitation work.

Another implicit rule is not to do anything to anybody's body without getting their consent, whether directly or indirectly—a rule violated knowingly if desperately on pediatric wards when a child who resists a procedure believed necessary is forcibly held down, usually screaming, while the task is performed.

Of note also are some deeply felt *moral rules* or norms—usually implicit unless challenged—which when broken arouse much passion, as in the case of the physician who kept working on a young child who had been socially dead for some days, despite the protestations of the mother who wanted the machinery turned off: the physician refused, saying that his job was to keep life going as long as possible—no matter what. In fact, there can be abrasive disagreements among staff concerning whether certain terminally ill patients who are now permanently nonsentient should be kept alive artificially by medical means. The more important point is perhaps that patients have been known to "pull the plug" themselves or to jerk out their IV tubes, only to have the staff keep them alive against their moral protestations (Glaser and Strauss 1965, 1968).

Building Trust

Another generalized work rule is that trust needs to be built so that work can get done, or done with efficiency, unless, perhaps, the work is of an emergency nature. Of course, if a task is simple and the work brief, then the person doing the work may not bother with establishing trust but go directly—if politely or pleasantly—about his or her business. The establishing of trust can be simple, involving merely an air of competence as well as concern for physical, interactional, or personal sensibilities. But, as we all know, gaining someone's trust can be a very complex task, involving much time, much talk, demonstration of competence, many subtle gestures, and the like.

When staff members unavoidably inflict pain on patients while doing necessary procedures, there are implicit contracts: "must do but will do as fast and painlessly as possible," providing patients will endure pain as best they can (see the discussion on pain management in chap. 5). Of course, the contract can be explicit, as when a patient thought possibly to be terminally ill told his physician, "If you decide I am dying, then you must tell me. Although I recognize you will need to tell me at your own pace, you must tell me. You must not withhold my dying from me." The patient is essentially saying that he knows the physician can be trusted to carry out this injunction, given the relationship already established between the two of them. The self-conscious building of trust is perhaps not usually as explicit a task for ward personnel as for physicians, who know that patients will place great reliance on their competence and concern. Otherwise rejection of their services is likely. However, whether explicit or not, it is such a necessary ingredient that when this vital task is neglected or bungled, then patients will complain or even sign themselves out of the hospital.

Even in the one-shot, brief situations defined by patients as near-emergencies, where the building of trust can be relatively negligible, still it may be implicit in those situations. When trust is not established, then:

> I was sleeping and my wife was getting ready to go to work. It was a cold day. She leaned over me, said goodby, and kissed me: off she went. Next thing I knew, she was back crying. She had slipped on the ice and hurt her lower back. So we went quickly to the university hospital, right into emergency. The doctor came and led her to a small room. "Ok, undress, I'll be right back." That room was very cold. She sat in this bare room with her bare skin, waiting. After fifteen minutes we said, "To hell with it," and left.

The resident not only broke his promise of a quick return, broke trust, but, of course, shattered another interactional taken-for-granted rule: it is unreasonable, even cruel, to leave someone shivering in the cold.

Composure Work

The great number of procedures and machine-related tasks done to and for patients exposes them to potential loss of composure, whether poise, face, or self-control. During these work sessions, much of the sentimental work done will consist of the staff, usually the nurses, helping or enjoining patients to keep their composure. This is done not merely for reasons of compassion but to insure that tasks get done with maximum dispatch and efficiency. Handholding or a touch on the brow or soothing sounds of empathy or encouragement "hang on, it will soon be over") will often help to pull someone through a painful or frightening procedure. Failure to make those reassuring or helpful gestures can be consequential for completion of tasks since patients may cry, scream, change body position, collapse in panic, or refuse to go on. Of course, this sentimental work is all the more important when procedures are to be done repeatedly, for once bitten twice shy. Obeying the more implicit interactional and work rules helps to further the patients' maintenance of composure, but explicit composure tactics and techniques are of additional utility in getting the requisite medical tasks done. Composure work is indeed, probably the most usual and the most visible type of daily, run-of-the-mill sentimental work.

Biographical Work

Biographical work is a rather special type of work, primarily intended to achieve only medical purposes per se, but which sometimes has a more intense psychological component bearing on those purposes. The ordinary diagnostic interview, with which we are all familiar, is an instance of biographical work that is done but not necessarily with any special regard for its sentimental-work aspects. The physician endeavors to elicit information bearing not only on symptoms but on past medical and social history and perhaps, too, on life-style as pertinent to possible relationships with symptoms and disease. This kind of interview is generally carried out in a rather matter-of-fact style, with rapid-fire questioning. The difficulty of doing diagnostic work without at least minimal biographical information is highlighted by what happens in emergency rooms when gravely ill persons who are brought in cannot give any medical or personal details because they are unconscious and there are no kin or acquaintances to supply those details. The physician makes quick diagnostic guesses, judging from symptomatic cues but also from age, gender, and life-style cues: Is the patient likely to be in a diabetic coma, having an MI, or . . . ? (Some assessments are very strong, like "he's drunk" or "she looks like one of those women," for moral judgments are very frequent and severe in emergency rooms [Roth 1972]).

Compare this with the style and complexity of the evolving interaction between an oncologist and a patient suffering from cancer. The physician needs to know a great deal about the patient's pattern of living, even his or her relationships with next of kin or with supportive close friends, in order to pace the prescribed therapy. The physician will need to keep tabs on the impact of the therapy, not merely on physical functioning but on the patient's capacity to endure, on the "will to live," and perhaps also on life-style. This kind of biographical work inevitably leads to some degree of mutual give and take in which the physician may reveal or answer questions about some features of his or her own biography, given primarily to further the therapeutic work. (Our thanks to Fritz Schuetze, University of Kassel, for these observations made at a cancer clinic and for the idea of biographical work.)

On the wards, nurses may do biographical work in order to make relationships between themselves and patients smoother, thus facilitating their trajectory work. Of course, if a patient is periodically hospitalized on their ward, they are likely to learn more and more features of his or her life and can utilize those in getting the sick person through difficult moments and days of illness. The hazards of ignoring a patient's personal history or ignoring biographical work are that trajectory tasks are impeded or resisted and that a downward cycle of mutual or staff retreat may develop, to the detriment both of ward morale and trajectory work—let alone to the patient's moods and medical care.

Identity Work

Empirically speaking, biographical work can move imperceptibly into identity work, but it is useful to keep the two analytically distinct. The former pertains mainly to getting personal and social information (health personnel sometimes call this "social history"). Identity work, in our definition of the term, refers to working with the patient on matters of personal identity; what is sometimes referred to as "psychological problems." We are all familiar with the psychological work, whether on deep or more passing issues, that is and should be done by kin and close friends to help ill persons maintain and improve a sense of identity in the face of extended and difficult illness. Hospital personnel engage in this kind of work, too, but usually with more distance and perhaps in a more calculated fashion in order to maximize the effectiveness of their trajectory work. We are not referring to kindly or compassionate gestures made because of empathy but to the *work* which staff members do in the service of their other trajectory work. Naturally, efforts which support a patient's identity can be spontaneous, situationally elicited, but overall they merge into the longer-range work itself. The many hours of conversation that nurses sometimes spend with terminally ill patients, even if enjoyed for their own sake, are designed to keep spirits up and to further the patient's closure on his or her life. The tactics of getting less gravely ill persons to face the realities of their physical conditions and to prepare them for their posthospital lives are other instances of identity work. On the other hand, in desperation difficult patients may be turned over to the hospital's liaison psychiatrist, since the staff's identity work has been to no avail: "Let's hope he can do something with (and for) her" (Fagerhaugh and Strauss 1977).

Increasingly, especially in the nursing and social work professions, there has been a proliferation of ideology that emphasizes working with patients psychologically and in professional modes. Chaplains who work with the terminally ill are also increasingly influenced by psychological literature as well as by traditional religious philosophies in their very special work with the ill. Some take great pride in what they have been able to accomplish, helping patients to gain better emotional equilibrium and satisfaction with or closure on their lives. This work and these ideologically oriented workers are likely to be found on certain types of wards working with certain kinds of trajectories. But whether ideology or common sense directs the identity work, its failure can contribute to the blocking of trajectory tasks, ineffective trajectory work, and the disintegration of the patient in the face both of physical deterioration and seemingly ineffective medical interventions. We should add, of course, that the few instances of identity work given above only scratch the surface of what is a very complex category of work. Our purpose here is only to distinguish it from other types of sentimental work, so that we can specify when each is done, by whom, why, with what consequences, and so on.

Awareness Context Work

There is another type of work, done partially in the service of protecting and maintaining a patient's identity but also for helping the patient to maintain composure, which we term "awareness context work" (Glaser and Strauss 1965, Strauss, n.d.). It is sufficiently important to warrant separate discussion. This work is done whenever staff withhold information which they believe will be difficult for the ill person to handle, such as probable physical deterioration, or will be really devastating, as in terminal cases. This work can, of course, also be done in the service of the personnel's comfort and composure but often is grounded in the philosophy that the less a person knows which would be psychologically harmful to him or her, the better. Moreover, the thinking goes, if patients really want to know, eventually they will ask or flash the proper cues. This kind of sentimental work can pertain to any kind of undisclosed information, but it has been fully described for dying patients who are unaware of the staff's belief in their impending death (Glaser and Strauss 1965, pp. 34–39). To sustain the unaware patient's belief in their version of his future, the staff members must control his assessments of those events and cues which might lead him to suspect or gain knowledge of his terminal state. Their attempts to manage his assessments involve them in a silent game played to and around him; meanwhile they use tactics intended to encourage the patient to make his or her interpretations inaccurately optimistic and to reduce spatial, verbal, and nonverbal cues that might arouse suspicions or to give those that will allay them. This strategy requires continual wariness and control by the staff members.

Rectification Work

One other type of sentimental work should be mentioned, for it, too, can be quite important. When patients express aggrievement or a sense of insult during or following the disregard of interactional or work rules by rude or thoughtless personnel or when their composure has been shattered by them, then one can frequently observe another staff member "picking up the pieces." An example from the field notes:

> I was following the resident who entered a woman's room, accompanied by five or six medical students, to do a cervical examination. They all stood closely observing the resident do his examination of her vagina. It was done with scarcely an introduction, with little explanation or attention paid to her reactions. A nurse did hold the patient's hand. The resident did vaginal scraping, demonstrating to the students how to do this right. Then they all exited without a single word, only a passing nod from the resident. After they left, the patient burst into sobs, while the nurse consoled her.

Such rectification work can include apologetic or caustic remarks about the brusqueness, inconsiderateness, or callousness of the offending staff member. Nurses often do this rectification after patients have been visited by technicians or after they have visited machine sites for diagnosis or therapy and also after a host of physicians with residents, interns, and students has breezed through the ward on daily rounds. But rectification work can perform a deeper function than helping patients to recapture poise; the helpful staff member may actually be reassuring the patient: you really *are* a person, despite being treated as nonperson. Without such rectification work, patients' resentments would doubtless mount, bodily or psychological insults rankle more deeply, and they might finally resist certain further treatments and procedure.

Summary

Among the subtypes of sentimental work, then, are: interactional work and moral rules, trust work, composure work, biographical work, identity work, awareness context work, and rectification work. Picture these types of work in dramaturgical terms: they are actions done during the medical scenes; sometimes they are front and center, more often they are at the margins of the main line (medical-nursing, technical) of action. Sometimes they are so marginal that they are barely discernible to any audience, because virtually the only actor who is aware of the sentimental action is the actor doing it. Now, we turn to describing some implications of that metaphor and of the foregoing discussion about the various types of sentimental work.

Explicit, Implicit? Accountable, Nonaccountable?

Around a patient who has been hospitalized for a few days, let alone been previously hospitalized once or twice, there builds up a thick dossier of documents which constitutes the medical record. This is the record perused by his or her physician(s), added to by physicians reporting their observations and orders, further added to by nurses, and still further added to by technicians reporting the results of various tests to which the patient has been subjected. This stack of documents bearing on the patient's case is a temporal as well as present-oriented record: it reflects the patient's condition over time, the medical interventions taken in relation to that evolving condition, as well as the monitoring observations continually covering both the illness and the results of the medical interventions (Freidson 1975; see also the discussion of information work in chap. 13).

For us, two features of that typical record are especially noteworthy. First, it is distinctly a *medical* record. Second, it constitutes a reflection of public *accountability*: orders must be entered in it, monitoring observations must be noted, drugs administered must be recorded, and so on. If aspects of the patient's behavior, attitudes, moods, and interactons seem relevant to someone among the staff, those might be entered into the official record, too, but not necessarily so, for these are not accountable items unless, of course, an order is given or an agreement is reached that those items should be monitored and then recorded. In short, the conditions and actions most related to sentimental work may not be considered important enough, medically related enough, to warrant orders for doing or reporting or recording them.

In relation to the medical record, two questions concerning sentimental work become immediately relevant. First, under what conditions is sentimental work explicitly requested or ordered and then recorded? Second, under what conditions does a staff member initiate sentimental work and actually bother to put this work in the record? These two questions can best be dealt with in tandem, for in a sense they represent the opposite sides of the same stream of events. When the sentimental work is explicitly agreed upon or officially ordered as part of the trajectory work, then if actually done, it should end by being recorded. That recording usually is done by the staff member responsible for performing the given sentimental tasks. When sentimental work is not ordered or agreed upon but is done voluntarily by someone—done implicitly rather than explicitly as part of the arc of work—then that person may decide to record the accomplished task. If so, then it has been made officially visible to others. Any further action prompted by that recording will become an accountable aspect of future trajectory work.

On the other hand, explicit orders or agreements about future sentimental work—just as with other kinds—may involve many tasks and ward interactions which are neither spelled out nor reported back because they are just assumed or involve too much minutiae for anyone to bother with. Said another way, the ward's machinery can be relied upon to carry out certain lines of work without the necessity for detailing the items of work or accounting for them. Furthermore, it should be readily understandable that the mix of explicit and implicit sentimental work—as well as types of that work—will vary enormously with the anticipatable line of work foreseen for particular trajectories or their phases.

High and Low Accountability

Generally speaking, either the explicitness or the accountability, or both, of sentimental work is rather limited within many specific arcs of work. (Edward Davis, doing research in a general hospital, has noted [verbal communication] that when he reviewed the medical records of patients who had checked themselves out of the hospital, there was virtually no information there to suggest why they had done that—whether, for instance, they were angry at the staff for not doing sentimental work or for doing it badly.) True, there are moments and phases in trajectories when the staff knows this work to be very pertinent: the physician knows he has to build and maintain trust; the social workers may be required to obtain biographical data bearing on the patient's personal background; a nurse may be requested to try to raise a patient's spirits "in any way you can figure out." And, as already noted, for certain trajectories explicit sentimental work is a built-in feature of the anticipated line of work: thus, during the last phase of terminal care, nurses quite explicitly do what they call "comfort care" (Glaser and Strauss, 1965, 1968).

There is, however, one condition which does greatly enhance the explicitness of sentimental work. This is the existence and operation of an ideology that emphasizes its salutary role. A striking instance of this is reflected in the writings of Futterman and Hoffman (1973), who reported on how, in a specially organized pediatric ward, the staff worked closely and self-consciously with children and parents on managing physiological and psychological states and on coping with physical deterioration and impending death. Ideological considerations, in fact, prompted both the organization of that ward and the highly experimental sentimental work done by the staff. Ward ideologies can be less directly rooted in medical specialties like psychiatry or disciplines like psychology. They may derive more directly from work experiences on the ward itself, as did the aforementioned comfort care, or the interplay between staff and patients described by René Fox in *Experiment Perilous* (1959), where all worked together in a specialized hospital and where nobody knew what the medical outcomes might be. Sometimes ideologies that affect the explicitness of sentimental work even spill over from social worlds that are not immediately associated with the world of medicine, for instance, the incorporation by personnel, especially the nurses, of holistic medicine or of women's movement themes, which may engender quite conscious attempts to "work with" the patients in new and not strictly medical modes. On the whole, however, there is limited accountability or explicitness of the sentimental work done in hospitals, given the dominant focus of personnel on acute illness and the medical interventions which it entails (Fagerhaugh and Strauss 1977, Kassenbaum and Bauman 1965).

There are at least two institutional forms that permit or even encourage exchanges of information about recently performed sentimental tasks, as well as about any other tasks that probably need to be carried out. There are staff meetings and briefing sessions at which nurses exchange information about the conditions of various patients on the ward. During both types of convening, staff are likely not only to discuss the more technical matters related to the patients but to report, or complain about, or gossip about, or just tell stories about aspects of patients' attitudes, moods, and psychological states, thus precipitating discussion about "what we should do." Sometimes the projected line of sentimental action proves effective, but sometimes so ineffective or even disastrous that the personnel throw up their collective hands in disgust or despair. That is when the psychiatrist is likely to be called in. Or kinsmen appealed to!

Division of Labor and Mixes of Work

There are some interesting questions concerning who actually does what kinds of sentimental tasks, and when and why. *And* how does that sentimental work intersect with other kinds of work? Any blunt assertions about physicians only doing medical work while nurses are left to do all the psychological work—which one hears occasionally from nurses—are either an expression of ideological and perhaps professional bias or perhaps just an overstated generalization. Physicians, for instance, may not bother with much composure work, but they do it when it seems they cannot help but do it, or when they see it being done badly, or when they are carrying out procedures that clearly call for composure work. It is the intern or the resident who often is most continuously in contact with a patient hospitalized for emergency diagnostic work and who really engages in the most sentimental work done by physicians. Even busy surgeons will under certain conditions perform identity tasks which otherwise they rely on nurses to do (if they think of that work at all). An instance is that of the chief surgeon on a ward for kidney transplant and dialysis patients who allowed himself finally to be drawn into an extended discussion with a patient about the patient's marital problems. The surgeon did not wish to spend time or energy on that topic but recognized that this work was probably necessary for the patient's medical welfare and that he was the one who must do it because this patient was so trusting and respectful of him. In general, however, the relative nonaccountability of sentimental work furthers a somewhat flexible division of labor around that work.

Contributing to the more-than-occasional softening of the strong tendencies in hospitals toward a division of labor based on occupation are the varieties of ways in which sentimental tasks get intertwined with other types of tasks. The former get fitted in and around the more medical and technical work, which is apportioned in accordance with familiar occupational bases. This means that either everyone may do some sentimental work in relation to carrying out technical tasks or—more radically—everyone may undertake or have sentimental tasks forced on them regardless of occupational position. Before or while performing a procedure, the physician or the assisting nurse or the technician may reassure an overtly anxious child or adult and may urge the patient to endure a bit longer until the procedure is completed.

Nonetheless, there is a high probability that the sentimental work will be closely associated with the standard work of the personnel. Thus, Mr. Einshtein (see chap. 2), hospitalized for a myocardial infarction, forced biographical and even identity work on his physician during the bedside visit, not on the nurses or technicians, concerning especially what might be anticipated now about the impact of illness on his life-style and his longevity, too; and the intern did composure and rectification work, reassuring him that the IV would balance out any possible danger from the diuretic given in error. Again, a psychiatrist or chaplain may be doing most of the "death talk" and other identity work with dying patients, while the nurses are likely to focus more on helping them to maintain their composure.

It is during the procedural work that an observer is most cognizant of the complex interplay between the standard occupational assignment of tasks and the subtle weaving in and out of occupation-based sentimental work—largely implicit, situational, but in any event not recorded as performed in the patient's otherwise detailed medical record. A couple of excerpts from field notes should be helpful in illustrating that important point. They will also reflect the kin's part in this division of labor and in carrying out sequences of mixed types of tasks. The patient, too, may enter into that division of labor.

1. Here is the case of a very sick 9-year-old girl, with renal disease plus complications:

> She is lying flat on her bed, a nurse working over her, bright and alert, while the mother is holding the child's hand. The nurse has marvelously gentle hands. The work had been going on probably for some time. Both nurse and mother are cuing the girl about "another thing" (a procedure) yet to be done—perhaps they even said what that was, but I could not hear. Nurse begins to pat the girl's chest with a cupping instrument, to loosen phlegm, doing this gently but persistently. Child evinces pain, mother tells her they must do the procedure. Mother holds her hand tightly. Tells girl to take her hand away from her chest. Explains that although she has been spitting up the phlegm, she must now throw it up. (The child had been relatively nonsentient for many days and this is her first day of sentience.) After about ten minutes of the cupping procedure, the child is examined but asks for her book. Mother props it up in front of her almost closed eyes. After a minute or two, both women tell her that now the tube must be put down, explaining its necessity and agreeing that it will hurt. Nurse carefully measures the tube, threads it through the girl's nose and down into her bile. A physician appears: he and the nurse pump a vile-looking green liquid from the bile, examine it, pump down antibiotics. During the threading scene, the mother is intensely holding her daughter's hands: this is the peak miniphase. The mother cannot watch the threading of the tube (later I learn that she knows this procedure can be dangerous, can cause an abscess). Mother kisses the child's hands, her head down, during the time it took to actually get the tube down.
>
> Meanwhile the patient has exerted immense control over herself, not uttering a sound nor a complaint or moving unduly. The mother is intensely involved in promoting the girl's self-control. The nurse's gentle overall presence also must help, creating trust. She makes no abrupt, potentially frightening movements.
>
> To my consternation, two nonward personnel have moved a huge bed scale into this small ward and are now waiting to weigh the child. They lower the vertical table,

> moving it to the bedside, and mother and two nurses now move the child to the scale. The girl says, "It's cold," and the nurse nods agreement. Then they move her back to her bed, making encouraging noises ("we know it hurts"). One additional point: during the giving of antibiotics, the mother was called to the telephone; I overheard the conversation and talked with the mother afterward about it. Her daughter had been told she would be in the hospital, alas, during Halloween, but that there would still be "trick or treat" there. So the girl had asked for an elephant mask, and the mother was saying to whoever was on the phone that she had a job for him or her: to find the mask she had promised her daughter.

In sum: the nurse's gentleness seems vital to the accomplishment of her medical work, being sustained by her careful handling of the patient, her continued fulfillment of two implied promises, not to hurt her more than necessary and not to perform more procedures than necessary. Moreover, the nurse's verbal gestrues involve cuing and explaining—all of this sentimental work overarching all phases of the medical work. The mother's presence is also vital and never more so than when she is sharing her daughter's worst moments during the painful tube procedure. The mother is also doing much explaining and alerting the girl to the next steps of the procedures. Maintaining her own composure, she is also working hard to help her daughter maintain her composure, too. Her unspoken but clear signals to the child to be courageous, to endure the necessary suffering, involve more than an expectation of the child's situational bravery, going deeper with an appeal to and expectation of appropriate behavior from a "brave girl." If that is so, then the girl is doing more than simply maintaining her composure: she is surely doing identity work with herself.

2. The next case especially reflects the need with children or infants to pace all the tasks throughout the session, as well as the way sentimental tasks (also paced) are allied with the standard work "roles."

> Grandmother is playing with infant boy in crib. Carries him over to a scale so he can be weighed. Two nurses are waiting there. Grandmother puts him gently on the scale, caresses him, stands aside. The surprised infant sees his mother peering over the scale, wiggling her fingers at him. She records his weight in her own book. The nurses record his weight in the child's chart. Grandmother then carries the child back to bed. Mother diapers child, grandmother helping to move the child's body and diverting its attention with a toy. A physician appears and does his stethoscoping as quietly and unobtrusively as possible over the mother's

> shoulder (she is now holding the child). Glances between physician and mother and a word or two. Physician next takes out an instrument with a built-in light and makes a toy of it for the infant, passing the instrument before the child a couple of times. Then peers through the instrument at the infant's eyes, from a distance and again unobtrusively, the others having turned the child's face in his direction.
>
> Next there is a convergence of bodies; the nurse to hold a soon-to-be squirming child down; the grandmother the same, but making frequent caressing movements while holding the child down. Mother bends down to the child's face and "makes faces" at the child. Child is yelling because the physician is poking the lighted instrument into the child's ear, looking through it. Scene soon accomplished, and we are then back to grandmother, mother, and child interaction, playing, with his toy put near him.

In sum: There are unnoticed procedures and highly invasive procedures and an expected difficult miniphase handled skillfully through sentimental work. Presence of kin and their gestures are helpful in to get weighing and in doing examination tasks. Kin work is periodic and frequent and, of course, intense during the expectedly difficult examination time. Placing a toy near a child is "familiarization work." (We are indebted to Christa Hoffman-Riem, University of Hamburg, for both the observation and the term.) At the cost of much kin work, there is a relatively smooth flow of medical tasks and minimal disturbance to the child. Note the clear division of labor, which is quite explicit although not "planned."

In short, the two cases bring out how—along with the main procedural jobs to be done, involving as they do a sequence of tasks—the sentimental work is woven in and out of these jobs. Sometimes the workers are quite aware of their sentimental work, sometimes not. This work may become such an integral component of a staff member's style that possibly he or she is not always self-reflective when doing the sentimental work, especially as the procedural work is usually salient. At any rate, during procedural work the sequential interlacing of different types of work can be complex—their separateness perhaps only noted by an observer who has both an eye for them and analytic purposes for finding them.

Focus and Visibility

That last sentence has buried within it the implication that only under certain conditions does sentimental work come into clear focus, moving from the margins to the center of attention. A number of conditions affecting its salience have already been alluded to: when the personnel are beginning to establish trust and again when there seems a need to reestablish it or confirm it; when rectification work is done, for then awareness of its desirability bears in on the consciousness of the rectifier; when the line of medical work calls for explicit accomplishment of given sentimental tasks; when ward ideology guides the style of care given to patients; when an ideological position derived from sources external to the ward itself (an occupational, professional, or extramedical movement or social world) influences the stance toward tasks of individual personnel; when a patient overtly proffers or forces the challenge or the burden of sentimental work; and closely allied to the last, when a trajectory goes radically awry both medically and otherwise and the staff finds itself in a no-exit situation where more, and more effective, sentimental work is inescapable. To these conditions might be added a related one: when a patient rejects the style or mode of a staff member's carrying out a sentimental task, thus bringing into sharp focus either how badly the task was done or the need for it to be done differently.

Under all such conditions, the person doing the sentimental work is more likely to be aware of doing this work. That does not mean, however, that others are similarly aware. Indeed, the work can be quite invisible to other personnel. (Thus, a nurse once complained to us that the many emotional-type things she did with patients during their dialysis sessions were simply not understood by the physicians or even by the social worker. She was, in our terminology, saying this part of her work was invisible to nonnurses, so that its true value was not appreciated.) Since much sentimental work is done interstitially, on an individualistic, ad hoc basis, inevitably it is invisible to others unless they happen to be on site or the work is reported back verbally or in written form to co-workers and supervisors. Even if the sentimental task is performed in plain view of other personnel, they may not notice: they are busy with their own tasks or they may look on those sentimental tasks as secondary and also take them for granted. Hence, the work slips by, going unnoticed even when fully visible.

A final important condition relating to invisibility of patients' own sentimental work, or that of their kin, is that the staff quite literally does not see this work. Not only may the staff not be present when kin are doing identity work with a sick relative, but even fairly obvious work may be misconstrued; this it is not uncommon for nurses to miss the grief and closure-on-life work done by spouses and dying patients (sometimes by both) during the last days, because the spouse's presence at the bedside is defined merely as a normal desire for wanting to be together near the end (Glaser and Strauss 1965, 1968). Surely, too, many patients prefer to do their own sentimental work (perhaps especially identity work) silently, invisibly, for it is their lives that are threatened by illness, their lives that must be reworked, their biographical stakes that are being gambled with by even the best-intentioned of medical interventionists.

Consequences

The most specific statement that might be made about the consequences of doing sentimental work is that they vary in accordance with the type of sentimental work that is done: composure work has an immediate impact; identity work has a longer-range and deeper impact. A more general statement is that a great deal of nonsentimental work could not be carried out as easily, efficiently, or at all if the requisite sentimental tasks were not done. Conversely, when the sentimental work is not done, or is done badly in someone's judgment, then not only the main line of medical work but also many interactions, moods, composures, and identities may be affected. Patients' feelings of humiliation, insult, invaded privacy, physical and mental discomfort, and resentment at being treated like an object are related to failures of sentimental work.

Much current complaint about the depersonalization of modern hospitals and hospital care is unquestionably related to such failures of sentimental work—often also compounded with failures of comfort work. (A colleague of ours, hospitalized for the first time in his life, recounted in amazement how in the entire week he was hospitalized for acute care, everything was "so instrumental" that only one intern acted toward him like a living, breathing, human being. To everyone else he seemed only to be something that gave out "blood, piss, and other products.") Even when a staff member has done the sentimental work competently, it can be construed quite otherwise by a patient. Contributing to that perception are not only the professional-lay differences between staff and patient but also the ethnic, generational, gender, and other disparities between the two parties in what is, after all, a rather subtle form of human interaction. One person's authentic gesture can be judged as wholly inauthentic by the other or simply inadequate to the occasion, or it may seem completely inappropriate. Depersonalized feelings spill over into malpractice suits, for probably most are related not merely to definitions of staff negligence and incompetence but also to the staff's failure to establish and maintain trust, bridge the gap between humans, and generally make effective sentimental gestures in the service of the medical work.

Failure to do adequate sentimental work may also negatively affect the ward's "sentimental order": "the intangible but very real patterning of mood and sentiment that characteristically exists on each ward" (Glaser and Strauss 1968, p. 14). (One instance among many given in that earlier publication was, "Sometimes a patient announces that he is dying, but the staff members do not think so. If he is correct, he dies alone, with no farewells to family members. Such a death shatters the sentimental order of the ward" [p. 199].) Of course, the sentimental order characteristic of a ward is a very complicated interactional phenomenon, and its maintenance is certainly not dependent only on sentimental work. Three deaths in rapid succession can be devastating to the sentimental order, quite independent of staff-patient relationships or failure of either sentimental or technical work. Nevertheless, when sentimental tasks are neglected or done badly or ineffectively, then the sentimental order is negatively affected. How can it not be? Such cases also show that the organization of a ward's total work (its "work order," Glaser and Strauss 1968, p. 40) can also be profoundly and negatively affected. Conversely, successful—even if implicit—sentimental work contributes positively to the ward's work order as well as to the sentimental order. Of course, it also contributes to staff members' gratifications over their work, as well as to their own sense of identity as related to their work.

7

Articulation Work

Managing and shaping a trajectory involve calculating and carrying out numerous lines of work, which, viewed closely, are constituted of clusters of tasks. Tasks and lines of work together make up the arc of work anticipated for the given trajectory. Both require "coordination," for they do not automatically arrange themselves in proper sequences or with proper scheduling. In other words, further work—*articulation work*—must be done to assure that the staff's collective efforts add up to more than discrete and conflicting bits of accomplished work. In common parlance, the physician arrives at an overall plan—a kind of trajectory blueprint, the head nurses guide its implementation, while the other health workers, including nurses and technicians, carry out the requisite operational tasks with more or less competence and dispatch. The central figure in the planning is the physician, but the key actor in the articulation drama itself is the head nurse. Without her, the trajectory work would come to a grinding halt, a fact of hospital life that physicians appreciate and hospital administrators can scarcely overlook.

Difficulties of Rationalizing Medical Production

The articulation of medical work in hospitals may or may not be more complex than industrial, engineering, legal, military, or other kinds of work, but that articulation certainly looks different when examined closely. One quick way of demonstrating such differences is to consider, first, some characteristic features of industrial production. At its most sophisticated—for example, the production of computers—it involves the application of scientific discoveries and engineering principles during an experimental developmental phase in which numerous options are weighed, put on trial, and "bugs" eliminated as far as possible. Only then does the actual production begin. This can encompass the coordination of an incredibly large number of lines of work, require resource arrangements of great complexity, and the meshing of thousands of tasks. Unexpected problems, which are internal to the production process, can disturb its smooth flow, but ideally at least the major obstructions have been anticipated and can be handled with relative efficiency. Only external contingencies of large magnitude (a rapid decline in the market for the product, say, or the disappearance of funds necessary for the production) will profoundly alter the envisioned or ongoing production process.

In short, many elements of industrial production are almost fully rationalized, while the remainder are rationalized as far as possible. Articulation is built in as part of this rationalization. All of that can be done because goals are clear, tested means for reaching them are available, and evaluation of results all along the course of work is both possible and feasible.[1] Indeed, it is only for this kind of production that models describing both ideal and actual forms of the process have been formulated, not by social scientists but by production engineers. Medical production has received very little such analytic study.

What then does the latter look like when scrutinized closely? To begin with, some tasks do approach full rationalization, since various implicated parties reach out for standardization that will reduce costs, hazards to safety, blocks to resources, barriers to effective clinical action, and the like. The rules of pharmaceutical testing and final release to markets are regulated by the FDA; other safety regulations are laid down by federal, state, and county agencies; hospital administrators are much concerned with rationalizing the hospital's purchas-

[1]In an unpublished paper ("Rationalization and Varieties of Technical Work," 1977), Elihu Gerson (Tremont Research Institute, San Francisco) lists as the elements of rationalization: (1) clear, unambiguous, mutually compatible goals; (2) predictable inputs; (3) component tasks which are articulated in an unambiguous manner; and (4) "in every situation, the conduct of the activity is unambiguously evaluated." He argues that there are four basic classes of inherently nonrationalizable tasks: (1) policy tasks in which there are multiple, vague, or conflicting goals; (2) engineering tasks in which the inputs are inherently unpredictable; (3) managerial tasks in which the articulation of component activities is ambiguous; and (4) evaluative tasks in which the relationship between means and ends is not perfectly clear, hence outcomes cannot be evaluated. Medical work has large numbers of all those nonrationalizable tasks, as he recognizes.

ing, supply, recruiting, and other requirements; and on the wards themselves, as we have noted, these are standardizing strategies for increasing the probability of successful clinical accomplishments.

Alas, a number of conditions affecting medical production mitigate against its rationalization. We have met those conditions before, but their recapitulation will help us to visualize what health workers (patients and kin, too) are up against in their attempts—within the hospital, let alone at home—to manage chronic illness trajectories successfully. Our focus should not be merely on sets of disruptive conditions: the several *sources* of those conditions are even more striking evidence of the magnitude of hazards besetting the "good coordination" of medical work.

First, let us begin with trajectories themselves, for they constitute a prime source of potential disruption. An illness, as we all know, however simple in appearance, however experienced the health personnel in handling it, can prove unpredictable. The patient develops a postsurgical infection or other complications and proves to be allergic to a tried-and-true drug. No matter, such contingencies are easily met. Others, coming in the wake of more uncertain courses of illness, are more difficult to handle. As remarked so often in this book, the trajectories associated with chronic disease can be very problematic. They have been stretched out as never before; they have new and unknown phases; they affect in unanticipated ways others of a patient's trajectories; and in general—even on purely "medical" grounds—they set major problems for those who so dearly desire smooth sailing in their trajectory management.

A second source of potentially disruptive conditions is part trajectory and part organizational in nature. Each ward tries to minimize the diversity of its medical product by having patients with similar diseases or conditions. The more heterogeneous they are, the more varied the requisite kinds of work and the more varied the resources necessary for doing those kinds of work. It is immensely difficult, however, to standardize by disease and condition: realistically, only very specialized wards can have "just one type of patient here." And even they are different from an industrial site where, let us say, just one kind of automobile is being produced but each of the twenty worked on there is at a different stage of production, for even on the specialized ward, each cardiac or dialysis patient will be at a very different stage of the trajectory. So, because trajectories are being worked on—whether multiple or diversely phased—a host of potentially disruptive conditions will threaten the articulation of work for each trajectory.

A third source is related to the second. There is actual or potential competition among patients for available resources, notably the staff's time, attention, and skills but also occasionally, if temporarily, scarce resources like equipment and drugs. If there are many resources, then the competition may be hardly discernible; if there is a shortage of any, then that competition may be visible even to the patients. The more important point here, however, is that such competition for resources can produce a host of contingencies which intrude upon unplanned or assumed articulation of work.

The patients themselves constitute a fourth source of potentially disruptive conditions. We have in mind here not simply a patient's behavioral responses but his or her unanticipated and unlooked for entrance into the staff's self-circumscribed division of labor, for that entrance may immediately or eventually confound the staff's order of business as they conceive of it. The degree of disruption and the kind will depend on the contingent aspects of how, when, and where the patient entered the division of labor. The entrance of the patient is what makes medical work *fundamentally* nonrationalizable.

A fifth source is medical technology, which harbors a host of conditions that can spawn contingencies affecting the articulation of the trajectory work. There should be no need to spell out those conditions, since we have only to turn back to the chapter on machine work (chap. 3) for them.

A sixth and very potent source of disruptive conditions is the hospital's organization, for coordinated trajectory work relies on supplies and services from many departments and on the scheduling and meshing of their flow into the ward and into the staff's clinical work. Again, there seems little need to elaborate on those organizational conditions since they are implicit or explicit on virtually every page that has preceded this one.

A seventh source is the interaction of the various types of work (machine, clinical safety, comfort, sentimental), for some of this interaction will threaten effective articulation. The importance of this source is easily overlooked unless one already understands that there are different kinds of trajectory work and that each may play its part in the total arc of work. The staff readily recognizes that a monkey wrench can be thrown into the coordination of their work by a patient's becoming impatient or angry at the way a procedure is being carried out or depressed by the implications of the necessity for that procedure, or that a patient's discomfort might need to be handled quickly because it can directly affect physiological functioning, which in turn can limit the effectiveness of ongoing therapy. The articulation of medical work is assuredly made quite complex by this possibility of untoward interaction among types of trajectory work. In the broadest sense, the point here is that work on a given trajectory may involve various kinds of work, but they may not run smoothly when the tasks are performed, or one or more of those work types may not be written into the staff's script yet may affect the work drama. Trajectory work with sentient persons can never escape those possibilities.

An eighth source of potentially disruptive conditions is the thorny problem of how to evaluate work performed in the service of the trajectory—work all along the course of that trajectory. All parties in the division of labor may agree, but then again some may disagree. They may disagree mildly or strenuously, openly or covertly, with authority or with little power to change the situation. Contingent on these and a number of other possibilities, evaluative dissensus leads in more or less degree to the disarticulation of the trajectory work.

Finally, over the course of the trajectory there may be a ninth source: an explicit or implicit reconstruction of the patient's self. Thus new "outside" commitments, biographical developments, and the like are very likely to intrude upon the staff's trajectory work.

In summary, the articulation of the lines of work and their implicated tasks conceived as necessary to the management of a course of illness is immensely difficult to rationalize. Too many conditions mitigate against rationalization to permit more than some proportion of component segments of the arc of work to be standardized—and then they, too, are subject to potential disruptions. Work on and with people adds a dimension of hazard to the articulation of work; if to that are added those hazards that flow from organizational, technological, and illness sources, then "coordination of care," for which personnel are constantly striving but know they are not often attaining, is something of a mirage except for the most standardized of trajectories. Its attainment is something of a miracle when it actually does occur. Nevertheless, as we shall see, a measure of articulation can be achieved for particular trajectories or for segments of their total arc of work, although that measure of articulation takes special work to accomplish.

Levels of Articulation Work

In analyzing what goes into the articulation of clinical care, it is useful to think of at least three levels of articulation work. On the first, topmost level is the articulation work of the main physician in charge of the case. It is he or she who has the largest view of the course of illness, especially if not too problematic, and what interventions are necessary to manage that course; that is, the physician has the big picture. This picture includes the main features of the arc of work: what major jobs will need to be done, when, more or less in what sequence or simultaneity, etc. As noted earlier, the physician can rely on much standard operating procedure (SOP), involving various departments—X-ray and clinical lab—as well as those elements of SOP under the aegis of the head nurse on the ward where the patient is housed. At the second level is the work of the persons who are organizing, setting up, supervising, and monitoring the physician's requested or ordered jobs. Most of that administration of jobs and lines of work is done by the head nurse (one on each daily shift), and especially on the day shift when so many diagnostic and therapeutic activities swirl around the patient's body. On a third level, there are the actual jobs, which consist of task clusters and sequences; for instance, to get an Xray taken requires alerting and sometimes physically preparing the patient for the session, arranging with the radiology department for scheduling of the shots, bringing up the gurney or wheelchair, transporting the patient back to the ward and perhaps getting him or her back into bed. There are many potential hitches in those sequences of tasks, and since more than the head nurse and the radiologist are involved in them, each person may be involved in lower-order operational articulation work. (The physician may engage in some third level work, too, when he visits the bedside or when he or she moves trajectory work along by conferring with the radiologist about the X-ray films taken for his patient.) The potential for misarticulation of minitask sequences can easily be grasped, even for such simple ones as measuring blood pressure or taking blood from a vein, and it is the nurse's or the technician's responsibility to keep those sequences moving, that is, to rearticulate them when they become affected by one contingency or another.

These three levels of articulation are not so separate in all occupations as in hospital work. For instance, in Barney Glaser's study (1976) of how a patsy articulates the work of various subcontractors when getting a house built, the patsy is seen as having the big picture in his head (i.e., the arc of work to be done for the construction trajectory), but the patsy is also doing supervisory work comparable to that of the head nurses and also doing a certain number of operational tasks which include operational articulation. Similarly, when fund-raising for a voluntary organization, the fund-raiser does both level one and level two articulation but engages also in a larger share of third level articulation than does the patsy, the head nurse, or the physician. (Our thanks to Frances Strauss for this information.)

Returning now to the medical scene: in relatively nonproblematic trajectories, such as that involved with simple surgery, the surgeon can anticipate and outline for the staff the lineaments of the overall arc of work and will need to do very little articulation work himself or herself. That articulation will be done mainly by the head nurses, who can rely on much SOP. Nevertheless, they will need to get tasks into motion, monitor them, assign proper nursing personnel to them, and the like. A stuttering of the operation machinery may still occur, however, indeed is very likely to occur, at some point before the patient leaves the hospital. And, of course, the expected trajectory may go slightly awry; a mild infection, for instance, will call for additional nursing or medical work, which now requires rearticulation action.

In problematic trajectories, the physician is playing the game more by ear, having only a rough blueprint and so is being forced to consider each phase as it develops. Aside from the physician having to juggle his or her other tasks along with those that are developing for this particular patient, the articulation of the trajectory work requires that the physician calculate next steps in medical intervention or diagnostic location, that is, what steps, in what sequence, at what rate, and the like. The head nurse will still be responsible for the administrative articulation of those next steps, as are other personnel for segments of the operational articulation of those steps.

The three levels of articulation are, in fact, sometimes not so sharply distinct as delineated above, since under certain conditions the physicians will do second-level work or head nurses will do third-level work. For instance, a physician who is dissatisfied with how the trajectory tasks are being carried out may not only complain to the head nurse but go into supervisory action himself. Residents and interns may engage in administrative articulation just "to get the show on the road" or to enhance the morale of the nursing staff by sharing their work. Head nurses will get involved with operational tasks, hence with the associated articulation work, under such conditions as when there is a shortage of staff, a snafu in carrying out tasks, a flagging in the mood or morale of the nursing staff, and under fortuitous circumstances as happening to be on the spot when a task needs to be done. (On the other hand, administrative articulation is ordinarily not assumed by nurses or nursing aides except under quite fortuitous conditions.) Furthermore, when the technology is quite new, especially when a new unit is being set up that embodies novel technology, then there is more likelihood of a blurring in the division of labor with respect to the three levels of articulation: physicians and house staff engaging in all three and the head nurse in at least two. (With changes in the nursing profession nowadays, too, new statuses are emerging, such as that of the primary-care nurse who is responsible for the "total nursing care" of given patients and who may be doing the administrative and even some of the operational work of the head nurse and assisting nursing personnel.)

For our purposes, a discussion of specific details of administrative and operational articulation work is unnecessary. Suffice to say there will be many different styles at each level and even greater diversity of tactics for getting the requisite work accomplished. It is generally true, however, that there is a strong tendency toward maximizing the use of SOP and toward constructing some of it when it is not already established. We have already noted generalized strategies for doing that, as well as the necessity for doing it, especially for the head nurses since there are so many contingencies and trajectory complexities that destroy her easy reliance on SOP. Tactically, the articulation work is likely to get done case by case, depending at least on the nature of the trajectory, its phasing, the organizational conditions bearing on articulation possibilities, and the individual styles of the articulating agents on the ward itself. Doubtless there are patterns of tactics, but we have neither studied them nor believe it is necessary to detail them here. So we turn next to the veritable hurricane of disarticulation issues associated with highly problematic trajectories.

Generalized Articulation Strategies

There are several articulation strategies that if properly realized help to further the rationalization of the trajectory work. We shall discuss these only briefly, since they are different only in detail from those used in nonmedical settings.

First, there is an attempt to standardize the flow of necessary resources, whether work force, skills, time, energy, supplies, or equipment. We have seen many of those efforts in the previous chapters. Of course, an adequate flow of resources may involve much "pressure," confrontation, discussion, persuasion, and negotiation, but once agreements are reached they may evolve into standard operating procedures. A great deal of resource flow rests, however, on established procedures whose origins are lost in the mist of organizational history.

Second, the SOP covers many other aspects of trajectory work. The physician and the head nurse, notably, call on this operational machinery without too much concern for potential hitches in getting requisite tasks accomplished. SOP includes scheduling, allocation of jobs among personnel, and so on. Reliance on SOP is not, however, without its difficulties. Its proper functioning requires some notion of what the needed resources are and what everybody's work normally is. The head nurse, for instance, needs to know a tremendous amount about what resources are actually available and where and how to get them, about the scheduling of key persons and servicing departments, about requisite paper work, and so on. Even to learn the SOP—as new personnel generally will recognize—may take a lot of time, energy, and teaching by old hands on the ward. One sees this with nurses, interns, and residents new to a ward and its routine operations. Some of the SOP involves knowledge that is quite local to the ward or the specific hospital, so that even experienced physicians or nurses who are new to the locale must acquire quite a bit of its local knowledge before they can successfully navigate through the otherwise hazardous stream of organizational events. The annual influx of residents and interns—as an instance of this—presents the receiving nurses with the necessity for cuing them in and sometimes with the necessity for repeated teaching of recalcitrant, inattentive, or perhaps not so bright newcomers.

The situation is further complicated because even established physicians may have different conceptions of SOP from those customary for the ward. Thus, the physician's philosophy may lead him or her to order different drug dosages from those most of his colleagues would order. For the physician, an order may represent SOP, but for the ward personnel, and especially the head nurse, it will be unusual the first time around and thereafter may call for repeated communications to (and persuasion, perhaps, of) noncued in or disbelieving personnel. Eventually a special SOP for this specific type of physician's order will be developed and transmitted to any personnel who may be involved in carrying it out. If a strong resistance develops against the physician's idiosyncratic practice, then the staff may revolt or try to negotiate or persuade him to change his mode of operation. They may even pressure higher authorities in order to obtain that change.

Moreover, a physician may not know what it takes to articulate the tasks requisite to carrying out an order. The nurses have to operationalize the request or command, but they, too, may not realize how complicated a chain of tasks must be coordinated to get the necessary work done. This is especially true if the order, for a procedure, say, is a new kind. But this can also be so if the responsible worker does not anticipate organizational snags, principally, perhaps, because he or she does not recognize the organizational problems of other workers or departments. For instance, the physician may request a faster report on an X-ray than is usual, and so the head nurse puts in her request marked STAT (i.e., immediately). The X-ray personnel may get angry because, as they say, everything is now ordered STAT! If they object or drag their feet persistently, then a head nurse may attempt to cut through the possibility of their cry-wolf discounting of her request by calling down and saying "for this order I do really mean right away." That is, she attempts to reassert the SOP status of her request.

Or the conflict between X-ray department and ward may result in negotiative conferences. Or the higher administration gets pulled into the fray, counseling to "be careful" or mediating to obtain a compromise. Eventually there are attempts to build these agreements into

SOP, thus rationalizing this aspect of the work—say, some kinds of orders become really STAT, while others are not unless special argument is made for them.

Third, there is a generalized articulation strategy of constructing an effective system of communication (see chap. 13 for "information" work). After all, many people and tasks are involved in managing a trajectory, and those people and tasks must be coordinated over several departments and over three daily shifts of personnel. Since many communications are informal, made in face-to-face situations, and often, and made between only two people, those do not necessarily get recorded. Hence, other personnel may not get to know about a particular communication, an oversight that can bring about an unfortunate lack of coordination, especially when the other persons are directly involved in carrying out the relevant tasks. More general transmission of the communication may occur when it is reported orally, as to the next shift, but the worker may not report it even then, or may wait until the next day or the day after if he or she happens to be off duty in between.

Before leaving this section, we should emphasize the important point that articulating the trajectory of a specific patient is quite a different phenomenon from articulating the short-term work of the unit across many patients simultaneously. Both kinds of articulation work are complex, but employ many of the same tactics. The next section will be focused on the first kind of articulation.

Articulation in Cumulative Mess Trajectories

To bring out vividly as well as analytically the articulation work required when a trajectory proves immensely difficult to manage and shape, we offer next a case history and an analysis of such a trajectory. The case will illustrate, of course, more than the articulation issues, but the analysis will be focused on those as they evolved over two months. The story will be recounted sequentially, accompanied by comments pointing to the continued round of articulation, disarticulation, and rearticulation called forth by contingencies derived from illness, technology, organization, and patients. The articulation work involves sentimental and comfort tasks as well as clinical safety and other medical ones. Our comments also point to relevant agents, including patient and spouse, and their relationships to segments of the total articulation of the trajectory work and to whether or not the personnel could rely on standard operating procedure or needed to make novel arrangements involving negotiation, persuasion, uncommon types of personnel, or unusual action. Then, at the close of this section, there will also be an analytic summary of this "cumulative mess" trajectory. (This case, of the woman with lupus, was discussed more briefly, for other purposes, in chap. 2. We use it again because it so ideally suits our analytic points about articulation.)

The Case

The case of Mrs. Price is characteristic of a type of illness trajectory found more and more frequently in our hospitals (Fagerhaugh and Strauss 1977, pp. 251, 268–69, 253–67). We call it a "cumulative illness trajectory" for reasons that will soon become apparent. Its chief features can be summarized chronologically. In order to keep a complex chronic illness under control, physicians utilize a variety of therapies, sequentially and in combination. These may or may not work for a while, but they inevitably add to the complications produced by the illness itself. To handle the complications and the new turns in the illness, additional tests, drugs, procedures, and therapies are utilized. Few of these are really experimental or untried, but their impact on the symptomatology and illness of the specific patient may be relatively unpredictable. Over time, as in the case of Mrs. Price, the patient's physical condition can become more and more unbalanced, with increasingly varied medical interventions becoming necessary to manage the imbalance. Pain may or may not be present during or at any point in such cumulative trajectories. Often, of course, it is present, even constant. Sometimes, as with Mrs. Price, it is an integral part of the cumulative trajectory.

The case of Mrs. Price illustrates vividly and dramatically the constant rebalancing of multiple considerations that accompany cumulative illness trajectories. We shall follow a course of illness that not only moves progressively downhill but also arouses anger, frustration, and desperation in everyone involved, not merely because of the worsening illness, but because of complications setting in from the interplay of the disease and the various technologies utilized. Morale plunges. Personnel, including the various medical consultants, move in an out of involvement; many eventually withdraw psychologically and indeed even in terms of giving conscientious patient care. Fears of narcotic addiction are prevalent, and the sense or senselessness of the risk of addiction is debated by people with very different moral and medical philosophies. Ethical issues are raised, fought over, and left unresolved. "Coordination of care" goes to pieces, periodically being patched together only to disintegrate once more.

Mrs. Price, the 45-year-old wife of a physician, was in her fourth hospitalization. She had been diagnosed as having lupus erythematosus two years previously. Since then she had three acute episodes requiring hospitalization, the last two occurring within the last year because of bleeding gastric ulcers, which required surgical intervention. The ulcers were complications from steroid treatments to control the lupus. In both episodes there were flare-ups of lupus, so that hospitalization was extended for two to four months. Moreover, the uncertainty of Mrs. Price's condition together with her low tolerance for pain resulted in narcotic dependency. There were conflicts between Mrs. Price and the staff over drug control. Weaning her from the drug proved difficult.

During this period of two years both the treatment and the disease had drastically altered the quality of her life. For example, Mrs. Price could not engage in her one great pleasure, gardening, because sunlight exacerbated the lupus. By her fourth hospitalization she had come to realize that her illness would eventually be fatal, that the treatment created other problems, and that the future was highly uncertain. At the time of her fourth admission she had a variety of disorders. As a result of her lupus she had (1) pericarditis, (2) pleuritis, both of which caused pain, (3) cerebritis, which caused some personality changes and a tendency toward tremors and convulsions, and (4) chronic obstructive lung disease from the lupus and her heavy smoking. As a result of the steroid treatments she also had (5) gastric ulcers and (6) Cushing's syndrome.

With each hospitalization she returned to the same nursing unit, a unit primarily for surgical patients where stays tended to be short. The nurses anticipated problems of pain management with Mrs. Price because she arrived on the unit with a previously formed reputation for being "manipulative" and "uncooperative."

Mrs. Price was readmitted to the hospital because of continued chest pain. The lupus specialist, Dr. Nagel, suspected a pleuritic flare-up from the lupus and recommended hospitalization for reevaluation and readjustment of the steroid drugs. Mrs. Price informed the reseacher that she couldn't tolerate the idea of hospitalization after the long siege of the past year and so delayed coming to the hospital, hoping the chest pain would decrease. With the increased pain and general worsening of her condition, and after several days of persuasion by her husband and her attending physician, she finally consented to hospitalization.

Trajectory location required

Necessary work for getting hospital trajectory started

The nursing staff members anticipated that this patient would become addicted and therefore decided to "set limits." They reasoned that in the past, since the numerous doctors on the case wrote conflicting drug orders, the nurses were caught in the middle. With only one doctor responsible for the pain drug order, they would avoid the patient "manipulating" the doctors for increased pain drugs. Dr. Power, the house staff member and assistant to Dr. Nagel, would be responsible for the patient's general care and the pain drug orders. Dr. Nagel would be out of town for two weeks for an important medical conference. A decision was reached that the patient be given 50 mg of Demerol and Talwin to control the pain, and these two drugs would be alternated every three hours. All the nurses and house staff were alerted to this schedule.

Discussion and negotiation (based on past experience with patient) about main articulating agent for pain medication

Attempt to articulate all in the immediate division of labor

The house staff was busy evaluating Mrs. Price's illness status during the ensuing three days. This involved innumerable blood studies, an electrocardiogram, and chest x-rays. Meanwhile, she was having increased chest pain.

Standard operating procedures (SOP)for diagnostic location

On the third day she refused to have a chest x-ray done at the time scheduled because she was too uncomfortable, and she insisted that 50 mg of Demerol was not holding the pain. The physician who was handling the pain drugs and the nurses refused to alter the drug order. Mrs. Price phoned the psychiatrist, Dr. Perle, and Dr. Abel, the cardiopulmonary specialist, asking each to alter the drug order. They decided to honor the decision that one person handle the pain drugs, reasoning that they could not risk another dangerous addiction problem.

Patient blocks segments of articulation

Patient attempts own articulation

Reaffirming staff's negotiated articulation decision

Later in the afternoon the researcher found the patient dressed an packed, ready to go home. She recounted her inability to obtain pain relief, said she was tired of hospitalization and simply wanted to go home and take her chances. The nurse caring for her described her as a willful patient who couldn't get her way (an increase in pain drugs) and

Patient breaks off the hospital trajectory

was using the threat of going home as a weapon. The nurse's attitude was that the decision, however, was up to her (going home), no matter how unwise. The husband visited the patient and confronted her with: "Alice, you can't go home in your condition. You know you can't manage at home. If you go home, I wash my hands of the whole affair." He left the room. The researcher spent some time with the patient, who talked about the quality of her life over the past year, the difficulty of living with uncertainty, and the pros and cons of remaining in the hospital. Later the psychiatrist persuaded her to stay. During the next two days she was relatively free of pain, although the drug order was not altered.

Sequential and multiple agent attempts to rearticulate the disintegrating trajectory

On the sixth day, Fay, the nurse who had cared for Mrs. Price during previous hospitalizations, stated that the pain problem was currently worse than it was during the last hospitalization. The patient was becoming more insistent that the 50 mg of Demerol was not holding the pain. She had been telephoning her husband and the psychiatrist to get an increase in pain drugs. Over the weekend she was able to persuade Dr. Abel to increase the Demerol by 25 mg for one dose. Fay described this doctor as being an "easier mark" than the other doctors for pain drugs. Fay feared the problem of addiction would "start all over again like the last time."

Patient's "deviant" revised articulation

On the previous day, Fay had been reassigned to care for Mrs. Price because the patient did not trust the new nurse, preferring Fay. This created some tensions within the nursing staff since the other nurses' work was disrupted. Fay also expressed frustration that previous methods of relieving the patient weren't working. An impromptu conference followed wherein other nurses expressed frustration about their inability to relieve Mrs. Price's pain. They were also concerned about her unstable lupus status. Some nurses stated that they would prefer her having cancer to lupus—that cancer would be less uncertain. Fay was criticized by some nurses because she

Revised articulation and consequential disarticulation of ward work could not separate her personal from her professional involvement with Mrs. Price. Fay was chagrined. She thought maybe she shouldn't take care of Mrs. Price. The next day she decided not to be assigned to Mrs. Price, in part because she found it difficult to see Mrs. Price deteriorate, but also because she wished to avoid the criticism of other nurses.

That evening Mrs. Price developed abdominal pain. In the following eight days not only did the abdominal symptoms increase, but new symptoms developed. The cause of the increasing abdominal pain could not be found easily; the early tests were all negative. A number of possibilities were posed: bowel obstruction, extension of the lupus, reaction to the steroids, or reactions to narcotics. During this period she had an episode of sudden, sharp chest pains. An electrocardiograph was taken, but it showed no pathology. Then one night she could not be roused from sleep. The staff was concerned. Did this mean she was overmedicated with pain drugs and sedatives, or was it due to further brain involvement? An electroencephalogram was done the following day.

Additional articulation work is necessary (but SOP for diagnostic tasks)

During the first few days after the appearance of abdominal pain, the staff took a firm stand that the pain drugs would be continued with not deviation regardless of the patient's objection. There were occasional flurries between the patient and the staff over drug control. Drug orders were changed; a tranquilizer was changed when it was discovered that the particular tranquilizer predisposed her to tremors and seizures. After an inability to rouse the patient, the phenobarbital (sedative) was stopped: it was restarted when the husband pointed out that the phenobarbital was necessary to prevent seizures and the patient was fearful of seizures, having had a convulsion in the past. Because of the abdominal pain, all drugs were administered by injection. Mrs. Price had little appetite.

Reassertion of negotiated agreement

Revised articulation (but SOP)

SOP revision

On the eleventh day she became very nauseated. Continuous intravenous infusions

Added (SOP) articulated tasks

were started because she was developing fluid and electrolyte imbalances.

Potential minor disarticulation and its management

Some difficulty was encountered while attempting to get into a vein because her veins were poor from the numerous venipunctures done for blood tests during this and previous hospitalizations. After three attempts the patient refused any more attempts but was persuaded to cooperate further.

Added (SOP)

With her continued nausea the house staff decided that a gastric suction would relieve the discomfort.

Patient blocks

She objected because she had received this treatment in the past and could not tolerate the gagging and discomfort from the tube.

Added (SOP)

Antinausea drugs were therefore added to her drug list.

Patient disarticulates

She now began to balk about having any tests when her pains were at peak.

Novel and additional articulation

Whenever possible, the staff attempted to bring into alignment the uncomfortable tests and the pain drugs, but quite often this was difficult to arrange.

Added (SOP)

Dr. Ambrose, a gastrointestinal specialist, was next consulted. He suspected other possibilities, among them pancreatitis. The staff all realized that pancreatitis was extremely painful; however, Mrs. Price's pain drugs were not increased.

Added (SOP)

Further tests were ordered: barium x-rays and a gastric analysis. The physician also recommended gastric suction. An intern attempted to put down the nasogastric tube but was unsuccessful because the patient had a hypersensitive gag reflex. Finally Dr. Ambrose convinced her of the test's necessity.

Patient disarticulates

Three hours after the tube was inserted, Mrs. Price pulled it out because it caused her much discomfort and did not relieve the abdominal pain. She reasoned that if the suction did not relieve the pain there was little sense in tolerating the gagging sensation.

Revised

To accommodate the possibility of painful pancreatitis, extra pain drugs were ordered whenever an uncomfortable test was done. "Give 25 mg Demerol now and revert back to the routine schedule."

Added (SOP)

With the appearance of numerous new symptoms the nurses began monitoring Mrs.

Price's vital signs more closely. Thus, all stools were monitored. The nurses were disturbed by her continued deterioration.

During this period the sister's many visits partially helped her to endure her pain. In the researcher's encounters with the patient, she frequently talked about the problem of not knowing the cause of her pain and about the unexpected symptoms. The psychiatrist continued to visit her daily but was not interacting to any great extent with the nurses. He was also much involved with the patient's husband who was often the victim of Mrs. Price's irritability, and he was looking more and more tired and haggard.

Trajectory relationships

On the fourteenth day a definitive diagnosis was made: she had developed a huge gastric ulcer. Also, a chest x-ray showed broken ribs. Both were attributed to the steroids, [which] could not be stopped because the lupus would get out of control. Of course, everybody was terribly upset at this news. To some degree the nurses blamed the patient because she had not been very "cooperative" about taking the antacid routinely prescribed for patients on steroids in order to prevent gastric ulcers.

Blaming patient for sending trajectory off course

Her order for pain drugs now read: "Increase pain drugs. Addiction is not the priority now. Increased tension, irritability re pain drugs increases gastric irritability." The order was changed so that she was to get from 50 mg to 75 mg every three hours.

Revised (SOP)

The patient was both relieved and upset when told the cause of her pain; she realized that treatment would not be easy. To the researcher's comment that she tolerated pain relatively well for someone who supposedly had a low pain threshold she answered: "What else can I do? The only thing would be to jump out of the window, and I haven't quite considered that."

Her reaction to it

The definitive diagnosis of gastric ulcers and the broken ribs, particularly the ulcers, posed immense treatment problems. The medical choices were limited. Ulcers and broken ribs were the result of the steroids, yet

Trajectory developments leading to next articulation steps

the steroids were essential to control the lupus. In the patient's current physical state she was a poor surgical risk. Yet the size and the location of the ulcer, unless immediately treated, had dangerous consequences. Thus, there could be erosion of the ulcer into the peritoneal cavity or it might cause pancreatitis, both of which could be fatal, and at the least extremely painful. Indeed, this pain could be more painful than the ulcer pain.

Numerous specialists were consulted. After debating pro and con, the decision was made to radiate the stomach to knock out the acid-producing cells and so prevent further extension of the ulcer. The radiation dosage would be low so that other organs, particularly the kidneys, would not be compromised. Concurrently, hyperalimentation treatment (special intravenous feeding through a tube placed in the subclavian vein, located in the neck) would be started in order to overcome the malnutrition. The physicians explained to the patient the limited choices, why the treatments were necessary, and that the radiation dosage would be extremely low. Hence the probability of compromising the kidneys should also be low.

Added articulation of division of labor

Revised

Added (SOP)

Added sentimental work

Mrs. Price reluctantly agreed to the radiation treatment. She could not be convinced that her kidneys would not be affected by the radiation, a skepticism based on experiences of friends who had had radiation for cancer, and her awareness that lupus could also involve the kidneys. Explanations by her husband and other physicians that the radiation for cancer could not be compared to this situation and that there were no alternatives could not resolve her doubts. Her disbelief was also due in part to the fact that the radiology resident, unfamiliar with the patient's complex medical and social history, informed her that her kidneys might be affected by the treatment. Throughout the radiation treatment she wavered back and forth, wondering if agreeing to the radiation was a correct decision.

Decisional articulation

Mistake that disarticulates

After the first radiation treatment, she informed her husband that she did not want any more treatment because of possible damage to the kidneys. Her husband answered that this issue had been discussed many times, that there were no alternatives, and that the radiation dosage was very low. Mrs. Price continued to disagree. Finally her husband responded: "Stop being stubborn. We have to control the ulcers to stop the pain. If you want to commit suicide there are easier ways to do it. If we don't stop the ulcers you can have peritonitis or pancreatitis which are both very painful. There are lots of easier ways to commit suicide and I don't think you're ready for suicide." Mrs. Price agreed she was not ready for suicide. (It must be pointed out here that her husband was well regarded by the hospital staff and known as an extremely gentle and kind man.)

Decisional disarticulation

Husband keeps this segment of treatment going

Aside from the doubts about the radiation, Mrs. Price dreaded the treatment because of the physical movement required to get on and off the stretcher and the radiation table, which increased the chest pains. The nursing staff made arrangements with the radiology staff to pace the pain drugs with the treatments in order to minimize her pain.

Additional (ad hoc) articulation

Just prior to the radiation treatments her sister returned home, which meant that Mrs. Price had fewer distractions which might help her endure the pain. By the twentieth day she was on 75 mg of Demerol every two hours instead of the previous every three hours.

Revised

On the twentieth day there was a change in house staff. The researcher informed the new resident of some of the psychosocial problems relevant to the case. He answered that at present he was more concerned with the difficult technical medical problems. Meanwhile the nursing staff informed the new house staff about the extreme uncooperativeness of this patient.

Cuing in to minimize potential disarticulation

In the ensuing 12 days, her nausea increased and she had several days of diarrhea, all related to the radiation. She would fre-

Patient disarticulation

quently resist the treatment, either because she felt too ill or because she doubted the wisdom of the therapy. Some days she would be persuaded by the staff, but increasingly she resisted. Or she would agree that the treatment was essential in the morning, but change her mind in the afternoon. The staff was becoming increasingly annoyed with the resistance. Finally, in desperation they gave her intravenous tranquilizers just prior to the test to make her very sleepy and less resistant. The resident and the intern took the stand that they could not put up with the patient's constant refusal of treatment—that the patient must either cooperate with the therapy or go home. The hospital was a place for treatment and not a nursing home. The nurses supported this position.

Novel articulation

Over the weeks innumerable specialists streamed in and out with no one person coordinating the patient's care. Dr. Osgood, the new resident, argued to the attending physicians that the complexity of this case required some agreement about who should be the major coordinator of care. Since the house staff was more aware of the day-to-day changes, and because the ulcers were the major problem, a decision was reached: the house staff and the gastrointestinal specialist would together be the major coordinators of care, and all new orders issued by the attending staff would be discussed first with the house staff. The nursing staff sighed in relief because at last the "mess" would be under control. However, the coordination continued to break down from time to time. When the patient could not get satisfaction from the house staff she would telephone attending physicians, crying pitifully. One physician in particular would telephone the nursing desk with orders based on his past experiences with the patient. This created much tension within the medical staff.

Potential disarticulation condition
Rearticulation

Rearticulation

Disarticulation conditions

Disarticulation

Blood studies indicated a low hemoglobin count as a result of the ulcers, as well as the lupus, so that blood transfusion was now done. Again hassles occurred between the patient and the house staff about both the timing

Added (SOP) but patient disarticulation

of treatment and the inflicted pain. (It must be noted that both the resident and intern were very competent and usually related well with Mrs. Price; Mrs. Price trusted them.)

Condition for potential disarticulation

During the period when the radiation treatments were given, the nursing staff was very busy with several othe critically ill patients. Also the staff was short because several members, including Fay, were on vacation. At the same time, with the hyperalimentation treatment given to Mrs. Price and the potential of many of her body systems going out of balance, the nursing staff had to engage in many treatment and monitoring tasks. The nurses were interacting more and more with her because of these tasks and when they were giving pain drugs. They were also becoming very weary of the daily hassles over the treatments.

Added (SOP)

On the twenty-seventh day the patient developed tremors of the hands and legs. Of course, she became very anxious since this was seen as a possible forerunner to convulsions, but because of her great anxiety the staff had difficulty making an assessment of her actual condition. The staff took the stance of "wait and see." The patient thought immediate action was called for. Again she phoned an attending physician who ordered drugs without consulting the house staff. The tremors did subside a few days later.

Disarticulation

Because of continued nausea, all drugs were administered by injections, which required some 30 injections a day. The injection sites were becoming fibrous knots so that the drugs were not being properly absorbed. The nurses were very concerned not only about the poor drug absorption but also about the possibility of infections because of the high steroid dose.

Revised (SOP)

On the thirtieth day the patient developed joint pains and swelling of her hands, elbows, feet, and knees—all symptoms of lupus. The steroids were adjusted. Fortunately in a few days the symptoms subsided.

Revised (SOP)

With each new symptom Mrs. Price became increasingly discouraged. From time to time she would tell the researcher that she

Trajectory relationships evolving

recognized she had a reputation for being uncooperative. She knew the staff was busy and all departments had their schedules, but: "There's only so much pain I can stand."

Early on the thirty-second day, the last day of the radiation treatments, she was exhausted from her cumulative pain and discomfort—chest pain, abdominal pain, nausea, and joint pains—and begged her husband to delay the treatment until another day. The husband acted according to medical protocol—he consulted the radiologist, asking if this was possible. The radiologist could predict no ill effects if the treatment were postponed. Although instructed to inform the house staff about all this, the radiologist forgot to do so. Hence, when the nurses called the radiation department saying that the patient was premedicated as arranged, they were informed that the treatment had been cancelled at the husband's request. The radiology technicians, of course, did not know the full or correct details. Consequently, the house staff and the nurses became very irritated, interpreting all this as meddling by the husband. The staff members—having had daily hassles about the treatment—complained that if she didn't have the treatment that day they would have to repeat the hassle tomorrow. The decision was made that Mrs. Price was to receive the radiation treatment. Intravenous tranquilizer was given to overcome her resistance to the procedure. Everybody sighed in relief when this last treatment was finally completed!

Potential disarticulation

Disarticulation

Coercive rearticulation

In chatting soon afterward with the researcher, the husband [a physician] stated he was trying very hard not to interfere with the therapy. The psychiatrist's advice—that he "act the husband and not the doctor"—was very helpful. However, this was often difficult because his wife constantly confronted him with medical questions.

On the thirty-third day the patient developed burning during urination and began to run a low-grade fever. More tests were ordered. The test results were not definitive, and the symptoms subsided in a few days. In

Added (SOP)

spite of the new symptoms, the patient was in a better frame of mind, if only from the relief of having completed the radiation treatments. She has less nausea and she complained less about pain. Food taken by mouth was now possible.

On the thirty-fifth day a staff conference (which included the psychiatrist, house staff, and nursing staff) was called. The conference was to decide the course of therapy and clarify the situation, so that the new house staff, due the following week, would avoid some of the "coordination" problems. The psychiatrist sketched the psychosocial background of the patient, and the resident responded that he wished he had known about this before. Decisions were reached. Now that the radiation series was completed, and the hyperalimentation treatment had controlled the nitrogen imbalance (patient had gained 20 pounds), and because she was now taking food by mouth, they would discontinue the hyperalimentation treatment. They agreed that there was a risk of infection with continued hyperalimentation. Medically, the patient now was fairly stable. They did not think they should try any more "heroics." It was now up to the patient to eat. They would do not more forced feeding. They were optimistic that the radiation would have its anticipated effects. An x-ray would be done within the week to check the effects of the radiation. Since the patient was now in a relatively stable medical state, the psychiatrist would be responsible for weaning her from the narcotic drug. There was considerable speculation about the possibility that the patient would try to starve herself. Physiotherapy would be started so the patient would begin to regain strength. Both the psychiatrist and the resident would inform the patient about the decisions. The house staff and the nurses agreed that the hospital was an "acute-care treatment center," a place of treatment and not a convalescent hospital.

Attempts to minimize potential disarticulation

Revised (SOP)

Articulated division of labor

Revised (SOP)

The staff took an optimistic stance, anticipating that the patient would be going home. She was placed on oral drugs, except for the

Revised (SOP)

pain drugs. The psychiatrist attempted to lower the dosage of the latter but met with little success. Everybody anxiously awaited the results of the stomach x-ray scheduled within a week.

Trajectory developments

For a few days after the patient began to take food by mouth, she had diarrhea. The staff thought this might be a reaction to the sudden intake of food after three weeks of nothing taken by mouth. In spite of the diarrhea, the patient attempted to eat. Eating was not easy because sometimes the pacing of drugs and tranquilizers was such that she was too sleepy and groggy at the scheduled meal times. For two days prior to the day the x-ray results were known, she was relatively pain free; that is, she complained less about pain even though the drugs were not delivered on schedule. The staff talked about the patient going home. Meanwhile, the patient was informing the researcher that she didn't think the ulcers were healing because her pain had not decreased.

Blaming patient for disarticulation

On the forty-first day the x-rays showed no decrease in the ulcer's size. There was much troubled discussion among the staff. The patient was blamed for her uncooperativeness in taking the antacids and for her chain smoking, which had increased the gastric secretions. The patient, of course, was upset. With great irony she remarked to the researcher: "I knew all along the radiation wouldn't work. All I probably got out of the radiation is kidney damage."

Revised (novel)

During the next days there was a great deal of discussion about the next course of treatment. A decision was reached that the only alternative was a subtotal or total gastric resection. There were, of course, surgical risks and unpleasant consequences from having no stomach, but without intervention there would be the danger of peritonitis or pancreatitis and hemorrhage. The decision was to wait another week or so, at which time a gastroscopy test and an x-ray would be done for reevaluation. The general estimate was that with the surgery the patient might live for several more years. She was informed of the recommendation. The staff realized that her decision to accept surgery would be a difficult one.

Trajectory developments

For the next three weeks, she agonized over whether or not to have surgery. Her husband was of the opinion that it was the only alternative. The psychiatrist thought the patient, if discharged home, would "drive the husband crazy," and that she would not consent to a nursing home. So surgery, they reasoned, should be done.

Revised (SOP)

Added (novel)

Because of the danger of addiction, Mrs. Price's tranquilizers were increased instead of the narcotics. Also, the narcotics had made her groggy, which meant she often fell asleep with a lighted cigarette. Because of a shortage of staff on the night shift, a sitter was hired to watch the patient so she would not burn herself. Mrs. Price told the researcher that she shouldn't smoke, that it aggravated her chronic obstructive lung disease and pleuritis. But she had given up so much in the past year, and had so few pleasures, that she was going to continue to smoke. She didn't have long to live, so what difference did it make?

Trajectory relations continue to evolve

In the ensuing days there were more confrontations between patient and staff about increasing her drugs. The staff's and husband's explanations that she would become dangerously addicted only infuriated her. "What difference does it make?" she would angrily answer. (It must be pointed out here that Mrs. Price never lost her polite social manners: she would thank staff members for small favors and was polite in making requests.

Novel (sentimental work)

The patient increasingly talked to the researcher about the frustrations of living with uncertainty, and her wish that she could die. She said the same things to her husband and the psychiatrist. All three wondered how seriously she wanted to die. Although the psychiatrist and the researcher encouraged the patient to talk about wanting to die, she could not pursue this line of talk beyond a certain point.

The psychiatrist, husband, and researcher were having more and more discussions among themselves about her sad dilemma and how to help her. She did not burden the nurses with her dismal thoughts. The researcher spent more and more time with her and less with the staff. The staff had difficulty in talking about as well as interacting with Mrs. Price.

Disarticulation of staff sentimental work

On the fiftieth day a great qualitative change in the patient's mood was noted. She was very subdued and talked at length about what her illness was doing to her husband and herself and of her ambivalence about dying. She commented: "I wish I could tolerate pain better." Both her husband and the psychiatrist were very pleased that for the first time she could talk openly of her anxieties about dying. When the researcher asked the nurses if they noted any mood change in Mrs. Price, they said "no."

Trajectory relationships evolving

It is worth noting here that during the early days of the hospitalization, when the patient would resist treatments, the nurses would have troubled discussions about the ethics of euthanasia. At one point, having difficulty in persuading the patient to take the gastric suction, one nurse had commented: "I know it's the right of the patient to take or not take treatment. And the patient has the right to make the decision to live or not live. But where is it the patient's and staff's responsibility?" The nurse became very teary. This type of troubled discussion was a frequent occurrence throughout the patient's hospitalization.

Trajectory accompaniments

On the fifty-fourth day a gastroscopy showed continued acid secretions. For 24 hours following the gastroscopy the Demerol was increased from 75 to 100 mg but was later reduced to 75 mg.

Revised (SOP)

For the next four days the patient wavered back and forth on whether to have the gastric surgery; it was becoming more evident that the surgery was required. Mrs. Price frequently stated that she had been saved from death two times, and she didn't know if she wanted to be saved agin. She would take her chances with no surgery, and so hemorrhage and die. She was weary of all the uncertainty. In the past year the lupus remission had been very short. In periods when she did not have pain she would talk less of wanting to die; in periods of increased pain [she] would talk more about wanting to die. At times she would ask the researcher to chat about "something nice, to get my mind off myself."

> Sentimental work articulation

Now she was eating less, in part because meal times did not coincide with the pacing of the drugs. The tranquilizers were altered so she would be less sleepy. The staff members were becoming concerned with her continued weight loss. They wondered if she was trying to starve to death. Her eating and not eating alternated, depending upon her nausea, pain, and mood. The intern wrote an order to start the hyperalimentation treatment again, but it was canceled. This was due in part to the staff's earlier decision that they would not force-feed her and in part to the infection risks; also the husband threatened that if she didn't eat they would start the hyperalimentation. She decided to eat rather than suffer the discomforts and general nuisance associated with the treatment. Because she had difficulty being alert enough to eat or had pain at the scheduled meal times, she was ordering foods like sandwiches when allowed greater temporal flexibility than hot foods. This meant she was eating at odd hours: 10 P.M. or 2 A.M., for example.

> Revised (SOP)
>
> Disarticulation
>
> Rearticulation
>
> Patient articulation

She was talking more about wanting to commit suicide. Often the discussion was wistful and flavored with fantasy. The psychiatrist consulted a suicide expert, who stated that the probability of this patient's seriously considering suicide was low. Still, the staff could not dismiss this possibility. As a precaution, her clothes were taken home and money and drugs were removed from her purse, because she was talking about taking a taxi and jumping of the bridge. The psychiatrist requested

> Novel articulation
>
> Added sentimental work

that the nursing staff make closer observations and record them. Fay was now back from vacation and was assigned more frequently to Mrs. Price. With the exception of Fay, the observations made of Mrs. Price were quite sparse. Fay spent much time talking to the researcher about her frustrations in managing Mrs. Price. Other nurses did not want to talk about Mrs. Price. For example, during coffee break Fay began a discussion with the researcher about Mrs. Price; the nurses requested that we discuss Mrs. Price elsewhere. They were on a coffee break and wanted some peace.

Added articulation

On the sixty-seventh day the x-rays showed an increase in the size of the ulcers. There was total agreement among the physicians, including the psychiatrist, that a gastrectomy was required and this should occur while the lupus was stable. Two days earlier, the lupus specialist had discussed with Mrs. Price the possibility of trying new drugs to reduce the steroids. Mrs. Price was positive about this possibility.

Decisional disarticulation

For the next seven days she agonized over the decision to have a gastrectomy. The surgeons, husband, and psychiatrist tried to answer as best they could any questions she might have. Mrs. Price consulted other attending physicians. They all agreed that a gastrectomy was essential. Her husband was looking tired and haggard. A relative visited in this period and persuaded her that surgery would be the only solution. She finally signed the consent slip for surgery. But, having signed, she wavered until the very last minute. She was transferred to a gastrointestinal surgical unit.

Sentimental work rearticulation

Added (SOP *and* novel)

Our account of the hospital episode will stop here. The surgery was successful, and the patient was weaned from the hard drugs, but not without considerable interactional difficulties between staff and patient. Indeed, the surgical-pain trajectory orientation of the staff maximized the interactional difficulties. On the one hundred twelfth day, she was discharged home.

Analytic Summary of Case

As noted in introducing this case, coordination of care is a central issue when managing and shaping cumulative mess trajectories. The simplest component of rearticulation, which is a continual necessity, consists of decisions to *revise* protocols (drug dosages mainly) or to take *additional* action (mainly tests and precedures, but also surgery)—"simplest" because they depend on SOP. Staff then takes familiar action, draws on usual resources, and follows established forms of making arrangements with servicing departments. The *novel* arrangements, however, rest on ad hoc conferences, much negotiation and persuasion among the staff—even between staff or husband and the patient—calling in consultants, dovetailing the division of labor of a psychiatrist or the special personnel (the sitter who will watch over potential fire hazards from the patient's smoking), and setting up unusual articulating actions.

Revisions in physicians' orders and the derived protocols (mainly changes in the medications) are called for mainly because of reassessments of new developments (positive or negative) in the course of the illness, although some revisions are precipitated by the patient's actions. Additional tasks are called forth by other kinds of illness developments, which are conceived as necessitating further diagnostic tests and treatments not originally envisioned. Each of those diagnostic and treatment tasks require further articulation into the ongoing stream of staff work. Novel arrangements are called forth when the trajectory work is percieved as drastically out of whack, when staff believe they must seriously reconsider their articulation strategies. Often the staff is, at this point, upset or highly annoyed or even desperate over how disarticulated the coordination of care has become. Unlike the revision or the addition of tasks, novel arrangements are designed to rearticulate the disarray in the trajectory work. Over the staff's novel work of rearticulation there hangs the dust of battle—battle with the patient but frequently also among the staff members as they debate what to do next.

The patient also engages in novel work (usually regarded as improper by the staff) designed to get things done as the patient believes they should be done: that is, first to *disarticulate* the ongoing work patterns so as to rearticulate them in a more appropriate fashion. It is precisely the patient's rearticulation work that most disrupts the staff's plans and operations. However, the patient's spontaneous refusals to undergo or continue with specific procedures or drug dosages will also temporarily disarticulate the procedures or operational tasks that seemed otherwise to be under no particular threat. Repeated disarticulation of this kind ("hassles") leads to staff's annoyance, disruption of their flow of work, and if it continues long enough will result in the staff's withdrawal or other consequences negative to their work and their medical and nursing care of the given patient.

All of this *rearticulation* work involves not merely revised, added, and novel medical, nursing, and technical tasks, but also tasks pertaining *to the other types of work* discussed in previous chapters, namely, machine, clinical safety, comfort, and sentimental work. So analytically one must take into account a very complicated interweaving of several modes of work, and their implicated tasks, when thinking about trajectory articulation. This can be true even for relatively standard, easily managed trajectories; it is all the more true—and striking—of more complicated trajectories, of which the cumulative mess ones are perhaps the most dramatic instances.

This type of trajectory illustrates at least two further important points bearing on the complexities and difficulties of articulation work when trajectories go awry. First, as the trajectory evolves, the work appears to become increasingly complicated and so more difficult to articulate. New tasks are required in fairly rapid succession, not only because of revisions but because of additions. Usually the latter come in clusters. They are quickly accomplished, but some may require repetition over many days. Both additional and revised tasks may require doing simultaneously or in quick sequence, adding to the clustering of new tasks to be done. Sometimes the rate of revision or addition is fairly rapid, further burdening the overall task structure.

The second point is related to the staff's heightened feeling that they have lost control over the evolving trajectory. Their experience is like that of the small boy whose rubber ball had a soft dimple, which when he poked it vanished but then appeared in another spot, and so on and on. Mrs. Price's symptoms may vanish only to appear again, or different kinds of symptoms appear, or more of them appear. The staff's query, "How can we get this illness under control?" gradually gets transformed into the increasingly weary and desperate "Will we ever get this illness under control?" Part of the staff's response is certainly related not just to loss of control over the illness itself but their inability to keep coordinated even the associated medical and nursing work, what with all the tests, treatments, consultants streaming in and out, Mrs. Price's minor and major interferences with their medical and nursing plans, and the obvious disintegration of interactional and work relationships with her. As the trajectory moves inexorably along, a complex tissue of interlocking events adds up to a downward spiraling of staff mood, morale, and staff-patient interaction, which in turn reduces the amount and effectiveness of sentimental and even comfort work offered to the patient.

All of that contributes, too, to the personnel's sense that the coordination of their work—their care of the patient—has been shattered. Their sense of the disintegration of coordination is, of course, different from what may have actually occurred. Our observation of cumulative mess trajectories, and of others somewhat less problematic, is that the staff members are working so persistently and hard at maintaining and reestablishing the articulation of their work that they believe eventually their coordinative control has slipped away. Yet we note also that precisely because the medical, comfort, and sentimental work are so closely entwined, articulation, in fact, does become cumulatively more difficult. In turn it negatively affects both individuals' moods and collective morale (the "sentimental order" of the ward). Then, this in turn cumulatively influences staff members' ability to keep the trajectory work effectively articulated.

It is not unusual for that downward cycle to be broken by a literal disappearance of the patient from the ward: through an operation which takes him or her to another ward, through placement in a nursing home, or through death. Such patients (whom we call "patients of the year" because they so dramatically stand out for the staff for so long) are remembered for many months. A principal feature of that memory is, to summarize the staff's feeling, "what a mess things were during that time."

Safety Articulation Work

To fill out the foregoing general picture—to give more conceptual density to the analysis of articulation work—we turn next to look at both the difficulties (which are many) and the mechanics of articulating clinical safety work with the usual run of patients in the hospital. We shall build here on readers' memories of the extended discussion in chapter 4. Also we choose to discuss the articulation of safety work because that work is almost always within concentrated focus of hospital staffs, is of such great moment for patients, and is such a complex business for everybody including the patients.

The safe management of a patient's trajectory ultimately rests on the alignment of numerous subtypes of clinical safety work. The extent to which those can be articulated depends on the degree to which various dangers and risks associated with the trajectory phases and miniphases can be mapped out and anticipated. This determines the extent to which the required total arc of work, including the bundles of implicated tasks, can be coordinated. Safety articulation work can thus be conceptualized as an effort to rationalize the work of maximizing clinical safety.

Sources of Disarticulation

The difficulties encountered in this articulation are embedded in the nature of hazard in medical work, which results in much overlapping of safety work among various kinds and levels of workers. As noted in chapter 4, the dangers and risks can come from multiple sources: from the patient, both as a disrupted physical body system and as a person, from varieties of clinical interventions, from the personnel, and from the environment. These sources of hazard are highly interactive, so that an increased hazard deriving from one source can affect many others. Of course, attempts are made to rationalize the safety work and its articulation, as by the environmental safety engineers attempting to manage and control the environmental hazards and the various technicians attempting to control and manage those arising from the use of machinery. However, because the sources are very likely to affect each other as well as the patient, there necessarily is much overlapping of safety work, as done by the personnel and the patient, too. All of that presents them with problems of articulation.

Work

The subtypes of safety work include: *preventing, assessing, monitoring*, and *rectifying* dangers and risks. These overlap at several levels of work, involving: (1) the overall trajectory (arc of work), (2) the managerial and organizational work, and (3) the various implicated tasks. A peculiar property of the subtypes of safety work is that they are inextricably linked. Misassessing a danger or a risk can result in a staff member's mismonitoring, mispreventing, and misrectifying. And one subtype of work may dominate during different phases of a trajectory, but the others are always integral to the total safety work. Then, too, at each of the levels of this work, multiple kinds of hazards are sequentially and/or simultaneously being assessed, monitored, prevented, and rectified. Some of those may be carried out by a single person; others require different types of workers. This articulation work, then, involves the linking and ordering not only of the work types, but of the various kinds and levels of personnel. So, whenever there is disruption of the preventing, monitoring, assessing, and rectifying, then rearticulation of kinds and levels of worker is likely to be involved. Also, the extent to which disarticulation can be effectively rearticulated depends not only on the degree to which hazards can be anticipated—during the various phases and miniphases of the trajectory—but also on the degree of hazard, plus the associated numbers and levels of resources required to rearticulate the disturbed arc of work.

Illustration: Pre- and Postoperative Surgical Phases

To illustrate this complex interaction, we shall discuss the work of preventing and handling respiratory infections, which patients undergoing certain types of surgery are very likely to get unless carefully "managed." During the preoperative phase, the prevention of potential respiratory infection—among many other potential but preventable risks—is a major responsibility of the attending nurses. This risk-prevention work is recognized by other personnel as directly in the nurses' province. The work involves helping and encouraging patients to cough up phlegm and to take deep breaths at periodic intervals. These tasks are relatively simple and straightforward. Indeed, much of this prevention work can be done by patients themselves.

So what is there to articulate in these uncomplicated tasks? Although the work is simple, patients often find it difficult because taking deep breaths, particularly when combined with coughing up phlegm—and most of all when abdominal or chest surgery has been done—can be quite painful. This means that to carry out the prevention tasks, it is necessary to coordinate those with the comfort tasks (see chap. 5 for comfort work): that is, to schedule the former at a time when the postoperative pain is not at its peak. Since the patient's cooperation is essential, a set of information tasks concerning the potential risk of respiratory infection is explained to the patient during the preoperative phase. Patients are informed that although the tasks are likely to be uncomfortable for them, it is extremely necessary to carry them out. They are also shown how to do the tasks and taught about the measures to be taken later for the control of pain. Therefore, the staff generally believes that the pre-, rather than the post-, operative phase is the more appropriate time for "teaching the patient" since in the later phase the patient is often less able to absorb the information because then he or she will be heavily medicated and they physical status will be lower. In the process of preventing respiratory infection, a nurse must assess the patient's potential for developing those infections: the criteria will include age, types of surgery, and general cardiovascular status. These assessments will determine how frequently and vigorously the tasks of prevention are carried out. Moreover, monitoring specific signs and symptoms is done to determine whether the current prevention tasks need to be altered.

Compared with other kinds of articulation of safety work, that done during the preoperative phase of surgery is not ordinarily considered especially complicated. However, the safety work then can be readily disrupted. Why? First of all, diverse kinds of contingency may disrupt the work order all along the course of the trajectory. Quite often the exchange of information with a patient can be omitted, because it is forgotten by the responsible nurse under the pressures of other tasks, or the surgery may be an emergency and there is little time to do it, or the patient may not be mentally alert because of his or her illness. Consequently, this omission of tasks may result in great resistance being offered later by the patient to doing coughing and deep breathing. Second, as noted earlier, prevention work is linked with comfort work, especially that of dealing with pain. Thus, disruptions in pain assessing, monitoring, and preventing can disarticulate the safety tasks. Unexpected pain-medication allergies can also occur, including nausea and vomiting. They can also disrupt fluid and electrolyte balance, which then requires being assessed, monitored, prevented, and if necessary rectified. Moreover, the physician's assessment of pain may be off the mark and so the prescribed medication may fail to control the pain. In other words, the comfort and safety work involves overlapping levels of work—the physician's, the nurse's (several of them), and probably the patient's, too. Rectifying the rearticulating the comfort-safety work will require exchange of information among all three. If the patient cannot be persuaded to do the prevention tasks and also has a past medical history indicating a predisposition to respiratory infection, then both medication and a respiratory machine will be used to loosen the plhegm. This latter work then calls for the articulation of the respiratory therapist's tasks with the nurses' pain tasks. The therapist has safety jobs to do with regard to the machine and also with respect to the patient's care, and some of the therapist's work also overlaps with that of the nurses. Hence, machine failure calls for still other types of rearticulation. And if the patient does indeed develop a respiratory infection, then the physician must reassess and alter the trajectory scheme. That, again, affects the alignment of safety work at the task level. Moreover, another characteristic of safety management is the constant ebb and flow of disrupted safety work. Safety priorities are constantly shifting. Therefore, for any given group of patients on the ward when there is a religning of work for one particular patient, this will bring out a realigning of work with other patients.

Effective articulation work then rests not only on being able to anticipate how various subtypes of safety work interact, but also how a given hazard or goup of hazards may increase over time. Usually safety work is organized around degrees and phases of appearance of hazard: (1) might go wrong, (2) going wrong, and (3) gone wrong. At each of these phases, or with each degree of hazard, the kinds of safety tasks will vary. More often than not, as degree of hazard increases, larger numbers of different kinds and levels of workers are involved. In consequence, the chances for disarticulation of safety work will increase. To make matters still more complicated, recollect also that the staff can vary widely in how they assess dangers and risks and how they balance them. Remember, too, that the new technologies that are constantly being introduced make the articulation of safety work more problematic. With the changing technology, new workers are introduced, and it takes time to determine where their tasks overlap with those of the traditional workers and what the limits of their task jurisdictions should be. All in all, safety articulation presents to the personnel and patients—and to us as reasearchers also—an immensely complicated picture. So how does the articulation ever get done? For, of course, it does.

Articulation Strategies

Despite all the sources of disruption a majority of patients leave the hospital in a less hazardous physical state than when they entered. Of course, many complain of disarticulated care, and yet most of their angry stories pertain to comfort and identity, stories often categorized as reflecting depersonalized care. (The reasons for their complaints will be addressed later.) An overriding premise that fosters the articulation of safety work is this: clinical safety has priority, one shared by large sectors of the personnel, since hospitals are primarily organized around handling acute phases of illness.

It is true that clinical safety may conflict with legal and financial risk and with the patient's comfort and identity sensitiveness or it may negatively influence staff's identities and their interaction, which in turn can contribute to disarticulation of the safety work. Concern for clinical safety, however, assures that when comfort or identity safety tasks are important for getting the medical jobs done, then (as remarked in chap. 4) they tend to get built into the task structure. On the other hand, when such tasks are not perceived as directly relevant to the patient's trajectory, then they may be neglected.

Related to this dominant concern for clinical safety is the fact that, by and large, the personnel tend to subordinate financial concerns and concerns about their own identities. This is especially true when major clinical hazards are involved. Staff who place their own personal concerns over clinical safety, thereby endangering the patient's clinical status, are severely criticized on moral grounds. Indeed clinical, along with legal, safety is a powerful leverage in fostering articulations through explicit accountability. For instance, when ICU nurses were unable to articulate safety work adequately because of old cardiac monitors frequently breaking down—not being replaced because of financial reasons—they were able to negotiate successfully for new monitors only by using the combined leverage of clinical safety and legal risk. In their argument for new monitors, they listed the clinical risks, which they linked with potential legal ones, as well as time and money lost in repairs, and only at the bottom of the list their own lowered staff morale. Or again, a physician on a committee for allocating hospital resources remarked that he was troubled by the demands of the respiratory therapy department. However, loath to pursue this both becasue he did not understand the technical issues involved and because he recognized this department dealt with life-saving machines, he voted in their support so as to avoid potentially major clinical hazards.

Tied in with clinical safety then is a concerted effort to articulate those tasks related to assessing, monitoring, preventing, and rectifying major hazards. Work associated with anticipated ones, and their potential complications, are articulated through explicit accountability. Thus, clinical safety is usually assured. But in the process, comfort and identity impact may be quite negative. Patients may be angry at this failure but often will forgive the staff because safety is also their own priority. Interpersonal incompetence is forgivable, providing staff is clinically competent; but clinical incompetence is not forgivable.

Process of Safety Articulation

The safety articulation is constantly changing because of the new technologies and trajectories, for those require assessment and management of their associated and still unexplored hazards. Thus, some aspects of safety work are well articulated while others are less so. In the early phases of a new technology or trajectory, there is concerted effort to identify the major and minor hazards—their safety limits, the criteria for preventing, assessing, monitoring, rectifying those hazards, and the necessary materials and skills to do the safety jobs. Since the probability of unexpected hazard is high, great attention generally is paid to safety details. Through experience, trial, and error, eventually the requisite knowledge piles up, so that during the later phases fewer major hazards need to be rectified. Attention now can be directed to better control of minor hazards. Eventually the necessary resources and various tasks become rather precisely identified and articulated into a clear task structure. Many of the tasks become routinized, while organizational articulation becomes standardized. Safety checklists and precise procedures covering task sequences are developed and thereafter teaching can be done. Programmed tasks concerning safety information for patients and programmed tasks for teaching the staff become articulated. Clinical hazards usually get first priority. When these become controlled, then risks to the patient's identity get identified and the corresponding work gets articulated with the major safety work.

Some hazards may eventually be discovered to be widely distributed throughout the hospital. Then organizational arrangements are instituted for handling them, such as infectious disease control, or product evaluation for assuring safety in equipment purchase, or forming various types of crisis teams for handling major hazards.

When articulation is particularly complicated, as when several departments are involved, then a special intradepartmental articulator (liaison position) is appointed. Frequently this occurs as a consequence of either formal or ad hoc committees being brought together to study particular safety problems. Indeed, the latter are very frequently found in acute-care hospitals today.

Aside from the special articulators, every staff person is more or less an articulator. The range of what they coordinate may be narrow or wide and may be an implicit or explicit part of their work. But the fact that the preventing, assessing, monitoring, and rectifying of hazards actually overlap both as processes and across levels of workers means that, somehow, major disarticulations get noted and then rearticulated. As mentioned earlier in this chapter, head nurses are key articulators because they know the immediate resource requirements and how to align them. That articulation work is assisted by ward secretaries, unit managers, and the like. As in any work place, there are persons who are important "trouble shooters." They are essentially rearticulators of disarticulated safety tasks. The work is sometimes shared, sometimes specifically assigned. Patients and kin are, of course, important articulators, too. They are instructed to apprise the staff of specific signs and symptoms, but aside from that they are watchdogs of suspected or perceived disarticulated work. Indeed much of their effort to get staff's attention is really an effort to rearticulate work which they have defined as something gone wrong. Quite often, of course, that behavior may be defined by staff members as demanding or complaining.

Currently, under the rubric of quality control, efforts are being made to delineate criteria and work arrangements for assuring maximum safety. This concern cuts across efforts to standardize and rationalize safety work for specific kinds of diseases and hazards, as well as efforts to match resources to hazards at different work sites, and so on.

Informational articulation is also a major type of safety work. Part of this is highly routinized, like the reporting of accomplished work from shift to shift. Each may even tape information, a practice that is becoming rapidly accepted in many large hospitals. Charts always accompany patients as they move from one part of the hospital to another. The key kinds of hazard information which must be transmitted within the team are taught. As hazards become controlled, special recording forms are developed so that key observations and measures can be monitored. In fact, such forms are proliferating, even to the extent that standing committees evaluate and standardize the forms. Of course, the legal risk of improper transmission and recording of information is an incentive to accurate record keeping and transmission of information.

Some safety tasks are common to many clinical procedures, and some hazards are common to many trajectories; hence, there exist industries which produce multitudes of standardized informational labels for alerting staff to safety tasks that help to avoid safety disarticulation (see chap. 4). These are plastered on charts and beds and are easily seen.

Personnel are fully aware that clinical safety work can be all too easily disarticulated; thus, there is an effort to standardize and rationalize it as best they can. This is accomplished by a constant process of negotiating which involes amany levels of workers. (This negotiation will be discussed shortly.)

Despite the standardization and rationalization of the work, there is always a danger that even the SOP can become disarticulated. Indeed, many disarticulations occur because the work is standardized. Thus, a paradox can arise: attempts to control major hazards are so strong that the staff does an excellent job of coordinating safety work (like the extensive informational work done with cardiac surgical patients), whereas someone who comes to the ward for run-of-the-mill surgery may have some safety tasks overlooked.

Insider-Outsider Articulation

Safety also depends on companies that produce the technologies, which in turn are influenced by numerous regulatory agencies, which in turn affect hospitals. Hence, the disarticulation of safety work that occurs within any of them, or among them, can contribute to disarticulation of safety work in the hospital. Here again, work external to the hospital rests on the central safety processes (preventing, assessing, etc.).

Finally, a major disarticulation problem also occurs when patients move from hospital to home or from home back into the hospital. Much has been written about the poor coordination of care. A central problem flows from the acute-care orientation of the professionals, who generally do well at articulation during acute phases of illness, but who generally are not well equipped to articulate trajectory concerns when identity and safety are so intricately intertwined during the less acute phases. That is what the anger around depersonalization is mostly about.

The Importance of Negotiation and Persuasion for Articulation

We wish now to put special emphasis on those ranges of action that lie outside of standard procedures for getting the trajectory tasks done. Under the conditions—so frequently found in hospital work—where SOP cannot be drawn upon, where tasks and their coordination are not easily routinized, then other kinds of action are needed to fill the gap between medical purposes and their fulfillment. Into that gap, as indicated obliquely throughout this chapter (and others, too), the personnel will move, seeking to maximize the articulation of their work. Their attempts may eventually be perceived by them as requiring coercive threats or even commands backed by authority. But those tactics usually are used in extremis, as last-ditch articulation mechanisms. Ordinarily the personnel, at every level, resort first to discussion. They talk things over trying to reach reasonable gounds for action. Or they work at persuading each other to their viewpoints of what such action might be. Or they negotiate differences between themselves which derive from positional or ideological dissonance.

Earlier in this chapter, we laid the groundwork for understanding why trajectory work could not be rationalized as easily as, say, industrial production. The structural considerations outlined there bear rather obviously on what is predominantly the negotiated order, which characterizes the hospital as an organization (Strauss et al. 1964*a*, Strauss 1978*a*). Negotiation, persuasion, discussion, and teaching are the dominant modes of attaining maximum articulation because of —to put it succinctly—the problematic character of the trajectories themselves and the host of technological, organizational, and client-derived contingencies that beset all those who are doing the trajectory work.

Of course, different actors in the drama possess quite different degrees of skill, sagacity, influence, and situational or positional power for affecting the evolution of the trajectory work. Yet that work could scarcely get done if one or more of the less institutionalizes modes of articulation were not resorted to by the personnel, by the patient, or by the kin.

Apropos of these less formalized, institutionalized, and perhaps less immediately visible modes of action, two sociologists, Peter and Dee-Ann Spencer Hall (1982), have offered some hypotheses about negotiation based on a comparison of our research on psychiatric hospitals (Strauss et al. 1964*b*) and their own intensive study of two schools. They suggest that: (1) an expanding and growing organization will evince more negotiation than one that is declining; (2) a successful one will show more negotiation than a failing one; (3) activities that are routinized, standardized, show less negotiation than activities that are variable, individualized, publicly performed, and involve teamwork; (4) the greater the size and complexity of the organization, the greater the degree of negotiation; (5) equality and wide dispersion of power are conducive to negotiations; (7) a system undergoing proposed or planned change will show more negotiation than one tending toward tradition; (8) and an organization whose leadership delegates authority, tolerates individuality and development of semi-autonomous programs, favors compromise over confrontation, and defines itself as a mediator will show more negotiation than one that centralizes authority, stifles creativity and development, prefers domination or conflict. These hypotheses certainly fit the complex and fast-changing character of American hospitals (or various of their departments). (See also for business firms, Burns and Stalker 1961, and for scientific laboratories, Latour and Woolgar 1979.)

As we have noted, actual negotiation is supplemented by discussion, teaching, and persuasion (even by actual coercion and coercive threat), and to that one must add the manipulation of people and elements of institutional structure. In a general sense, we would term all that the negotiated order of the hospital. Without it the trajectory work would never be accomplished, the effective articulation of that work would be impossible, and the hospital as a working institution would simply grind to a halt (see also the discussion of negotiative work in chap. 10).

8
The Work of Patients

All of the types of work discussed in the preceding chapters are also engaged in by patients. They have been seen working to insure their own comfort, to catch staff's errors, as with drugs and IV drips, working hard, too, at maintaining their composure during procedures, making decisions about whether to go through another operation or to die, and monitoring the dialysis machines and other equipment. Patients, however, are not employees of the hospital and have no status as health professionals or other kind of health workers, and so they are not easily conceived by the personnel as actually working and certainly not as a literal part of the division of labor in managing and shaping their own trajectories. Indeed, much of their work is quite invisible to the physicians, nurses, and technicians, because that work is not actually seen, is kept secret, or if it is seen, is not defined as work but just as patients' activity or general participation in their own care. Ironically, patients are expected to be "cooperative," in common hospital parlance, while the staff is working hard on their care—meaning not merely that patients should be passive or pleasant, but should do the things they are supposed to do in the service of their medical and nursing care. Doing the things they are supposed to do certainly can involve putting time and effort into the requisite acts or activities. In

Earlier versions of this material appeared as "Patients' Work in the Technologized Hospital," *Nursing Outlook* 29 (1981): 404–12, and also as "The Work of Hospitalized Patients," *Social Science and Medicine* 16 (1982): 977–86.

short, the sick work, but their work is not necessarily conceived of as more than acting properly or decently in accordance with the requirements of their care by professionals and assisting personnel.

The larger theoretical issue here, for the sociologist at least, is that whenever a client is worked on or with by any servicing agent, then that client can become part of the division of labor in getting the work accomplished, even though neither may recognize the client's efforts as constituting work (Davis 1980). This is another way of stating what was noted earlier in the book: implicit in the fact that patients are worked on is the possibility they might not merely react to what is being done to or for them but might indeed enter into the very process of being serviced. (Clients or customers may be involved in working even when they are having objects, rather than themselves, serviced, as when they bring radios or cars or hearing aids to be fixed: they may have done preliminary diagnoses, they may give useful information.)

In this chapter, we intend to trace some of the ramifications as well as the peculiarities of how patients participate in the managing and shaping of their own trajectories, whether that participation is seen by themselves or others as actually being work. The relevant questions here include:

1. What types of work do patients do?
2. How does that work relate to various trajectories and their phases?
3. What is the relation of that work to staff work?
4. Under what conditions is the work visible or invisible to staff?
5. Under what conditions is the work appreciated or not appreciated by staff?
6. What are some consequences of patient work for staff work, for trajectories, and for the patients' own medical and biographical fates?
7. How does patient work at the hospital relate to trajectory work done at home?

In beginning to answer those questions, it is quite necessary to consider again the familiar triad—chronic illness, technology, and hospital organization—discussed so often in previous chapters.

Sources of Patients' Work

The classic picture of the patient—whether painted by a discerning Dutch realist or more recently described by Parsons (1951) with "sick role" imagery—is of an acutely sick person, hence temporarily passive and acquiescent, being treated by an active physician and helped by equally vigorous caretakers. That is hardly an accurate depiction of chronically ill persons except when rendered helpless during the most acute phases of an illness. Although interrupted by occasional or even frequent acute episodes, most of the business of their lives is transacted in and around whatever symptoms bedevil them. If the symptoms, or the recommended rigimens, are quite intrusive then those will in varying degrees present problems for "normal" living, which in turn necessitate a more or less complicated juggling of how life is lived. If the trajectories produced by medical intervention are stretched out or have novel phases, or if the illness affects other physiological systems, then the maintenance of patterns of normal living may be further complicated.

The general point here is that the chronically ill are engaged, unless altogether helpless, as with victims of severe strokes or people who utterly disregard their symptoms and regimens, in managing and shaping their lives in the face of physiological impairment and medical intrusion. They work more or less successfully at controlling symptoms and disease processes and at carrying out their regimens. Think of diabetic patients arising in early morning to clear their urine, later to test it for sugar, to take or give themselves their insulin shots, to work also to resist the temptations of potentially dangerous but inviting foods (Benoliel 1975). Or think of people with ulcerative colitis who everyday must frequently and minutely monitor their wastes and record this monitoring (Reif 1975). Of course, both kinds of illness necessitate that those who suffer from them engage in varying degrees of sentimental, comfort, and clinical safety work, as well as in the more procedural medical work. Time, effort, and patience are integral elements of this work done at home and in public places.

So, too, must those who suffer from them gain varying degrees of knowledge and craft about medical technology, whether pharmacological, procedural, or involving the tending of machines. Patients may be taught initially by hospital personnel how to handle those technologies, but they add to it through their own experiences. The chronically ill become vary knowledgeable, also, about the interplay between these technologies and their own unique bodily reactions; often they become very skilled in managing those reactions. Only they can possess, even earn, this specialized knowledge. When they become very acutely ill or need a more complicated technology, they may enter a hospital: yet they do not leave any of their experiential knowledge behind them, however much the staff may regard them, as sometimes the staff does, as medically innocent.

In the hospital these patients are expected to act appropriately while the personnel go about doing the medical interventions and the other acute-care activities called for by the illnesses. A traditional acute-care philosophy still lies embedded in the medical-nursing care given in hospitals, as noted in chapters 1 and 6; this assumes a patient in a state of illness rendering him or her relatively helpless, dependent on trained professionals and technicians, who through their resources and skills will sooner or later effect improvement in the patient's condition. The latter's job is simply to cooperate with the personnel to whom responsibility for care has been delegated. So there is the paradox that involves chronically ill persons whose heads, and often hands, are well endowed with experiential knowledge and skill and who now become wards of the health personnel, presumably delegating all responsibility and caring tasks to them. Actually, of course, every medical intervention involves the possibility, often the probability, that the patient will have to do something, hence not be completely inert during the intervention. Given the organization of hospital work, it is easy to see that these knowledgeable patients may sometimes attempt to prevent or at least catch staff members' mistakes, seeking to have those rectified, or rectifying the mistakes themselves; may enter into the articulation of tasks whose sequences might otherwise go awry; may provide some of their own so-called continuity of care through the daily three shifts and in the face of staff rotation—and so on. To repeat then: patients find themselves in a paradoxical—ironical is, perhaps, the more accurate term—situation wherein they do delegate responsibility for care to the staff, but . . . .

Patient Work: Explicit and Implicit

Some work done by hospitalized patients is explicitly recognized by the staff as genuine work, primarily because it duplicates or supplements the staff's. On dialysis wards, nurses expect patients, unless very sick or inexperienced, to monitor both the machines and their bodies during most of the repeated dialysis sessions. On physical rehabilitation units, the therapists recognize fully the work that patients do in order to endure an carry out the sometimes painful or otherwise difficult exercise. And when patients are taught how to manage regimens and machinery just before discharge from the hospital, the work that must now be done at home is perhaps quite likely to be recognized as genuine work.

Associated with this explicit recognition of patients' work may be a quite clear and even elaborate staff philosophy about how much and what kinds of work the patients are allowed or requested to do. One particularly striking ideology which places special emphasis on patients' efforts is the Simonton method advocated for people suffering from cancer (Simonton 1974). A central idea in this fairly complex philosophy is visualization therapy, in which the person visualizes his or her internal body, the cancer itself, and the immunity system. The visualizations promoted are rich in personal imagery; for example, the patient imagines his or her immunity system as an army of warriors in the bloodstream attacking the enemy cancer cells. The therapist works at changing the belief system of the patient (and kin and personal physician even), but the patient also works very hard at changing his conceptions of himself and his cancer—works with kin, too, and sometimes hospital personnel after rehospitalization.

On the other hand, most patients' work when at the hospital goes unrecognized: it is taken for granted. Among the unrecognized tasks are nonmedical ones pertaining to personal housekeeping: going to the toilet, putting out the bed light, combing hair, getting out of bed if ambulatory, feeding oneself. Then there are certain things which it is assumed that patients, unless they are infants or nonsentient, can and will do: give information during the entry and diagnostic interviews, for instance. Patients are also expected to report discomforts and untoward symptoms or bad reactions to drugs. Then, there are expectations of them during various tests, as when cardiacs are put on the treadmill. They are instructed to report when angina appears. Certain other patients are instructed how to do necessary things and are expected to do them—to cough postoperatively, for instance. Other tests require patients to put out considerable effort in order that their performance levels can be measured; indeed the staff member may encourage the patient to perform to his or her utmost, often giving approval for successful efforts, as with someone who is having respiratory outputs monitored. And, of course, there is much informal and even recognized teaching of patients how to monitor machines or bodies. When they are deemed responsible and experienced, they are more likely, naturally, to be trusted with the monitoring itself and with reporting the results.

Still other work done by patients is not so easily recognized as work, either by the staff or by the patients themselves. It may involve expenditures of effort, even resolve and courage, especially if the patient is very ill or in severe pain, though it is so taken for granted that it slips by relatively unnoticed. Managing body position is an instance. The X-ray technician requests the patient to turn now to the right, now to the left; the patient moves his or her body as requested. Immobilized patients or infants must be positioned because they cannot be expected to follow orders to position themselves. Again, the physician, nurse, or technician says "this procedure will hurt but it is necessary," and the adult or older child is assumed to be capable of refraining from any interfering movement. Children and occasionally adults who refuse to follow requests about body movement or lying still may be forcibly positioned or restrained.

Moreover, there are a few body tasks that require patients to do other things with their bodies: they must swallow barium or "take a big breath now and hold until I say let it out" or "hang on to this rail with your right hand and walk, but keep up with the treadmill" or "blow into this as hard as you can." Even when it is necessary for the patient to hold something so that the technician can do something else, and the latter literally says, "Help me," thrusting an electrical connection into the patient's hand, that does not necessarily mean the technician is thinking of the patient's work as anything more than just cooperation. Finally, there is another kind of body work familiar to us all: giving on request various body substances—urine, faeces, sputum. Patients who have just gone to the toilet may conceive of this as work, but surely the staff does not!

Referring now to a point touched on earlier: the staff expect patients to be cooperative during procedures or other interventions. Cooperation refers often to behavior that involves endurance, fortitude, self-control in the face of discomfort, pain, or potentially humiliating medical intervention. Persons who are normal, intelligent, and self-disciplined ought to be able to restrain their impulses to scream, shriek, pull their bodies away, refuse to undergo any more of a procedure, or take any more of a drug. When somebody breaks the staff's implicit, though sometimes clearly recognized and explicitly stated rules about these matters, then the staff will attempt to get him or her to adhere to them. The staff may cajole, tease, scold, empathize, but insist on obedience, thus attempting to persuade the patient. Or the staff may attempt to negotiate: "if you endure it, then we will do it as fast as possible," or "only one more time," or "let's skip the drug or procedure for now but do not skip it next time, ok?" If the patient remains recalcitrant, or worse yet persistently recalcitrant, then a negative reputation will rapidly build up. These staff judgments about cooperative or uncooperative patients very often have a strong moral coloration insofar as they involve not simply someone's capacity to endure but whether he or she chooses or has enough character to endure—or to lie still, or to do whatever is being judged in a positive or negative mode (Duff and Hollingshead 1968, Lorber 1981).

We are not especially interested here in spelling out the frequently important consequences for patients who are so judged or for their care or fates (see Strauss and Glaser 1970), but in emphasizing that patients are judged on their carrying out of *tasks*. These are not usually conceived of by staff as tasks (or jobs or work) but in terms of patients' participation in the staff's work—contributory actions rather than work, which have an implicit moral core. Patients, too, may morally evaluate their own actions, and themselves as actors, being proud or ashamed at their endurance or fortitude. Ordinarily, however, they do not conceive of their actions as work, as contrasted, say, with their monitoring of equipment. It is worth adding that the medical literature is replete with commentary, and studies too, about patients' lack of compliance (usually but not always concerning not following regimens when at home), replete, too, with a full lexicon of terms, ascribed motivations, and personality ascriptions for explaining why certain patients, or populations of patients, fail to adhere to regimens that so obviously are designed for their own medical good (Strauss and Glaser 1975). "Uncooperative" patients are often thought of as recalcitrant about submitting to medical intrusions which are believed necessary by those to whom they have delegated their care.

There are more subtle kinds of patient work, which if not done, or not done properly, get patients into trouble with the staff. We have in mind, for instance, the complex situation which can arise when the staff knows that a terribly ill person now knows he or she is dying. The patient is, in our terminology, expected to do certain (unrecognized) work involving maintaining reasonable control over reactions which might be excessively disturbing for the staff's medical work, for its composure, too, and, perhaps, even disruptive also of other patients' poise.

> Once a patient has indicated his awareness of dying, the most important interactional consequence is that he is now responsible for his acts as a *dying* person. He knows now that he is not merely sick but dying. He must face that fact. Sociologically, "facing" an impending death means that the patient will be judged, and will judge himself, according to certain standards of proper conduct. These standards, pertaining to the way a man handles himself during his final hours and to his behavior during the days he spends waiting to die, apply even to physically dazed patients. Similarly, certain standards apply then to the conduct of hospital personnel, who must behave properly as humans and as professionals. The bare bones of this governed reciprocal action show through the conversation between a nurse and a young dying girl. The nurse said, "Janet, I'll try as hard as I can"; and then when the youngster asked whether she was going to die, the nurse answered, "I don't know, you might, but just keep fighting." . . . Patients known to be aware of death have two kinds of obligation: First, they should not act to bring about their own deaths. Second, there are certain positive obligations one has as a dying pa-

tient. . . . People are supposed to live correctly while dying, providing they understand that they are dying, but Americans have no clear rules for their behavior. . . .

Nevertheless, in our hospitals staff members do judge the conduct of dying patients by certain implicit standards. These standards are related to the work that hospital personnel do, as well as to some rather general American notions about courageous and decent behavior. A partial list of implicit canons includes the following: The patient should maintain relative composure and cheerfulness. At the very least, he should face death with dignity. He should not cut himself off from the world, turning his back upon the living; instead he should continue to be a good family member, and be "nice" to other patients. If he can, he should participate in the ward social life. He should cooperate with the staff members who care for him, and if possible he should avoid distressing or embarrassing them. A patient who does most of these things will be respected. He evinces what we shall term "an acceptable style of dying," or, more accurately, "an acceptable style of living while dying." . . .

The contrasting pattern—what the staff defines as unacceptable behavior in aware dying patients—is readily illustrated. For instance, physicians usually honor requests for additional (or consultants') opinions, but object to "shopping around" for impossible cures. . . . Other types of unacceptable behavior emerge vividly from our field notes. Thus the next quotation involves a patient's serious failure to "cooperate" in his medical care, and it shows the extremes to which a physician will go to get such cooperation:

> The patient had been moving his arm around a lot so his intravenous needle was in danger of coming out; he is very testy at all such rigmarole. The doctor got irritated, apparently, at his lack of cooperation and said that if he took that needle out of his arm, he'd die. The nurse: "that's what the doctor said to his face—that this is what is keeping you here; you pull it out and you'll die."

. . . Patients who do not die properly . . . create a major interactional problem for the staff. The problem of inducing them to die properly gives rise, inevitably, to a series of staff tactics. Some are based on the patient's understanding of the stiuation: staff members therefore command, reprimand, admonish, and scold. . . . These negatively toned tactics . . . are supplemented, and often overshadowed, by others through which personnel attempt to teach patients how to die properly. (Glaser and Strauss 1965, pp. 82–83, 86, 90–91)

In short, patients are expected to do, and certainly often do, a great deal of implicit work, especially sentimental work, while dying; conversely, the staff, whose medical-nursing and composure work is often shattered by patients who break the rules of dying, finds itself engaging in the additional and mostly unwanted work of persuading or teaching conformance with those rules.

Patients' Work: Visible or Invisible, Legitimate or Illegitimate

Another condition for the nonrecognition of patients' work is when it is not visible to the personnel. Sometimes the work is done when they are not present. Sometimes, although a staff member and a patient are together, the latter's work is literally invisible, as with some kinds of comfort or sentimental work. In either event, the patient may elect not to tell what he is doing or has done. Patients may not indicate their work for a variety of reasons: because it could be defined as illegitimate or done wrong, or because it involves criticism of the staff, as with monitoring their competence, or because it is altogether too personal, as with much identity work and so on.

Some of this work—but not defined as such even perhaps by the patient—may become discovered. If then regarded as legitimate, it may be responded to variously: with gratitude, dismay, amusement, empathy, indifference. If defined as illegitimate—as when a patient in pain takes medication carefully secreted away—then the staff will attempt to prevent future transgressions (Strauss and Glaser 1977, Fagerhaugh and Strauss 1977). If the illegitimate work seems foolish or crazy, as when a patient in pain keeps elaborate records of when pain medications were given, then the staff may merely scoff at or denigrate the patient among themselves. The last illustrations suggest, of course, that patients and personnel can hold very different definitions of legitimate and illegitimate work done by the patients (again not usually defined as work); this is all the more reason for a savvy or suspicious patient to keep the work hidden.

Here is a complex and frequent instance that involves the issues of legitimacy and visibility: a patient defines some activity as necessary (perhaps as work, even) but the staff disapproves, never dreaming of the patient's definition but only perceiving that he or she is disobeying instructions and refusing obligations, (for example, when a rather anxious patient a few days after a myocardial infarction is required to be ambulatory but is carefully working at "resting," as insisted on previously by the same staff. While the nurses may see the patient's immobility as an overcautious precaution, they are more likely to view this silent work as flagrant disobedience to the doctor's orders, prompted by a too generous dose of anxiety.

One additional and rather special condition for the invisibility of a patient's work is when the staff is working on a main trajectory while the patient is doing subsidiary work on other trajectories. Then the staff's focus hinders their noticing the patient's work or makes less probable that they will discover this work when he or she chooses not to reveal it; if revealed, it is still not necessarily understood as work in the service of another trajectory. As an instance of the lengths to which such work can go, here is a case involving a daughter as well as the patient, but also involving what we would regard as the staff's contributory comfort work:

> A very elderly lady came in for a standard cataract operation, ready to stay for three days. She and her daughter "came prepared" because she had arthritis, and also easily became cold because of circulatory problems associated with her age. They brought the patient's own pillow, also special underwear and blankets to keep her warm. Nevertheless she became cold, so the daughter explained to the nursing staff that her mother was extraordinarily cold. A heating pad was then brought. Everybody worked hard, also, at only removing her clothing when absolutely necessary. As for the EKG, the lady herself put her clothing back on, assisted by her daughter. Since there was no official restriction of her movement, she could get in and out of bed at will, something she needed to do since her arthritis made it difficult to remain long in one position.

Trajectories, Division of Labor, and Patient Work

The work that patients do is trajectory work in the service of managing and shaping aspects of their trajectories. So the particularities of their work, quite like the staff's, must necessarily relate to the specific trajectory in which they are so unfortunate as to be caught up. At this point in the book, that should not require much if any elaboration. It is perhaps well, however, to be reminded that patients' work is also connected with trajectory phasing. For instance, a young woman informed by her internist that her breast biopsy showed some malignancy and that she would require a mastectomy operation, engaged then in phased work. Aside from being plunged into composure work and some initial identity work about dying and a disfigurement, she systematically sought information that would allow her to make intelligent decisions about the next steps. What kinds of operations were possible and feasible? What were the rates of success and failure for each? What were the alternative modes of treatment? What was the reputation of the surgeon to whom she was referred? Who could tell her? To whom should she go for another consultation? Who would be the anesthesiologist and had he and the surgeon worked much together? What would be the impact of the various therapies on her life? Unless a prospective patient is extraordinarily passive, he or whe will ask some—or even more—of those questions; if as active and searching as this particular woman, much time and energy will be spent to get reasonable answers. As the trajectory moves along, the work will be different: in the hospital, this woman after her mastectomy decided not to take any pain medication, developed modes of minimizing body discomfort that came in the wake of the operation, refused to have her blood drawn by an untidy and fumbling technician, complained to the head nurse about that incident, worked too at keeping her "cool" when a friend anxiously inquired about the operation. Once at home, there would be still different tasks in accordance with next phases in trajectory management. Some who have had mastectomies confront the specter of cancer recurrence and possible death, which precipitates plenty of identity work that physicians, and husbands, too, seem loath to share with them.

If it is true that patients as well as staff enter into the work process, then an important theoretical question is posed. Just what, then, is their part in the total division of labor concerning trajectory management and shaping? It should be clear enough by now that there is no simple answer to that question. Undoubtedly hospital personnel tend to believe the bulk of patients' work—definitions of "work" per se aside—consists of handling composure and coming to grips with identity problems associated with the illness. If pressed they would agree that patients share in getting some of the more medical tasks done and must make some of the big decisions about undergoing surgery and other drastic procedures. In fact, patients engage in all the types of work discussed in this book. But that kind of global conclusion does not directly address the basic question of the division of labor.

A more specific set of answers to it would have to include at least the following notion of types of patient engagement in the trajectory process. First, some of the patients' work is the *mirror image* of the staff's work: patients give urine, the staff takes away the urine and sends it to the lab for testing. Patients obey commands to position themselves while staff gives the commands, then does the procedures. Second, some work by patients is *supplementary* to, but not exactly the mirror image of, staff's work, such as maintaining composure in the face of procedural tasks. Third, work by patients may *substitute* for work that staff did not do but either were supposed to do or patients believe they were supposed to do. Fourth, patients may do work that they believe is *necessary*, although the staff would disagree (if it knew), like monitoring for potential error or incompetence. Fifth, patients may *rectify* staff errors, directly by themselves or by reporting—or complaining—to responsible authorities. Sixth, patients may do the work that *staff cannot possibly do*, meaning not only their own sentimental work but more medically tinged actions like giving information about allergies to certain drugs or explaining they have other chronic illnesses whose symptoms may interfere with the staff's working on the main trajectory. Seventh, patients may engage in work that is *outside the range* of what staff may conceive of as the locus of their own work, such as coping with highly personalized, deep identity problems precipitated by the illness, or other work which staff may eschew even when aware of the patient's problem, like Mr. Einshtein's constipation problem or the postmastectomy people struggling with disfigurement and fears of impending death.

These various types of work, of course, can match, supplement, and fit in with staff work in very diverse ways. Combinations of staff and patient work are equally diverse, as are the relative complexities of their respective tasks. At the risk of overburdening readers presumably now aware of how complicated the interplay of staff and patients' work can be, a further elaboration of the point will be made through a few illustrations. We will have met them before, but not quite as fully spelled out in terms of the simplicity or complexity of the interplay between the respective work of patient and staff.

A subtle and complex situation first: immediately after a treadmill test—completed when the patient got considerable angina—he was moved to a prone position under a nuclear tracer machine, which for the next half hour or more would be recording the heart's performance. The attending physician occasionally asked "How are you doing?" And the patient responded "OK." He was, in fact, all right except he was uncomfortable because of his angina, which caused him to burp from time to time. In turn, the burping soon gave him heartburn, but he contained his dis-ease. Soon, too, his neck began to hurt somewhat, because he had a slightly bad back condition and the position in which he was lying aggravated it. That discomfort he also contained without moving or saying anything about it. From time to time the technician moved the recording part of the machine so that the patient found himself protecting himself by slightly moving his head to avoid the machine or to get away from its mild but discomforting pressure. All those were technologically induced, if essentially minor jobs. A more difficult and more important one was that he had to prevent himself from coughing, not an easy task, since he had bronchitis, and this happened to be precisely the time of day when normally and involuntarily he coughed up much phlegm. Just once he gave way, properly warning the technician beforehand, and then went back to his concerted control again. Except for the body positioning, none of this work was visible to the technician, physician, or nurse and ordinarily they would not become aware of it, yet it was all relevant to the success of the machine's accurate recording.

Let us turn once again to staff and patient work done during dialysis sessions, a very complex interaction. After repeated dialysis sessions, a patient learns and is taught how and when to work. Patients may be involved in setting up the machine or connecting themselves to it. (Some centers have self-care philosophies, so patients are expected to do much of this.) Some take great pride in tending the machine, setting it, as well as monitoring its performance. Men especially take pleasure in their knowledge of mechanics and can fiddle successfully with the machine when it is not working quite properly. Patients may also prepare the solution used in the treatment. During the periods immediately after getting on the machine and getting off, the users are much more in evidence, doing their tasks around the machine and in relation to the other patients. The long period in between involves much monitoring by the patient of both machine and body responses, since body and machine are in such potentially delicate balance. Patients are also monitoring each other and will call the staff if they see or believe another patient is in trouble. Personnel may put forward a philosophy of patient participation, prompting even reluctant patients to do more for themselves during the dialysis session, but the more experienced and responsible are trusted more by the staff, who can then be engaged in other work at the nursing station or with patients who need greater attention.

It goes almost without saying that dialysis patients do composure work: during the early weeks of being on the machine, some, at least, need to muster their courage to get through the sessions, their anxiety levels being high. Abetting the nurses' composure work with them, often, is the same kind of work by other experienced patients. Yet anxiety may never be quite eliminated in some patients: for example, one man told the researcher that he simply did not trust most nurses during the dangerous period just before the end of the dialysis session "when the bubbles that can kill you can appear if it isn't done right," so during this time at every session he does his self-defined most important work, watching the nurse's handling of the tube and machine like a hawk! Thus, while nurses are judging the patients' competencies, patients are also monitoring and judging them. In sum, while there is great variation in the amount of work done by these patients, we can appreciate the remark of one woman who jokingly said that "MediCal should pay me—I do all the work!" (Our thanks to Barbara Artinian, who is studying dialysis patients, for this quotation.)

And a third illustration to bring out the interplay of staff-patient work in a negative sense: the patients are doing collaborative work in the absence or failure of staff's work. For instance, a patient hospitalized for an eye operation noted both her own work in others' behalf and that of patients acting as a group. Being more "awake" than some of her roommates, she was the one who called the nurse, pointing out oversights such as with the patient whose drops for glaucoma had been overlooked. "Occasionally three patients would consult with one another about the best strategy for handling a problem—whether to complain to the nurse or wait for the physician. It was a sort of lame, halt, and blind collaboration. There was definitely a 'we' group feeling." Consultations among them often centered on IV monitoring; did the others think the drop was too fast, too slow, solution getting too low, time to call the nurse, did the nurse on duty seem to know or care about what's supposed to be happening? The strategy of the patients in a situation like this may be to ask for a particular nurse whom they regard as responsible or to complain to the physician when he arrives or to ask a family member to talk to either staff member.

To summarize this section then, there are, alas, no simple answers to the seemingly straightforward question: What is the patients' part in the division of labor? The principal reason is that the question is perhaps wrongly, if conventionally, posed. The question should be: How do the various types of patient work fit in with the staff's work, and in relation to their mutual shaping of trajectories? Undeniably, however, there is an official division of labor and some reality to this official version, since there *is* physicians' work and nurses' work and various technicians' work, some of it overlapping but some rather distinct. The patient, too, has a status, all too often felt as constraining or as involving powerlessness. Nevertheless, to achieve a realistic perspective on the division of labor issue, one must focus on the actual interplay of the work of the persons who embody those various statuses. (See chap. 10 for further discussion of this point.) In hospitals—whatever the staff, patients, kin, and even the critics of the medical scene believe—this interplay of work is a many-splendored thing. The more aggressive, fortunate, and knowledgeable patients surely understand that phenomenon.

Expecting, Demanding, Inviting, Negotiating, Teaching

The various illustrations of patients at work suggest different modes of immersion in a ward's division of labor. The most obvious mode is that staff *expects* patients to work (whether staff calls it work or not). Reluctant or recalcitrant patients are subject to the demand that they bear their responsibilities and get scolded or otherwise punished when they will not do their jobs—as with patients who fight the respirator or rehab patients who will not "put out." Patients who honestly attempt to do their tasks but have difficulty—as with one who kept ruining a breathing test on a respirator machine by choking up and coughing—may eventually arouse some annoyance, but at least they are trying their best.

Patients are sometimes also *invited* into the division of labor, tasks being proffered for a variety of reasons, including the following: the nurse must temporarily leave, being called elsewhere; she is very busy, and the task proffered has lower priority; she wishes to save herself a bit of work; she would rather not do that particular task; she believes that the patient will feel less depersonalized, feel less "worked on" or perhaps feel more secure if he does something. Also we have seen, the patient may be invited to do something on explicit ideological grounds, whether the philosophy is a professionalized one or derived from a wider social movement like "patients' rights."

Of course, patients may *offer* to do something, fix something, move something, watch something, not waiting to be asked or persuaded, just as they may demand to do one or another of those things. Another mode of entry by patients into the sharing of labor is through *negotiation*, where something is offered for something else in exchange. One sees this with the personnel's handling of young children, where rewards are given for cooperative behavior (composure work, body-positioning work) in enduring painful or discomforting or frightening procedures. The rewards may be tangible (one of the authors, when quite small, was promised and later given an ice cream cone and a quarter for enduring an operation). The rewards may also be more subtly symbolic, as when a physician warns a child of what he is going to do next, asking permission to work on her, showing solicitude, politeness, friendliness, generally acting "like a good guy"—trading all that for the young patient's cooperation. (We call this negotiation rather than persuasion because of the trade-off.) Persuasion refers more to talking someone into something, convincing directly, as when a child reacts to a portable X-ray machine, crying because "of the needle," but then is persuaded that there *is* no needle. Both explicit and implicit negotiations transpire around patient work, and either staff or patient may initiate the exchange. Some types of cooperative work, as in rehab exercises, with or without machines, are greatly facilitated by open and generous exchanges by both parties: yes, the staff member agrees, we can have a shorter session today providing you continue doing so well for the next ten minutes.

"*Teaching* the patient" is translatable into getting the patient either to work or to work more effectively in his or her own behalf, largely through negotiation and persuasion. (Demanding, manipulating, coercing that work are rarely appropriate to genuine teaching, at least by themselves.) The increasing complexity of drug and machine technologies, and the complex regimens that patients face when they go home, literally force on everyone the concept of the patient-as-technologist. In some part, surely, the rise of the liaison nurse (who bridges hospital and home), and the generally increasing emphasis on teaching the hospitalized patient, express the response of the nursing profession to the increasing prevalence and difficulties of managing problematic chronic illnesses and to the complex technology related to that management. One of our research assistants, a nurse-sociologist, expressed that point in a field note after her interviews and observations at a university medical center:

> One of the things that struck me in conversations with several nurses was their emphasis on patient teaching. A few years ago, commitment to patient teaching was primarily a preoccupation of nursing educators. Now, I was immediately struck by the preoccupation of the practitioners with this activity. What is more, it has become highly formalized and organized here, often with written protocols. It seems unrelated to the educational background of the nurses I interviewed: a nurse who was a graduate of Massachusetts General and who described herself as very technically and procedurally oriented, told in detail how she visits her patients prior to open-heart surgery or major bowel surgery and instructs them. Another thing nowadays is the complexity of these machines: on 8 West they use aortic balloon pumps, Swan-Gans catheters, A-Lines, you name it. The patient cooperation (even when very ill) is still helpful, even critical to working with them on these machines. So this is very complex and increasingly tricky work that the nurses have to do, and they need all the help they can get. If they can't get the patient's help, they feel better off if the patient is "out." So if patient teaching gets the work done better, they do it.[2]

(Our thanks to Roberta Lessor, School of Nursing, University of California, San Francisco, for these observations and our use of them.)

The old but now increasingly important function of the nurse as educator partly represents a turning away from a predominantly "medical model" of care, because staff members recognize the necessary social and psychological aspects of care (Redman 1976). The teaching emphasis, however, nowadays, also represents a more strictly technical focus on teaching patients and kin the basics of technology (whether drug, machine, or body monitoring) whose use is essential in home care. Without this reaching and its implementation by patient and kin, relapse may occur, the patient will be returning sooner to the hospital, and speedy death may even result. While much teaching is targeted at home care, increasingly nurses and other personnel (dieticians, physical therapists, etc.) are teaching in the hospital, either informally or with more official accountability.

The teaching perspective does have some weaknesses, when conceived in terms of the policies and potentialities of patients' work. Basically, the teaching perspective—regardless of the specific teaching model utilized—assumes the staff member is the teacher while the patient is the learner. Of course, the contemporary models emphasize room for sharing and learning together, but they assume that the primary flow of information is from teacher to student. A second drawback to the practice of health personnel as teacher is a tendency to focus on formal teaching, not to the exclusion of informal teaching or teaching in situ, but formal instruction tends to be given priority. Third, the teaching perspective often focuses too narrowly upon the medical, technological, and procedural aspects of illness management, omitting or underplaying important social-psychological and biographical aspects of chronic illness trajectory management. Fourth, the teaching orientation tends to employ a language of evaluation, assessment, and goals—all probably reinforcing the teacher-learner axis per se and giving the former both a hierarchical position in relation to the patient while also emphasizing unduly those aspects of the teaching-learning situation that can be clearly assessed or measured, that is, the more medical and procedural aspects of the teaching-learning. Fifth, the teaching perspective does pay attention to certain features of the hospital or ward setting which create impediments to teaching and learning, but the perspective tends to embody a relatively incomplete grasp of the hospital as an organization and what that implies for staff's care and teaching, patients' work and learning. Sixth, the teaching orientation tends to emphasize both the patient's needs and what the patient needs to know. On the one hand, the focus is on the teacher responding to presumed or known needs, and on the other, the patient is required to learn certain necessary things. Teachers may attempt to balance between those two poles *or* move toward one or the other. Meanwhile, a teacher can forget that her or his own needs and judgments about the requirement to teach specific materials can muddy the interactional waters, thus preventing deeper understanding of what is transpiring between oneself and the patient. A seventh and last point: the teaching perspective does not specifically emphasize the implications of prevalent chronic illness for the teaching-learning process itself. A steady focus on chronic illness allied with the teaching perspective would literally demand that the teachers seek sources for their own learning in patients' experiential work at home and in the hospital.

Problematic Trajectories and Decision Making

As noted in the second chapter when discussing trajectory options—large and small, policy and operational—problematic trajectories can involve patients in the decision making. Patients enter into that decision making, whether asked in , demanding their way in, or entering because contingencies make for facing the options directly. This would be true, even if the "patient power" movement were less of a force, because so many trajectories are quite problematic (Wiener et al. 1980). Nor need we assume that each patient necessarily wishes to participate in the decision making or that, being a long-time chronic sufferer, he or she knows a great deal about the options and their implications. The very open-endedness of many trajectories insures that patients will do the decision-making work. Some of this involves making choices on small operational matters. Some, of course, involves genuinely major choices.

Most options faced by patients are neither so fateful nor anguishing as in the case of the woman who hesitated between yet another operation and dying. The options consist rather of choices that they elect to make or have forced on them, at virtually any point along their trajectories. However, problematic trajectories beginning to get out of hand typically involve some very difficult choices. Thus, in cumulative mess trajectories virtually everything, medically and organizationally, eventually goes awry. Patients then cannot but be brought into the decision-making work that needs to be done at the critical junctures (let alone during the minor episodes) during these highly problematic, chronic illness trajectories. Much of their actual decision work is then explicit and highly visible to the staff—but not all of it—and sometimes not until after it is completed, as with unanticipated signing out from hospitals or even attempts at suicide.

We shall end this chapter by underlining the point that chronic illness trajectories flow from home residence into and through hospitals, and out again back to the home. When we consider such repeated cycles, it becomes apparent that patients are, as remarked earlier, working technologists, too, not only at home but in the hospital. They may overestimate their own expertise, but most have earned and use it. In future years, not to recognize this reality is likely to bring a considerable increase of conflict between patients and hospital staffs. The very rise of self-care groups signifies the current widening degree of recognition by groups of patients and kin of their respective expertise. (This is reflected in the words of one arthritic who exclaimed when given the informational, teaching pamphlet put out by a hospital's arthritis center: "It's so skimpy!") The future is very likely to bring an increasing challenge to hospital staffs from these patients over getting more share in the management of their own illnesses. Researchers like us wonder whether hospital staffs will recognize the source of patients' rising expectations: Will staffs wait until the challenge becomes overt and the tempers impossibly high?

9

Macro to Micro and Micro to Macro Impacts: The Intensive Care Units

All of the preceding chapters except for the first have been persistently focused on the details of trajectory work, and although larger structural conditions were brought into conjunction with those details, attention has been mostly on "microscopic" rather than "macroscopic" phenomena. Virtually all social science writing, if it combines macro and micro considerations, tends, as in the foregoing pages, to run the line of impact from macro conditions to micro consequences. But there can be feedback, with resulting two-directional impact. This chapter will elaborate that assertion more abstractly.

The Intensive Care Nursery

First, we shall discuss the birth trajectory as it flows through labor and delivery and intensive care nursery units, highlighting the macro-micro interaction. This involves the impact especially of changes in medical technology and medical specialization on these wards and the

A section of this chapter is based on a fairly extensive study of a labor and delivery ward and an intensive care nursery in a hospital located in a metropolitan area, over a five-month period, and rather less intensive fieldwork and interviewing at a comparable metropolitan hospital. An earlier version of this material, organized in somewhat different terms, appeared as "Trajectories, Biographies, and the Evolving Medical Technology Scene," *Sociology of Health and Illness* 1 (1979): 261–83, with Carolyn Wiener as the senior author.

reverse impact of that work and those kinds of wards on both technology and specialization; it also involves the lives of families and the children saved in the ICNs and the possible influence of the technological changes on the larger health issues. We shall discuss, too, the influence that ideologies and ideological debate (professional and nonprofessional) seem to have had on the premature-infant trajectory, and vice versa.

A Changing Technology and the Birth Trajectory

Labor and delivery wards are moving from what was considered the practice of an "art" (abetted by analgesic intervention) to heightened application of technology ("we are now more clinically definitive"). With the explosion of new knowledge and new medical technology in the last decade, a quasi-fatalistic attitude in obstetrics has been replaced by aggressive intervention in order to maximize the possibility of conception and to maintain formerly hopeless pregnancies. At the same time, goaded by a consumer movement that labeled hospital birth as too impersonal and technological and by the competition of a midwife and home-birth movement, hospitals have opened alternative birth centers (called ABCs), which offer none of the usual technology and no drug intervention. The rationale for acceptance of this radical change has been the closeness of emergency backup. To quote one doctor:

> Avoiding the hospital is not the answer; humanizing the hospital is. . . . The birth process represents the most dangerous day in the life of the newborn. . . . He has the best chance of dying on that day, and we're not only talking about death but about crippling and handicapping. That's the time that that baby ought to be very close to all care possible. (Fox 1979)

Alternative birth centers in most cases represent a philosophy rather than actually constitute a separate center. ABC rooms within the conventional hospital have been furnished in a homelike decor, complete with plants, stereo, and a double bed to serve for labor, delivery, and rest. Nurses, who are no longer identifiable by uniforms, remain with the mother the entire time, as may fathers, siblings, and others of the mother's choosing.

Well-baby nurseries have also undergone a change, being sparsely populated since babies now spend more time in their mother's rooms. But adjacent to a near-empty nursery, there is a beehive of activity in the highly machined and highly staffed intensive care nursery, where the radical survival techniques are being performed.

Machines have been to a large extent responsible for who goes to the ICN. But before turning to the ICN and its technology we shall briefly discuss continuous fetal monitoring, the simultaneous electronic recording of fetal heart rate and uterine contractions during labor, which developed out of the desire to assess fetal and/or maternal distress more accurately. Used during pregnancy by applying external electrodes or, if necessary, by adding an intravenous administration of oxytocin, this machine has been found to be a useful tool for gauging fetal capability of withstanding the stress of labor, thereby guiding the best timing and mode of delivery. For indicated cases (such as diabetes, hypertensive disease of pregnancy, intrauterine growth retardation, Rh sensitization, previous stillbirth or premature birth, low esterol excretions), a periodic oxytocin challenge test (OCT), or "nonstress test," as it is sometimes called, can be used to determine whether the respiratory function of the placenta is adequate. The goal is to keep the pregnancy going long enough to give the baby the best start, without endangering either mother or baby. This test is often used in conjunction with drugs and/or other techniques, such as ultrasonography.

A high infant mortality rate gave additional impetus for greater acceptance of the continuous fetal monitoring because of an effort to lower that rate. Moreover, current theory held that mental retardation and cerebral palsy were closely tied to oxygen deprivation during the time immediately before and after birth. Smaller family size, coupled with generous resources for frontier medicine, heightened the value placed on saving each baby. Intensive care nurseries, which started out focusing on babies, soon saw the advantage of monitoring the mother, preferably during pregnancy, but at least during labor, and that led to the expansion from baby transport to mother transport.

What started as a useful tool for high-risk labor, however, became routine in many hospitals, now evoking attack. Critics point to a sharp rise in cesarean births (a riskier and costlier procedure than vaginal delivery), which they attribute to panic readings of the fetal monitor. Defendants maintain that the problem is merely one of interpretation and skill:

> A lot of patterns we don't know completely, and sometimes it is difficult to interpret—even if there are late decelerations, it doesn't mean the baby is necessarily distressed. In major centers, where we have a lot of experience, monitor information can be put together with fetal blood samples, but smaller hospitals may not do that.

Participants in a national conference held in the late 1970s on antenatal diagnosis examined the arguments surrounding the growing routine use of monitors. They concluded that although current data were inadequate, no evidence could be found that electronic fetal monitoring reduces mortality or morbidity in low-risk patients (National Institute of Child Health and Human Development, 1979). Thus, the machine's biography has gone through research, development, and refinement to controversy.

Machinery purchased to aid such high-risk cases, however, takes on a life of its own. As stated above, unknowns abound in labor: a woman can evince optimal pelvic physiological construction and still not progress, just as the opposite can occur; labor can be slow for hours and suddenly speed up, requiring quick and pressured decisions. Not only do staff experiential biographies differ (varying degrees of competence at interpretation can lead to confrontations between nurses and physicians), but variability comes into play. Questioned about the routine use of the fetal monitor on low-risk laboring women, nurses answered that it is easier for themselves, that is, the nurse can leave the room, since presumably *someone* is watching the monitor at the central nurses' station (called the "slave monitor" by one nurse). Additionally, there is the ever present fear of malpractice suits. The machine's printout is part of the record and, to quote one physician, "If you've done the right thing, it will support you in court; if you've done the wrong thing, it will damn you" (Neutra 1979). Malpractice notwithstanding, the tyranny of this machine is that a compulsion has been set up to take all possible precautions against missing the signs of fetal and/or maternal distress: "You get afraid after a couple of bad experiences." The fetal monitor has become an evidence machine, by which staff make accusations of negligence or defend action or inaction. As expressed by a nurse, "The old philosophy was everything is normal until proven otherwise; now it's everything is abnormal until proven otherwise." In teaching hospitals especially, this monitor becomes part of the convincing process. As one resident put it:

> Because of studies that have been done, criteria develop, and in order to *justify* [emphasis added] what you have done, you have to go by these criteria. So even if you hear something with the fetascope and it is not on the monitor strip, somehow it is invalid. I don't know whether this is defensive medicine or a preoccupation with hardware.

As machines are assessed on the units—and this information is converted into improvements by industry—specialization and associated work and procedures become more sophisticated. Technological innovation and medical specialization proceed in a parallel and interactive manner (Fagerhaugh et al. 1980). What were the formerly relative static and low-status specialties of obstetrics and pediatrics are being sliced smaller and smaller to correspond with the technology of controlling the correspondingly smaller slices of the birth trajectory itself. Thus, there emerges both perinatology and neonatology. The first is the specialty defined as pertaining to before, during, and after the time of birth, time designation being arbitrary. Neonatology relates to the period immediately succeeding birth, and continuing, roughly, through the first month of life. Each of these medical specialties has spawned attendant clinical nurse specialists and a growing cadre of pediatric specialties in associated services like cardiology and neurology. Staff nursing, too, has become more specialized, requiring special ABC nurses, experienced nurses to accompany and care for high-risk mothers and babies on transports from outlying hospitals. Entwined with the growth of medical machinery has been the expanded knowledge of biochemistry and microchemistry, through which results can be obtained from an ever smaller amount of blood. In addition to juggling the tasks required of all nurses, the intensive care nurse must be an alchemist, striving to achieve and maintain a delicate balance of body chemistry based on sophisticated readings of blood gas studies and keeping an ear ever attuned to the beeping of the heart and respiratory monitor—a far cry from the nurse who rotated from labor and delivery to postpartum to the nursery.

Moreover, the drive for regionalization of services, in the interest of cost control and better utilization of skills, has divided hospitals into three classifications for the newborn: primary care (small hospitals with no support services for distressed babies); secondary care (minimal support, like oxygen, intravenous assistance); tertiary care (acute services). A medical dispatch center can direct the transport of at-risk babies to the appropriate hospital. These transports allow information to fan out from the medical center to the outlying districts. Since they are vital to the information flow and to the economic structure and prestige of the receiving hospital, staff are ever mindful of the public relations aspect of their work. Greater skill, knowledge, and experience are seeds for judgments of mismanaged labor and/or delivery out there; being received as the saviors from the big city (sometimes augmented by press coverage) adds nourishment to these seeds. The transport staff must be reminded constantly that an irritated and angry local hospital staff is not likely to remain a source of referrals and that effective teaching under these conditions must be tactfully presented in order to be effective.

Technologized Work, Ideologies, and the Birth Trajectory

Since delivery allows little or no time for quality-of-life decisions, such decisions move from the delivery room to the intensive care nursery. If the infant has a congenital defect, parents may decide they want no corrective procedures. Staff must then continue maintenance care, knowing the baby will not survive. The prolonged agony of such cases is a tremendous strain on parent and staff, and great effort is made to ease the effect on the infant.

With premature births, the staff watches closely during the first six to eight hours. If the baby is judged to be a 25- to 27-weeker, on 80 percent oxygen with oxygen support going higher and higher, the family is told that the outcome is highly questionable and asked if life-sustaining care should be continued. The following is a composite quote about this situation from one ward: "The response can be everything from the father who says 'Where are the autopsy papers?' to one who says, 'I don't care if he's blind and retarded, save him.' In most instances, the family will say, 'Withdraw support.' If we can't read the family, or if the family says they want the baby to survive, we will go great guns." Decisions must be made in rapid succession on the basis of various assumptions. The base of knowledge is recent, rapidly changing, and largely unpredictive. For example, it has only been since 1977 that knowledge about intercranial bleeding has become more conclusive. Now that a brain scan is part of the routine workup, bleeding has been found in 50 percent of the babies who are less than 1200 grams (usually the babies who have been transported). Occasionally the bleeding is massive or shows that major motor function has been affected. More often the results are ambiguous. In addition, it is not unusual for the baby to be too distressed to be subjected to a scan until considerable time has elapsed. Furthermore, a scan that indicates no bleeding does not rule out oxygen damage.

If the infant needs the aid of a respirator to ventilate, the delicate balancing begins: close monitoring of the respirator pressure to minimize lung damage, insertion of tubes to drain air, insertion of an umbilical line to monitor oxygen level through blood gas tests, anticoagulant drugs to correct clogging in the line, drugs to repress the normal breathing that would compete with the respirator, drugs to aid lung development, transfusions to replace blood taken for tests, periodic brain scans and X rays, insertion of a line to feed through the jugular vein (hyperalimentation), antibiotics to ward off infection. The succession is totally open-ended, as are the complications—from unanticipated, or anticipated but not fully controllable, contingencies—that can further snowball. Such babies may spend as many as six to nine months in the intensive care nursery, during which time staff members and parents may be asking at any point, "What are we doing?"

Faced with a parent who wants "everything done," staff is often unsure if that parent hears or understands what is meant by "brain damage." During this period there may be vast differences of opinion and judgment among staff, and they attend to different indications of improvement. When a physician focuses on trajectory and says, "She's doing well—she's off the respirator," the nurses may still be agonizing over biography, to wit: "What is her life going to be?"

In intensive care nurseries which place utmost importance on quality of life, although encouraging family involvement in life-sustaining decisions, the staff know that the family does not have the criteria to make such decisions. And they know their own criteria are weak. What sustains the staff is the understanding that as their knowledge base increases, it becomes possible to decrease the implicated assumptions. A baby who survives precarious months as described above (including a succession of some 40 insertions of chest tubes) and goes home breathing room air, showing no intercranial bleed, with eye problems that are correctable, becomes the rationale—despite ethical questions—for continuing treatment on future babies. Bulletin boards covered with snapshots of successes and a Christmas party for graduates serve this same purpose.

Going back to the topic of labor: identity work here also becomes paramount when there are strongly held ideologies. Many childbearing couples who question the hospital system do so on the instruction of theorists like Frederick Leboyer (1975), Fernand Lamaze (1970), and Robert A. Bradley (1974), who teach that birth is a normal process and that with attention to prenatal preparation and an appropriate atmosphere, parents and child can avoid the stress associated with the conventional hospital delivery (see also Arms 1975). For some of these couples, there are ideological stakes. Having reached this final moment of truth, this long-awaited delivery, they place accentuated and negative symbolic significance on each dimension of hospital intervention: enema, prep, drugs, forceps, episiotomies, silver-nitrate for the infant's eyes. Any of the above, if deemed necessary by the hospital staff, are potential points of contention. Conversely, staff, too, may have ideological stakes in the normal childbirth controversy (they may be critical of doctors who believe in responding to the patient's pleas, "Do something!" with, "We'll take care of it, honey") but may not have a choice in their assignment to specific women in labor. And while some prospective mothers have made a conscious choice regarding the camp in which they wished to be placed—some take a defensive posture ("I'm no pioneer"), while others are enthusiastic believers in the alternative birth center—many are not aware that in selecting a physician they may have placed themselves in one ideological camp or another. Most important, they are not likely to be aware of staff ideological stakes. Frequently, the situation will become clear in retrospect. The analysis of one woman ("I think the nurses lost interest in me when my labor was prolonged and it was necessary to induce; I think the challenge for them was gone") was given additional credence by the expressions of frustration voiced by a nurse:

> The mother is doing well. You close the door and cut off the world. Then there's a fluid stain, or the labor is prolonged, or she needs an analgesic. In comes the anaesthesiologist with the crash cart, a tray, a blood pressure machine, the epidural; we attach the monitor.
>
> And I feel a failure.

The course of each labor is totally unpredictable. As with ethical issues, the absence of clear-cut answers merely increases the rivalry of ideological positions. For every staff member who feels that drug intervention during labor impedes labor, leads to learning or motor disabilities, or detracts from a normal process, another can be found asserting that despite a reassuring physician, partner, and nurse, a significant number of women are going to remain anxious and are going to need intervention. Furthermore, the tone of many of the books about the Leboyer, Lamaze, and Bradley methods has contributed to public competition and peer pressure. (Nora Ephron, writing of her own experience with Lamaze, reflects perhaps a growing reaction: "The trouble is that it has the capability of being every bit as fanatical and narrow-minded as the system it has replaced" [1978].)

Another ideology that has had popular impact concerns parent attachment, labeled "bonding." This term—based on research spanning the last three decades but accelerated in most recent years—signifies the whole range of nurturing stimulation (stroking, swaddling, cuddling) felt to be necessary for the infant's emotional development. Marshall Klaus, whose research led to guidance on how the hospital can fulfill these needs, even in an acute-care setting, has stressed the "fantastic adaptability" of infants and warned against the danger of assuming that bonding must occur immediately at birth (Klaus 1979). Nevertheless, as with all such theories, popularization brings a certain degree of fanaticism. To quote one nurse recalling a "rough case":

> She was a 35-weeker, who wanted an ABC delivery and bonding, and was so freaked out by ending up in labor and delivery with a baby headed for the intensive care nursery.

> She had already been worn down, and accepted stirrups, draping. I had to convince her that doing an APGAR on the baby during the first five minutes was more important than bonding. [APGAR is a test done to determine the degree of asphyxiation of a baby at birth.]

Belief in the bonding ideology also complicates the imparting of information to parents of sick infants: "You don't want to scare them, and you don't want to affect their ability to bond, so you tell them enough to be concerned and not enough to divorce their feelings. It's hard to know what they understand."

The ward ideology also figures prominently. An intensive care nursery that believes in bonding, is mindful of quality of life, and encourages parent participation is opening up the possibilities of confrontations with parents. Access to the infant's chart may result in a deteriorating relationship between staff and parent, as the following case illustrates. An unfortunate characterization of the mother noted in the chart by her obstetrician both fed into the composite mother biography that staff was building and antagonized her to the extent that her behavior became increasingly withdrawn. A confrontation finally occurred when staff, fearful that the baby was not getting sufficient nutrition, encouraged supplemental bottle feeding. The mother, imbued with the necessity for breast feeding, which is part of bonding ideology, refused. This had been preceded by her accusations of negligence against a midwife and a premature delivery, which thwarted plans for delivery in the alternative birth center. A downward spiral was created which culminated in a mutually agreed on, but earlier than warranted, discharge of the infant. Staff and parent shared concern for the future biography of the infant. They differed on managing the course of the trajectory. Such confrontations arise when an ideology like bonding remains central for parents but, due to other considerations, recedes from staff focus. The emotional blow of an expected ABC delivery that has turned into the nightmare of a sick baby is apparent, and staff are mindful of this trauma. However, ABC parents are quite often assertive—questioning, and sometimes refusing, procedures.

Such behavior is often understood in retrospect but viewed as hostile when it adds to the strain of work. Staff is being called on to do identity work with the parent, when pure medical-nursing work would be preferred.

For the birth trajectory in general, expansion of perinatal and neonatal knowledge, skills, and technology and the ICN itself have made it possible to save babies who formerly were lost, with a paradoxical consequence. It is possible to move infant biographies farther and farther back, thus saving younger babies, who are more at risk by virtue of their being younger and having a less developed physiology. "We used to get excited at saving a 28-weeker; now it's 26 weeks." "Small" has moved from 1500 grams, to 1200, to 1000. This push back is not infinite; prior to 26 weeks there are no lungs and the eyes are sealed. However, there is some ambiguity even here, since each organism progresses at a different rate. Just when the neonatologists feel they have a partial predictive grasp about these babies, along comes a 25–26 weeker, 600 grams, who defies the odds and goes home in five weeks, gaining weight and breathing room air.

This stretching out of the birth trajectory has so far been continuous, for developments have been rapid and revolutionary. As already mentioned, brain scans have provided a tremendous breakthrough in predicting the infant's future. Another fundamental change has come about through the combined efforts of biochemical research and the development of a new technique, continuous positive airway pressure (CPAP). The discovery that surfactant, a detergentlike substance, is essential for normal lung function has led to the administration of hormones to speed the infant's production of this natural substance. CPAP is the application of continuous airway pressure; tubes through the mouth keep the infant's lungs inflated between breaths and can be used continually until the body begins to produce its own surfactant, and the lungs mature. For babies who are not so small and so sick as to need the aid of a respirator, CPAP has been a tremendous boon in radically decreasing the incidence of respiratory disease syndrome, formerly called hyaline membrane disease and formerly the leading cause of death among newborns.

Those who have been in neonatology for as few as five years describe the field as primitive when they started; one physician compared the pace of those five years to twenty in most specialties. During those years, ventilating techniques on the respirator have been vastly improved, in response to the discovery that a type of blindness that affected premature infants (retrolental fibroplasia) was associated with giving too much oxygen. The balancing fight against eye, lung, and brain damage still requires constant monitoring, which is why blood gases must be taken frequently. Hope is now being placed in the transcutaneous oxygen monitor, a machine that measures oxygen through a small platinum and Teflon sensor which is taped to the infant's skin. The sensor warms a small patch of the skin, causing the underlying capillary blood vessels to fill with blood. A current between electrodes in the sensor rises as the oxygen level goes up and is translated into a digital readout on the machine. Since the expectation that this noninvasive technique would replace the umbilical line or heel sticks has not been realized, reaction to this machine varies. What to the physician is a revolutionizing concept that will ultimately measure other values—carbon dioxide, acid-base balance—and with experience may detect an insult to the body like a pneumothorax before it occurs is still an unproven phenomenon to the nurse who now has an added machine to manipulate while still taking periodic blood gas tests. The machine's sensors have to be moved every two hours to avoid a burn; even so, they leave red circles, which recede in twenty-four hours, to be replaced by new marks. For parents, this is one more thing with which to cope. Yet this machine—its development still emerging and its production bursting in growth—is producing unexpected information. It has illustrated that the oxygen level drops when the infant is stuck with a needle for blood tests and, in a surprising tie-in to bonding theory, that just talking to the infant will cause a drop in acidity level.

Such discoveries are sustaining to staff, as when waterbeds, employed as a method of preventing depressed heads, surprisingly were found to decrease the problem of decelerated heart rate. On the other hand, many procedures remain controversial. For example, the administration of hormones to speed lung development is not used in some hospitals for fear of long-term effects. Some parents and staff are wary of subjecting these infants to a substance whose iatrogenic consequences, like those of DES,[1] may not show up for years. But to those working within this arena there is the constant challenge of new discoveries around the bend, new information that will enlarge the possibilities of saving more infants with hopes of better biographies.

So far the follow-up clinic is not yielding guidelines for continuance or withdrawal of treatment from doubtful cases, as hoped. The clinic's immediate value lies in imparting practical information to help parents. One parent's accidental discovery that running the vacuum cleaner was a substitute for the nursery noise which seemed to be needed for sleep, has been passed on to other parents. A grandfather's report of the irritability induced by the diuretic which both he and his infant granddaughter were taking is integrated with the evaluation of this drug. The liaison nurse, the follow-up nurse, and parents are learning together about the problems of coping with ICN infants and are forming family support groups to help parents while babies are hospitalized.

From the staff's perspective, the importance of follow-up care lies in the application of biographical information to the larger view of the

[1]DES (diethylstilbestrol) is a synthetic hormone (estrogen) which was used by pregnant women between 1941 and 1971. Problems of cervix and vagina are now being found in many DES daughters and minor genital tract abnormalities in DES sons.

birth trajectory. A $10,000 computer that stores information on all drugs and techniques used for each infant is being used to test hypotheses in the hope that over time the assumptions will be replaced by a firm knowledge base. Unit and hospital stakes are high, and a success rate is important justification for the whole enterprise.

The staff members themselves are being shaped by the extended birth trajectory. When the nursery census is high, the unit is hot and noisy with the beeping of machines. The work requires close attention. There is also a complication: since parents are both giving and not giving their child over to the staff, problems arise because of staff expectations and assessments of parents—judgments about parental qualifications for taking on this child, this artifact that the staff have sustained and nurtured by their skills and technologies. As hospital discharge approaches, further discordances appear; when parents have not conformed to staff values (frequency of visits, visible signs of bonding), staff will be much concerned over the social conditions of the child's future.

Today's birth-trajectory nurses are young and energetic, becoming bored when their learning begins to level off. They place high demands on themselves—how they should function, how much they should accomplish. Faced with the emotional strain and the intensity of the work on such a unit, these nurses are candidates for that technologically related work hazard, "burn-out" (Freundenberger 1974; see also Reichle 1975). Here, too, as for parents, the benefits and satisfactions of this work are incalculable, and individual, and as it is with parents, the staff response is complex. One obstetrical nurse expressed her mixed feelings regarding transport cases: "It's scary. The women may be sick and are terrified. Delivery of a premature or sick baby is emotionally traumatic. The nursing care is all technological—two ambulance sirens going. I, personally, get a kick out of it. It is exciting, intellectually stimulating to see these strange cases."

The effects of an extended birth trajectory are further evidenced in (1) new and expanded career lines, (2) changed hospitals, and (3) altered individual biographies.

1. *New and expanded career lines.* As already noted, the explosion in perinatology and neonatology has meant that new specialists have evolved and are involved with the increasingly smaller phases of the birth trajectory. Perinatologists rely during various phases on technical experts in specialties like ultrasonography and amniocentesis, as neonatologists do on specialists in radiology, ophthalmology, cardiology, and neurology. In order to qualify as a regional center, the labor and delivery unit must have a full-time obstetrical anesthesiologist who, as patient load increases, calls for increased staff and equipment.

Respiratory therapists are employed to help assess respiratory needs of infants, plan and execute this aspect of care, and upgrade physicians' and nurses' knowledge of respiratory function. Physical therapists are needed for babies who have had a prolonged stay in the ICN. These particular specialists help assess the infant's development; they exercise the baby, look at muscle tone, and watch for possible signs of cerebral palsy. Specialists on neonatal medical and nursing staff have evolved: they must be experienced, finely skilled, and attuned to every nuance in the given trajectory phase, since they are dealing with delicate bodies, and reversibility can be quick, unpredictable, and damaging.

Expanded services have led to a splintering of the role of the head nurse. Her new title, nursing care coordinator (NCC), is fitting since the major part of her work has to do with coordinating the many services that feed into the unit (for instance, in the nursery: laundry, X-ray, clinical laboratory, pharmacy, and central services for the massive amount of supplies). New middle-level administrative classifications, such as "staff development nurse," have been created to take over some of the former head nurse tasks, like the hiring and orientation of new nurses and their instruction on new equipment. In the labor and delivery ward a liaison nurse handles the administration of the alternative birth center and family follow-up; a master's-level perinatal clinical nurse specialist serves as resource person for transport and other high-risk patients and spreads new obstetrical knowledge to staff nurses and to outlying feeder hospitals.

The ICN has added a liaison nurse whose work also reflects the outward stretch of the trajectory. Families with babies who have spent long months in the nursery need support after discharge. Often these babies have immature nervous systems and are hyperirritable after months of continuous twenty-four-hour stimulation. Emotional adjustment places a huge strain on families:

> It's the isolation that gets to them. They are feeling trapped; they are afraid that the babies will get sick and be back in the hospital and they get to resent their responsibility. These were often first babies—the parents were active, young, vibrant people. If the babies are on oxygen at home, they can't be taken out of the crib. We do have a transport system, but it weighs 11 pounds.

The liaison nurse and the baby's primary nurse look for ways to make the parents' lives easier and contact continues long after hospital discharge. The liaison nurse also reflects the changed organizational structure brought on by regionalization of services. A large part of her job has to do with furthering the network of in-feeding hospitals and tactfully teaching staff nurses in these hospitals. Hers is a dual goal: to decrease mismanaged deliveries while maintaining good public relations in the service of an expanded referral pattern.

A social worker also assists in the support of families and, in conjunction with the above administrative nurses, in sensing and responding to the staff tension which mounts whenever ethical, quality-of-life issues arise. Because of the close interweaving of staff and family biographies, periodic "stress meetings" are held: one hospital's social worker holds weekly social service rounds, while another employs an ethicist, who holds monthly ethics rounds—an open acknowledgment of the need for identity work. Addition of a behavioral pediatrician to record and study infant behavior with computerized recording of a number of variables like sleeping and waking states, motor activity, color is another example of this felt need.

Further support is given to babies who are judged to require long-term evaluation by providing a follow-up clinic which is offered to all babies who fall within the following categories: those under 1250 grams; those with central nervous system bleeds; those who while on the respirator were given drugs to paralyze the musculoskeletal system; those who were given drugs to speed lung development; those who had cytomegalo virus, a respiratory infection that runs about 30 percent in premature babies; those with any other special conditions indicating a need for follow-up. This service is staffed by a nurse practitioner, a pediatrician, and a psychologist.

2. *Changed hospitals.* Since it is no longer economically feasible for every hospital to offer every service, in one of the hospitals that we studied the decision was made to focus on geriatric and newborn services. This was in keeping with two considerations. The hospital had a long tradition of support for family services, which could be continued by extending geriatric care and by encouraging family involvement in newborn care through open access to nursery, inclusion of siblings, rooms for parents when babies are hospitalized. The second consideration was economically realistic: reimbursement from the government is greater for critical care (including intensive care for the newborn) than for other services.

Intensive care nursery charges are high. In this hospital (as of 1978) beds were $472 for the most critical level, $333 for semi-intensive care, and $234 for recovery care. These charges covered physicians' and nurses' costs. The major impact on hospital biography lies in the generation of additional income. Every time a blood gas study was done, which could be as frequently as every 10 to 30 minutes, the charge was $35. Respirators cost $150 a day, a brain scan $300, and an X-ray $75. Then a new machine, the transcutaneous oxygen monitor, cost $50 for 4 hours, plus $25 every time the electrodes were shifted—every two hours. Chest tubes were $150 an insertion; suction catheters and gloves used, approximately $25 a day; hyperalimentation $100. "You can figure a baby on a respirator costs $1000 to $1200 a day, and that doesn't count extra procedures." Nursery charges represented a major part of the budget for X-ray and clinical laboratory services. What is more, the nursery provided enough income to cover other hospital losers: labor and delivery, the alternative birth center, postpartum, well-baby nursery, and pediatrics. The interdependency of these particular services may appear one-directional economically, but the needs are reciprocal. A skilled labor and delivery unit will funnel babies into the ICN through its management of high-risk mothers. In order to obtain residents to serve as house staff in the nursery, a full residency in pediatrics must be offered. Of course, knowing that one is being "carried by Big Brother" financially does not make for felicitous feelings: "We have a lot of pull in the hospital; there's resentment that we get a lot, like expensive equipment, which we do."

Other feelings are generated by this interdependency of services. Accusations of mismanaged deliveries—often not explicitly stated—are most often directed toward outlying hospitals, as already discussed. However, the accusations can be intrahospital as well. Disagreements may arise between obstetrical (perinatal) and pediatric (neonatal) staffs over subjecting a woman with a 24-week fetus to a cesarean birth—the former staff focused on what it will do to the mother, the latter on giving every child every chance. When the nursery census is low, wry comments are made about labor and delivery treating premature pregnancies with drugs and forestalling delivery. Conversely, transported mothers may be greeted happily by a labor and delivery unit that is experiencing a low census of patients or anticipated with groans by a nursery staff already under stress because of a high census.

3. *Altered individual biographies.* A third general consequence of the stretched-out birth trajectory lies in the shaping of various implicated individual biographies. These include the infant's biography, through the ICN's technology the infant has been given increased biographical time, but it is, in a sense, gestational time. The finished product is still unfinished—the nursery is, in effect, an institutionalized womb. Parents can get their child back at any time—in any shape. Logically, parents can say, "I don't like what you're doing," but structurally they are fatefully locked in. Nurses who remain in contact with these families are learning that the deep anxiety being experienced by parents, as well as any displeasure over staff management, is often suppressed

until the baby has been at home for quite awhile. Parental dependency is felt too keenly to risk disturbing the staff.

For parents of a premature or sick child the birth trajectory is of heightened relevance, forcing a new definition of their own biographies and what has happened to them—a realignment of expectations. The financial strain on them is substantial, sometimes causing bankruptcy. Only the very poor (for example, a four-member family making about $11,000 annually) qualify for state support. The rest incur liability proportionate to income before government funding takes over. Financial and emotional costs are interwoven:

> Some of these families are in turmoil. Their financial status takes a tailspin—they're having to live on a shoestring. One family lived in the country; they had birds and horses, lots of land, a nice home. They moved to be near the medical center. They feel trapped—their MediCal status is judged monthly. Only one of them can work, so they can keep their income down to qualify. MediCal doesn't count baby sitters. They express resentment and ask, "How long is this going to go on?"

Some babies are covered by private insurance, but obviously such coverage is not limitless. It is possible, as happened during our research, for a baby born at 27 weeks to be in the nursery for six months, coming close to a lifetime insurance limit of $250,000. In order to qualify for reinsurance, this particular baby cannot be readmitted to the hospital for two years, which places a tremendous, and probably impossible, burden on the family to keep her well. The resulting financial and psychological stress apparently drives some parents to the marriage counselor and perhaps ultimately leads to divorce. If the child is saved through medical intervention, there may still be months and years of turmoil and travail for the parents of a not altogether physically normal child.

Other Possible Large-Scale Consequences

What might be said, in addition, about other possible large-scale effects of the highly technologized ICNs and the extended birth trajectory largely produced by them? We dare to speculate a bit about this, since in fact nobody actually knows. What can be said is that there is increasing media coverage on how babies are saved through all this specialized technology, knowledge, and organization. And, correlatively, there is necessarily a heightening of public awareness, thereby, of the hospital as an increasingly technologized workplace and environment. Besides increasing the public's awareness, the media coverage is surely raising expectations of what can be done about babies, and more generally about illness, in these hospitals. ICUs, as we shall see in the next chapter, are very visible in the media and ICNs are undoubtedly central in their public imagery.

On the negative side, public distrust and antagonism to medical technology—perceived as contributing to depersonalized health care—cannot help but be fed by the experiences of parents who have had difficult and highly destructive relationships with ICN staffs (Stinson and Stinson 1979). Those particular parents are accusing these staffs of being so technologically, research-, and career-oriented that they are ultimately indifferent to parents' feelings and to the larger human implications of what they are doing.

> What sort of memories or thoughts could we have of Andrew? By the time he was allowed to die, the technology being used to "salvage" him had produced not so much a human life as a grotesque caricature of a human life, a "person" with a stunted, deteriorating brain and scarcely an undamaged vital organ in his body, who existed only as an extension of a machine. This is the image left to us for the rest of our lives of our son, Andrew. (Stinson and Stinson 1979, p. 72)

This kind of message cannot fail to have some impact on the public image of medical technology and of the ICNs.

The issue of equity is also raised by these wards and their work. Why should so much money be expended on so few births, rather than being spent on the nation's more pressing health needs (the United States, for instance, has an inordinately high mortality rate, contributed to mainly by our more poverty-stricken populations) or on illnesses that affect larger numbers of people? Questions are raised, too, about what kind of "ICN graduates" are being produced, since some proportion of them will be at least disabled and many will be chronically ill for their entire lifetimes. As one pediatrician said to us: "Somebody had better study that!" His exclamation points implicitly to a paradox, namely, that by saving infants the ICN staffs are contributing, in whatever measure, to the numbers of people who are chronically ill. These children constitute, in our terminology, persons whose trajectories have been very much stretched out. In fact these trajectories would never have begun or would have been quickly over if medical interventions had not been partly successful. If the halfway technology does indeed gradually produce visible evidence of its partial failure to a wider public, then, to return to the main theme of this section, this will be additional evidence that the work on those wards has consequences far beyond the narrow confines of the wards and hospitals themselves.

The Intensive Care Unit

The elucidation of macro-micro relationships will again be the major theme, but here those relationships will be sketched and analyzed more elaborately through discussion of the evolution of the ICU as an organizational form. Our intent is to bring out the complexity of macro-micro relationships and to suggest how that can be analytically ordered, focusing especially on actual or possible reciprocal impacts.

The section will take the following form: first, a very abbreviated list of changes in the ICU's organization and work over twenty years along with a few related changes in hospitals, machinery, and drug technology, the feed-in technological industries, the health professions and allied technical specialties, the federal government's actions relating to health care, and various extra-health industry social movements. This listing of this bundle of changes provides background illustrative material for sketching an analytic ordering of the above changes.

Our discussion requires conceptualizing social structure as not something "out there" or "above" the ICU as an organizational form, but as sets of structural conditions that (1) contribute to the patterning of events and processes and (2) also in some part are contributed to by those patterned processes and events. As remarked elsewhere (Strauss 1978, p. 101), the lines of impact can run either way. The name of the analytic game is to study changes over time—in the ICU case, over two decades—in an interactive/contextual fashion, rather than adhering to the more conventional model of one-directional causality.

1960: General Conditions
Health field
Prosperity
Lots of money for research
Health as a right beginning
Much faith in medicine
Developed medical centers—research and teaching, with government financing.
Explosion in drug innovation; big drug industry
Industrial and government money pouring into diagnostic technology
Machine industry rudimentary; small companies; many failures and consolidations
Heart machinery in forefront of innovation by engineers and physicians
Safety regulation emerging
Large hospitals
Specialties and subspecialties emerging, with appropriate hospital space
More support services emerging—(transport, maintenance, etc.)

Apparent deterioration of physical plant, many new hospitals built
Hospital administrators more professionalized, hospital administration more complicated
Government affecting hospitals through Blue Cross
Research, subspecialty surgery, general floor with different kinds of patients side by side
Sophisticated heart surgery
Knowledge base of medical specialization
Anesthesiology
Surgical techniques
Life-support systems
Pharmacological knowledge
Laboratory diagnostic technology
ICU
Lots of resources
High-risk patients: variety of types of trajectory, narrow range per type
Staff learning on job: nursing mostly unspecialized; chronic shortage of nurses; M.D.s, including residents and interns, with specialty backgrounds, but uncertain knowledge because of frontier medicine
Closed unit—inner sanctum
Sharp division of labor between ICU and surgical floor
Both LVNs and RNs staffing ICU
Not yet one-to-one nursing
Machines: discrete, bulky, experimental
Anesthesiologists and respiratory specialists the experts on life-support machines
Nurses' work: monitoring multiple machines and body systems
Physicians' work: monitoring periodically, backup and emergency; teaching-research involvement
Nurses learning from doctors
High morale
Tension between ICU nurses and nursing supervisors and central nursing administration
Life-saving syndrome
Impact of high patient mortality
Patients occasionally stay too long, sentient—which is awkward
Patterned interaction with kin, i.e., mostly avoidance.
1960–65: ICU Impact
Specialization
Cardiac specialization: knowledge, training, and procedures
Kidney specialization also
Nursing qua profession
Cardiac specialists
Some training in nursing schools
Professional organization (outside of American Nurses Association) exchanging information, workshops, etc.
Machine-tending anxiety
Tension about keeping patients alive too long—social death
Hospital
New hospitals, and old creating new spaces; impact on hospital architects
New procedures in ICN require new workers, then departments
New spaces for diagnosis and support services and various departments
Purchasing of equipment, tests of equipment, etc.
Procurement of supplies, machines; so many more com-

plex relationships with vendors, companies
Safety departments emerging (lots of accidents)
Government beginning to move in on ICU regulation
ICU expansion to smaller hospitals, specialization in larger ones
Range from acute to ambulatory wards; images of the future hospital
Outside services: increase of home care, visiting nurses, social services, etc., but fragmented

Industry
See above regarding explosion in development of cardiac machines
See also the changing hospital-company relationships
Drugs: innovation, improvement, stimulation of drug industry
Problematic trajectories require variety of improved drugs

General
Continuity of care issue: fragmentation regarding specialization concerns
Death and dying movement is only professional: nurses, social workers, ministers, a few psychiatrists
General growing awareness by public, with cardiac-kidney and ICU as consciousness-raising
Pacemakers and all the ICU equipment
Role of media
People talking about ICU
Health industry beginning to look different to public
Johnsonian image of battle: heart, cancer, stroke.

1965–70: Developments
Government war on poverty
Nation committed to health and payment for it
Money for medical indigents: impact on health industry, continuance of other conditions noted above
Professional nursing: psychosocial emergence; clinical specialists emerging; new modalities of nursing care experimentation; union movement now visible; continuation of professionalization

1970–75: ICU Impact

ICU developments
Diffusion of ICUs, spreading everywhere
Hospitals embracing them
Profitable
More specialized ICUs in the big hospitals
Every kind of surgery in them

Staffing
LVNs decreasing in big hospital ICUs, going into smaller hospital ICUs
Nurses and M.D.s trained in big hospital ICUs, then fan out to smaller centers
Nurses work in smaller and are recruited to larger
New technicians, such as respiratory therapists and other specialists, sharing nurses' previous work, also doing new work
Overlap in division of labor

More extensive knowledge base required of nurses
Highly specialized
Beginning to do increasingly interpretative work—major backup for the M.D.s: EKG, electrolyte balance, etc., i.e., junior M.D.s

Patients much sicker because of experimental surgery and neurological procedures—i.e., specialties doing more risky kinds of surgery
More research involvement as research assistants, keeping research records, etc.
Some work becomes SOP; always incorporating new things
Safety work; high risk constant
Psychosocial developments
Increasing number of coordinations for head nurse because of many new departments
Physicians
Highly experimental and research-oriented
Working with uncertain trajectories plus those produced by interventions
Finer specializations
Work with new departments increasingly complicated, consulting with many different kinds of personnel
As techniques improve, trajectories more risky, e.g., diabetic patients
Again increasing numbers of specialists working together
Medical specialties
Knowledge, training, procedures, and even operations
Cardiac transplant, kidney transplant
Machinery
All kinds of new machinery paralleling the teaching of surgical specialties and subspecialties
Environment of machines in walls, panels, etc.
Drugs
Continued explosion and increased range
Increasing hospital pharmacological specialization, professionalization, and departmentalization
Nursing
Growth of subspecialties; on-the-job training, also impact on nursing education
Nursing clinicians more specialized
Nursing administration: searching for new models of administration and move toward decentralization, but differentiation so marked, can't make any general rule: a nurse is a nurse
Need for upgrading of skills; in-service training now found everywhere
Hospitals
Small hospitals' ICU a moneymaker
Recruitment of new workers of various kinds
New departments
Recapitulation of larger hospitals ten years before on smaller scale
Large hospitals—competition for specialized space and resources
Administrators juggling additional problems
Larger hospital administrative departments
Larger and more specialized departments (safety, nuclear medicine, bioengineering, etc.)
More complicated relations with drug and equipment industries
Impact on the general scene
Patients' rights, informed consent: regarding research surgery and experiments

Bioethical issues now full blown, with specialization evolving
Public debate and awareness of bioethical issues
Death and dying movement now also a lay concern
Dehumanization and technology much more a public issue, with ICU and high technology imagery—and affecting public, flowing back to the professionals
Cardiac and kidney disease and cancer all hitting public awareness with their high technology and specialized hospital care
Increased medical costs
Alternate health care not just for hippies but a reaction to technological medicine plus the inability of technical medicine to handle many of the chronic illnesses

1975–83: The Larger Scene

General developments

Feminist movement
Nurses' autonomy movement increasing
Open wards
Patients' rights and kin rights
Crosscutting with consumer movement
Environmental movement and increasing focus on safety in general
Increasing antitechnological faith
Third World movement, affirmative action, although explosion of technicians not appreciably of Third World personnel; Third World employed in lower-order support services (transport, etc.)
United States still committed to health; increasing costs give rise to tension, constraints on expansion, etc.

Government

Safety regulation increasing
Technological assessment increasingly institutionalized
Cost containment now in operation
More scrutiny of hospital management and billing, etc.

Equipment industry

Continued small companies but some large ones
Giant ones for scanner, X-ray, etc., increased range of innovative feedback from hospital staffs
Larger range of equipment, with growth of specialization requirements
Computer and scanner the striking public image of high medical technology
Anti–government regulation trend

Hospitals

Location of multiple ICUs—whether centralized or on same floor or decentralized (i.e., cost versus efficiency and specialist control issues)
Architects' current hopeless dilemma of keeping up with innovation; also new philosophies of hospital architecture and reshaping of old space, juggling of space, constant remodeling, increased building costs
Plus more of the same conditions as during the last time period, but more intense and complicated.

ICU

Tripartite ICUs: graduated care, personnel and work to match

Constant production of new and problematic trajectories and sicker patients
Resources reduced, ICU patients sent quickly to other wards
Patients stabilized as quickly as possible
Patients less easily taught despite the teaching ideology; but need to teach patients (often coming from hundreds of miles away) about use of technology at home
Tremendous movement of patients in and out of ICU and hospitals, because they can be stabilized faster through technology
ICUs more expensive to run: staff, supplies, maintenance, etc.
Home care connections beyond the immediate postsurgical period provided
ICU and ICN type transport increased, systematized, networks formed with smaller hospitals
Public awareness of saving lives in the ICUs, people are drumming up more business for the ICUs. Nurses doing more teaching, liaison work

More of everything for nurses: research, interpretation, knowledge, specialization, clinical safety, coordination, maintenance
Coordination problems even more difficult
Increased phychosocial nursing, entering from feminist movement and internal to the profession
Nurses' monitoring of equipment and patients increasingly complex
"Burn-out" of increasing concern; high turnover of nursing staff
Some ICU personnel leave for home care and various kinds of patient teaching
Division of labor: nurses ceding tasks to technicians; also working together in an increasingly blurred division of labor.
M.D.s: more of the same as in preceding period; technicians taking over machine work and also interpreting results operationally. M.D.s increasingly dependent on technicians and specialist consultants.

Paradigm for Ordering Change

These data suggest rather clearly, then, not only that larger structural coditions affect the ICU as an organizational form, along with the work done on the ICU, but also that the reverse is true: the continually emerging organizational form and its work have a reciprocal effect on some of the macroscopic conditions. Having noted these phenomena descriptively, we ought to be able to take the next step of thinking about how this two-directional flow might be conceptualized. It is far easier, however, to argue how it ought not to be conceptualized than to suggest better alternatives. The following section represents our attempt to handle the obvious difficulties of providing analytic imagery that will do justice to the complexity and processual character of relationships obtaining between the ICU and the structural conditions impinging on *and* affected by the ICU.

There are various possible modes for examining the ICU data, none of them catching their complexity. For example, a linear, sequential description might be given of the ICU's development from 1960 to 1970, then from 1970 to 1980. Or an analyst might give sociological, political, economic, and ideological grounds for the sequential changes: thus a complex of structural conditions bearing on health care would have produced the characteristic organizational form by 1960, whereas a different complex of conditions produced the ICU of 1970, etc. (see Russell 1979, pp. 41–70).

In this kind of organizational analysis, the researcher tends to assemble a laundry list of formative conditions, each of which seems likely to have contributed to the organizational form in question. Sometimes ad hoc inferences will be made about the nature or extent of the contribution. Often the mechanics of it are not studied. Usually the contributions actually measured pertain to selected features of the organization such as size and types of personnel. This type of analysis may refer only to two phases (before and after) rather than three or more, let alone focus on a stream of relatively continual changes. Anyhow, these types of approach are definitely linear: one-way impact. The approach is also sequential: one phase after another or one set of changes after another. Such interpretative schemes, however, may include the concept of interaction among the determining conditions themselves, which then in turn act on the organizational form. (These characteristic analyses also apply to case studies of a single particular organization, such as a hospital or a business firm.)

Looking again at the ICU materials, one can begin by noting a series of *domains* (hospital, technology, medical specialization, etc.), each domain seeming to have an influence on the ICU. Most domains seem also to have interacted with each other. If we stopped with that analytic account, we would get a singularly oversimplified version of ICU changes, diagrammed as in figure 1.

A more complex scheme would involve breaking the unitary character of each domain into sets of conditions, as is often done in conventional sociological analysis. And, as in the latter, the conditions within each domain may interact. But in our paradigm, and as reflected in the previous description of ICU evolution, we conceive of them interacting in various ways. Condition *a* of domain 1 may affect condition *b* of

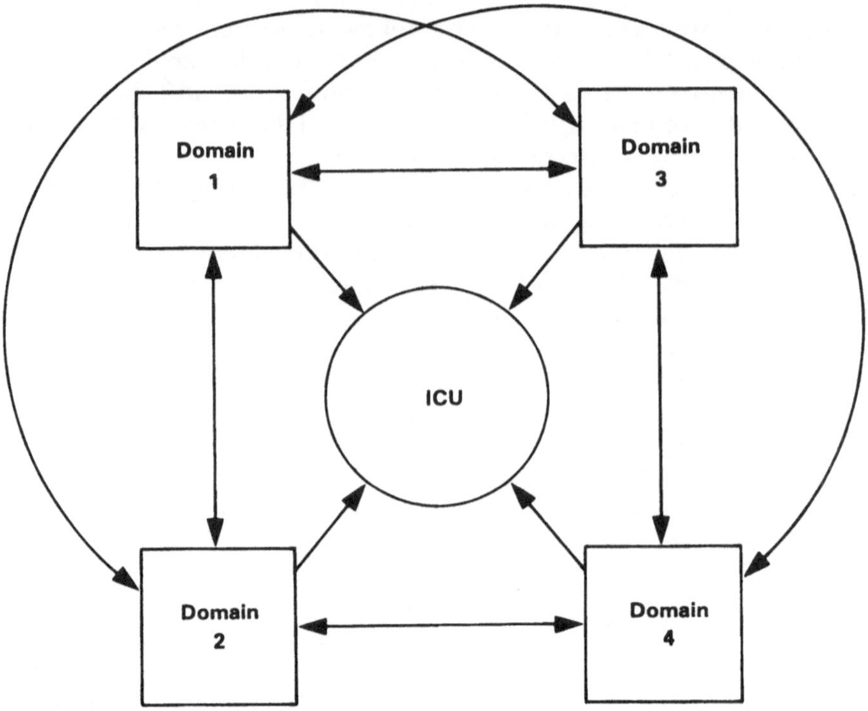

Fig. 1. Domain Influences

domain 2, or the impact can be reciprocal (same or different kind of impact). Or *a* and *c* can both impinge on *b*, but *b* only on *a*. Then, to make the picture more complex: domain 1 impinges on domain 2 not as a block unit; rather, different conditions interact or intersect, yet not all conditions do this.

The complexity indicated in figure 2 can be added to by noting also that over time the different conditions within domains will be changing at different rates: some relatively unchanging, some changing very much, some disappearing altogether, while others are just appearing. And why are they changing at different rates? Presumably because of the strength of various other conditions bearing on them in the contextual-interactive fashion diagrammed in figure 2. This differential rate of change is tantamount to talking about short-term and long-term changes.

But figure 2 needs to be modified again, since features of the ICU apparently have influenced various of the domains in return. Thus, the ICU also can be diagrammed as consisting of sets of conditions, with

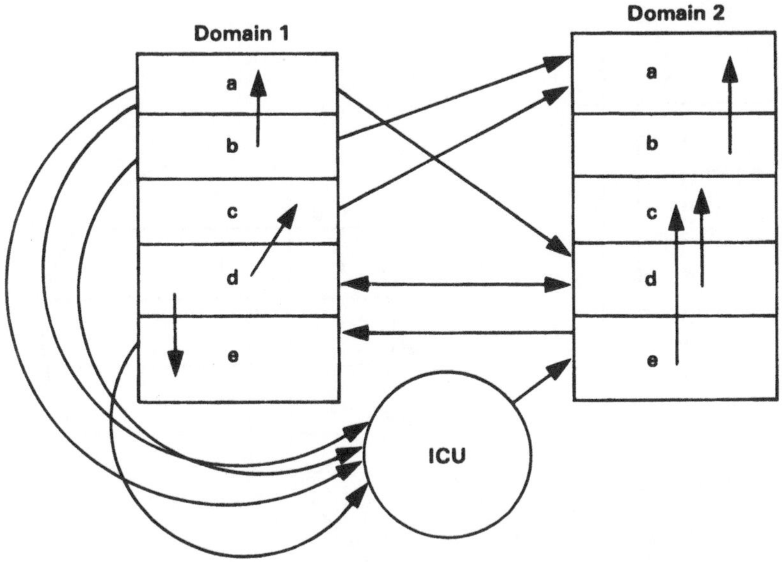

Fig. 2. Subdomain Influences

lines running to other specified conditions within domains 1 and 2 (see fig. 3).[2]

The two-way flow *over time* suggests a movement that is virtually "galactic"—the whole 1960 galaxy moving toward its 1970 state, and then to its 1980 state, and it encompasses all the interactions within and among domains, including the ICU domain.

Surveying this changing scene (looking not only at macro- but also microconditions), one cannot hope to grasp more than some of the contextual and interactive patterning. Into this amazingly complicated and disorderly reality, the analyst can expect only to put some modicum of analytic order. For our purposes, it is enough to suggest diagrammatically how the two-directional flow would need to be stud-

[2]In a similar observation Elihu Gerson (memo, April 1979, p. 3) has remarked that "a new organizational innovation . . . often requires new skills on the part of those who are to implement and carry out new arrangements. To the extent that these skills are rare, the diffusion of the new innovation will be retarded. In the world of organizations and technologies, schools may be founded to increase the supply of needed skills." Using an ecological metaphor, Gerson then notes that the schools "may in turn become the foundation of a new ecological niche in the system [and further illustrates that] the niche-creating and -defining activities of technologies, which may often as much run 'backward' in the resource chain as 'forward.'"

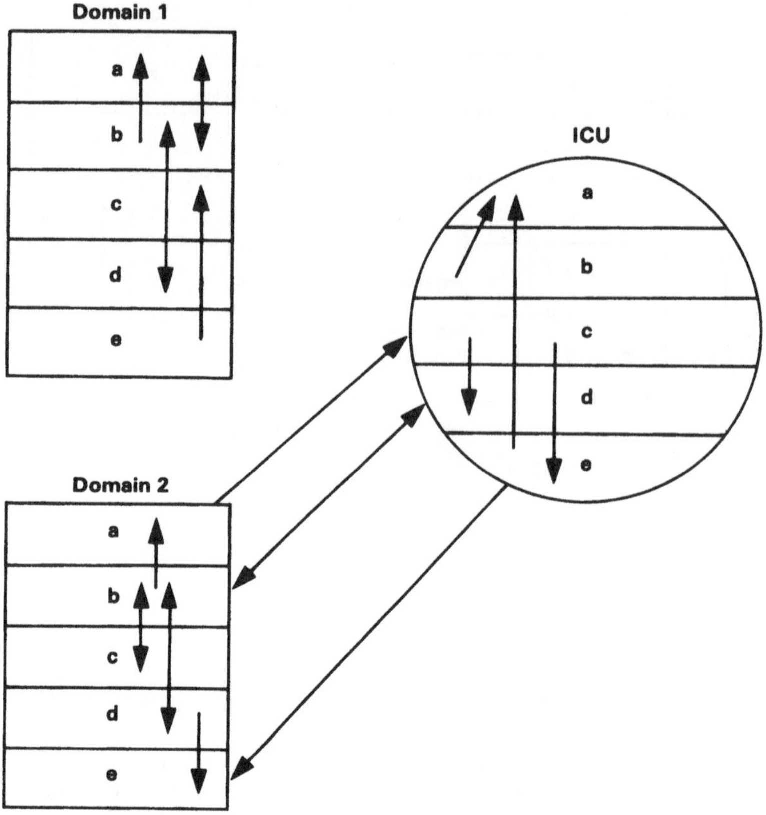

Fig. 3. Complex ICU and Domain Influences

ied, and its details specified, if one had that aim as a main purpose of investigation. For our own purposes, one of which is to combat the oversimplified notion that work is affected by larger structural (macro) conditions but not vice versa, we avoid, admittedly with relief, the difficult task of specifying exactly what impinges on what, under which conditions, how, and with precisely what consequences, in, assuredly, an extremely complicated interplay of relationships occurring over the entire two decades.

We can at least, however, assert this: whether looking at a type of organiation (*the* ICU) or a single organization (*an* ICU), the analyst is metaphorically quite like a movie-goer who is simultaneously watching several films and who must put together their events and story line in relation to one "main" film (ICU evolution). To do justice to the full complexity both of context and process, the analyst must absorb and integrate information from multiple domains. (However, those domains need to be discovered, their relevance specified and demonstrated as far as possible.) In the next chapter, in which several theoretical implications of our research will be discussed, we shall also note some implications of the "galaxy" metaphor for research into organizations and organizational change.

10
Theoretical Implications

In this final chapter, several important issues in the sociology of work and occupations/professions will be addressed. We can examine those issues in terms somewhat different from those found in their respective standard literatures because of implications resident in our analysis of medical work. The issues to be addressed are:

1. "Mistakes at work" (E. C. Hughes was the first to call attention to these)
2. "Dirty work" (another of Hughes's seminal ideas)
3. Information work
4. Body work
5. Clients: objects or participants in work?
6. Teamwork within organizational contexts
7. Negotiations and negotiative work
8. Division of labor
9. Temporal order and temporal matrix
10. Industries and interogranizational transactions
11. The sociology of work—but what work?

In addressing those issues, our aim is modest: we are concerned only with asking what happens to conventional perspectives on those matters when one looks at them not from the standpoint of occupations, professions, or organizational structure but of *work*. Our thesis here is that when work—conceived, planned, attempted, and sometimes accomplished—is taken as the path into those enduring issues, and into a few new ones, then additional dimensions, questions, directions for inquiry are opened up. Perhaps, too, work will seem somewhat different from its traditional forms. (See Hall's 1980 review of much of the recent American and French literature.)

Before taking up the issues themselves, it should be useful to list aspects of work especially emphasized in this book:

- collective or organized work done within organizational settings
- work done along a time line, with consequences for workers that in turn affect the line of work (i.e., trajectory)
- changing contingencies that alter the trajectory and its implicated work
- problematic trajectories and trajectory phases as well as routine, expectable trajectories and phases
- types of work entailed in doing the trajectory work, their relationships, their conditions and consequences
- work done on reacting objects (clients)
- work done on persons who may do some of the trajectory work themselves rather than merely responding to others' work
- work affected by arena disputes and by the ideological positions of the workers themselves

It will be useful to keep those points generally in mind throughout the following discussions since most approaches to the issues noted above emphasize occupation/profession, even when their authors indicate they are discussing work. It is difficult, of course, to talk about occupations without touching on their work: the question is one of relative emphasis and salience.

Mistakes at Work

E. C. Hughes's paper "Mistakes at Work" (1951) was instrumental in calling attention to the importance of this issue for the study of occupations and professions. Here are some of his points. Mistakes are found in all occupations since occupations are subject to contingencies contained in learning and maintaining skill. Occupations train their neophytes in proper skills so as to minimize the probability of mistakes at work. The mistakes made in some kinds of occupations (medicine) are more fateful than in others. Occupations build up rationales, collective defenses against outsiders (professionals against the lay world) in reference to the risk of their mistakes. Occupations are delegated certain things to do because other people (for technical, economic, psychological, moral or status reasons) do not wish to make the inevitable mistakes entailed in that work. A collegial group will stubbornly defend its own right to define mistakes and to say when one has been made—and the right to make such a judgment is jealously guarded. Hughes ends his paper by emphasizing, as one might expect from his emphasis on occupational rights, prerogatives, and jealously guarded terrain, that work is an object of moral rule, of "social control in the broadest sense."

The themes of social control and occupational/professional prerogative are carried over forcefully in writings and research on the medical profession by Eliot Freidson (1975), a student of Hughes's. But Freidson is considerably less trusting, much more pessimistic about, and also quite concerned about how outsiders can actually influence the professionals' deficient internal control over serious ("deviant" rather than routinely inevitable) collegial mistakes. Recognizing the lack of outsiders' expertise and arguing against the efficacy of external and especially administrative regulation, the weight of his argument is to advocate more effective and conscience-based internal controls. In short, he wants professions and occupations to be more responsible—more conscientiously self-regulatory—both for effectiveness (in minimizing mistakes and their consequences) and for moral reasons (for the good of the wider community).

In the same general vein, Bosk (1979), in a recent book (subtitled *Managing Medical Failure*), focuses on occupational behavior and self-regulation. He, too, finds that internal control over mistakes—though mistakes are difficult to minimize, manage, and even sometimes to define and evaluate—could be much improved if there were "corporate responsibility." As he says in his closing lines:

> the [professional] community needs some control of sanctions so that it is able to control malefactors within its own ranks. . . . At present, a physician's conscience is not only his guide but the patient's only protection. The patient deserves the protection not only of the individual's but also the collectivity's conscience. Beyond that the profession as a whole needs to raise its conscience about its public responsibilities. The collectivity needs to promote the structural changes that will build stronger accounting mechanisms into everyday practice. (P. 192)

In both Bosk's and Freidson's approaches to the issue of mistakes, distinctions are made between "inevitable" ones (routine and normal) and those that might well be preventable by better self-regulation. Stretching the point in the direction of political rhetoric: both men are saying that in a genuinely responsible democracy, the professions and occupations ought to be more conscientiously responsible to the rest of society. Neither man is primarily interested in the intricacies of "mistakes at work," but rather in showing contemporary deficiencies in the control of bad work—work so bad, so unprofessional, as to be potentially harmful, even fateful, to us clients (see also Millman 1977).

Occupational control aside, there are several other characteristics of the writings reviewed above, and also of a paper by Stelling and Bucher (1973) on medical trainees' acquisition during socialization of occupational rationales, which minimize identity damage to themselves when making mistakes associated with the uncertainties of medical work. To begin with only physicians are in focus, rather than the total range of actors in the medical drama. Their work is not examined in terms of the medical process itself, the trajectory, but in more static terms: mistakes at diagnosis or when treating patients. The impact of mistakes is limited in these writings to issues of clinical safety; generally ignored are the consequences for efficiency, efficacy, equity, cost, for the organization itself or for the workers (or for clients other than their safety). The lack of intense focus on medical work, rather than on the occupation, insures that mistakes associated with each of the different types of work (comfort, safety, etc.) are missed. The clients' minimizing, preventing, discovering, and rectifying of the professionals' mistakes are all missed, as are the many ways, both formal and informal, that professionals also do those things.

When sociologists focus on work itself in relation to the mistakes made when doing the work, that shift of perspective enables some correction of those limitations of the occupational approach. Two examples are provided by the writings of Riemer (1976) and Glaser (1976). The former has studied mistakes made during the construction of buildings, focusing on: (1) the structural conditions for different kinds of error, many of which are quite inevitable given those conditions; (2) the different types of error by phase of what we have termed the arc of work; (3) the workers' tactics to keep their errors secret; (4) the consequences of error in the decreased quality of the building; and (5) the clients' responses if, immediately or later, they discover the errors. Glaser's detailed examination of how a "patsy" supervises the home-building of subcontractors and their workmen represents a specifically processual approach both to the construction work and to the potential mistakes entailed in that work. His approach allows him to specify potential errors per phase of the arc of work, as well as consequences of errors (to structural design, taste, cost) and the patsy's strategies for, and difficulties with, minimizing or rectifying error. Furthermore, various structural conditions are carefully linked with all of those phenomena.

A third research example of focus on work, which also includes attention to mistakes, can be found in the writing of L. Star and E. Gerson (forthcoming) on scientific work. They note that when in the course of scientific inquiry an unexpected finding occurs, then the question is: should it be attributed to a mistake in the work? Or is it an "artifact" (attributable to defective instrumentation, etc.)? Or does it point to a genuine discovery? Deciding which of those three it might be entails, first of all, reviewing possible sources of error, and if indeed it is a mistake, then eliminating that source. Star and Gerson note that in deciding whether the mistake (or artifact or discovery) is genuine, "there is also room for differences of opinion"; "as a result negotiation" will take place within "this ambiguous context." This situation of unexpected mistakes-artifacts-discoveries is not at all unusual but is part of the customary business of scientific work.

The Glaser, Riemer, and Star and Gerson studies illustrate how a direct and detailed examination of work itself can focus analytic attention on features of mistakes at work other than that of noting the deficiencies of professionals' self-regulation for maximizing the safety of their work (see also Olesen and Whittaker 1968, pp. 176–77 and 248–49). Our own research as presented in this book incorporates those features and suggests additional issues to be considered in future research of mistakes entailed in doing work. Discussion of these probably need not be extensive since all of our points have already been mentioned, adumbrated, implied, or even illustrated throughout the text of this book (see also Fagerhaugh et al., forthcoming).

As a prologue to our discussion, we will introduce the term *error work* to refer to the various tasks involved in preventing, minimizing, defining, detecting, covering up, rectifying, estimating the consequences of, and so on, mistakes. Doing those things involves work, too!

Analytic consideration of mistakes begins with the central activity itself (whether that is caring for patients, constructing buildings, or manufacturing automobiles). What is its nature and what are its salient properties? What are the arcs of work—with associated kinds and levels of tasks—entailed in the activity? The central activity provides the context and conditions for probable mistakes, their types, when they appear, where they appear, who will make them, the degree of difficulty in rectifying them, the types of consequences of mistakes made or rectified; also what risks are balanced against consideration of various types of potential errors and their estimated consequences. Consequences of error will relate not only to types of consequences (see p. 000) and to where in the arc of work it occurs, but to the properties of error itself as defined by various participants in the work. These properties of error include at least: seriousness, predictability, frequency of occurrence, rate, number and kinds of persons involved, number and kinds of actions involved, discoverability, cumulative impact on other errors whether intentional or unintentional, and rectifiability.

Different trajectories will provide different conditions for potential errors, as well as for probable strategies in preventing, rectifying, and the like. Diabetic trajectories, cancer trajectories, and heart failure trajectories each involve quite different arcs of work, quite different kinds and sequences of tasks, quite different calculations of risks of medical intervention or nonintervention, of organizational resources necessary to maximize successful work. The same is equally true for Glaser's or Riemer's construction work: different kinds of error work are entailed in building small houses or high-rise buildings, for small houses on different geographical terrain or in different climates, and so on. Likewise, manufacturing small automobiles, large ones, or trucks each entails different potential errors, hence of error work. Calculating these potential errors, preventing them, or minimizing their occurrence, rectifying them if they occur or at least blunting their dire consequences—all call forth organized efforts that will certainly vary for different types of trajectories. And this specific further organization of work will also increase the probability of additional mistakes, hence of error work before or after the committing of mistakes.

Different trajectory phases entail different error work. This point hardly needs elaboration beyond noting that different kinds of trajectories have different phases, both expected and unexpected, with each phase potentially necessitating somewhat different error work. Of course, the same trajectory will have different phases, too, each calling for possibly different emphasis in, or kinds of, error work.

An especially important property of any trajectory which affects error work is its relatively problematic or standard character. The same is true of its phases. Highly problematic trajectories, as we have seen, entail uncertainties attending the constituent tasks; these uncertainties greatly increase the probability and even cumulative impact of certain kinds of mistakes stemming from the tasks themselves, from possible consequences of doing the tasks (e.g., administering new drugs), and even from the organization of error work itself, which can lead to unanticipated new mistakes.

Error work can be viewed as the mirror image of trajectory work. So far we have emphasized that error work should be viewed as an important aspect of trajectory work. But another way of conceptualizing the relationship of trajectory work and error work is that for every step and for every operation planned and done there are potential errors. Mistakes are inevitable, or at least probable, made by someone, at some time, during the carrying out of every single task. Alas, none are so simple, so easily done, as not to make error possible. And not only because of workers' lack of skill, knowledge, motivation, or because of boredom or tiredness, or other individual or aggregate-derived conditions but by structural conditions (indeed all the former conditions are ultimately affected by the structural conditions, too). The point can be illustrated graphically for work on illness trajectories by citing the instance of a brochure advertising "Nursing Care Labels," published by the United Ad Label Co., Inc.: this brochure includes about 250 message labels such as "on hypersensitive drugs," "allergic to penicillin," "reorder narcotics," "save all urine." There are also seven checklists of about a hundred items. Essentially these all represent things to be done or noted, and each can be the source of at least one mistake (and probably more)! Of course, these do's and don'ts represent only some of the actions that need to be carried out for patients, each action harboring potential "goofs."

Different levels of work along the total arc entail different task structures (tasks, sequences, relationships, and implicated organizational resources for carrying out the tasks); *hence error work will vary by level.* In this book, three levels were noted (chap. 7): first, work in planning, designing, redesigning when necessary, and generally overseeing the total arc, done by the physician or physicians in charge of the case; second, the articulating of operational work, most of it done by the head nurses; third, the carrying out of a host of operational tasks, done by all who are involved in each step of that work. (Of course, additional levels could be distinguished, depending on the researcher's analytic purposes, and lines of work in different industries involve various numbers and kinds of levels of work.) Clearly the level of work will directly affect the error work and, of course, the division of labor in handling that work.

The different types of work that form component strands or dimensions of the total arc of work—whatever that arc may be—are characterized by different error work. The latter can, of course, differ in kind, degree, preventability, rectifiability, ease or difficulty of definition or detection, and the like. Mistakes characteristic of machine work are rather different from those that arise in doing sentimental or comfort work; correspondingly their prevention, definition, detection, rectification, and other error management tasks will vary.

A corollary to the preceding point is that mistakes in one type of work, and their management, can impinge on other types of work. In this book, we have seen many illustrations of this phenomenon: errors in machine work having consequences for kind and degree of safety work, "snafus" in sentimental work having consequences for comfort work and vice versa, and so on. Since the types of work may vary for different kinds of activities (medical, commercial, manufacturing, or the like) the investigator needs to analyze the component types of work, the error work entailed in each, *and* the consequent salient interactions. Otherwise, the analysis will fail to encompass much of the actual complexity of error work that occurs in the realm of the activity under investigation.

Clients may participate in doing error work. This point follows directly from the consideration that clients not only react to work done on or for them, but, in varying degrees, may be involved in the work process itself. In this book, patients have been seen working hard preventing, minimizing, assessing, detecting, and rectifying—and debating about—the errors committed by staff. There is every reason to believe that the clients of other practitioners and service people do likewise. Of course *their* error work may produce further errors and so add to other people's error work as well as have consequences for the clients themselves, including the necessity for more of their own error work.

Error work can have multiple types of consequences, differently viewed by various workers or bystanders. One aspect of error work is an estimation (before) or calculation (after) of the impact of error work. But impact on what? Safety? On whose safety: workers, clients, bystanders, environment, the general public? Or is the impact upon cost? On quality of work? On worker efficiency? On the efficacy of the work? On individuals' or collective morale? On identity? On careers? Phrased that way, it is clear that different actors in the work drama may well be: (1) assessing error work impact along different dimensions, as well as (2) giving different priorities to the dimensions themselves insofar as these other dimensions are taken into account.

This tells us also that those assessments may be matters of debate—both in balancing whether risks are worth taking that may entail errors (and error work) and their consequences and, afterwards, in allocating blame for the perceived consequences. Those debates also must be viewed by the analyst as part of the total work engaged in by the workers. These are not merely debates, for they become woven into later sequences of work as conditions which affect that work. Debate can even be institutionalized, as in the instance of governmental commissions or inquiry boards that recommend organizational changes, which will minimize future potential error, and these changes then will affect future conditions of work.

It can now be seen that the Hughes, Freidson, and Bosk emphasis on occupational self-regulation is focused on concern with just one set of consequences—safety, particularly the safety of clients in terms of faulty practitioner work, and so ultimately the greater good of society. The direction of corrective error work suggested by sociological or other commentators may differ, but the focus of the commentary or critique is on client-to-society safety only. It is worth noting that even that portion of government regulation which is addressed to industrial or occupational safety issues actually covers a wider range of safety issues: namely, worker safety and environmental safety, perhaps even moral safety. So the sociological literature on "mistakes" is extraordinarily narrow in its analytic scope. Moreover, it is so entwined with political and moral considerations that in its recommendations for improvement of client safety it precludes enough detailed analysis even of this one consequence of error that it insures that its recommendations—as a rectification strategy—will not increase the errors or have other distressing consequences, such as decreased quality of work or increased cost to clients or government.

Dirty Work

"Dirty work" is another phenomenon called to our attention as worthy of study by E. C. Hughes (1971). Again emphasizing moral order and occupation/profession, as much or more than work itself, Hughes noted that "Dirty work of some kind is found in all occupations. It is hard to imagine an occupation in which one does not appear, in certain repeated contingencies, to be practically compelled to play a role of which he thinks he ought to be a little ashamed morally" (p. 343). And work becomes dirty perhaps when "it in some way goes counter to the more heroic of our moral conceptions." Hughes pointed to kinds of work that have low status in given occupations or professions, such as the practice of lawyers who handle "the less respectable legal problems of even the best people" (p. 326) and the hospital workers who "perform the lowly tasks without being recognized among the miracle workers" there (p. 307). Hughes also noted the phenomenon of a profession's being connected in some way with work not considered respectable in the larger society, for example, medicine's connection with abortionists and quacks. Hughes does make a twofold typology, but only in passing, distinguishing between work that is physically disgusting, as that of garbage-collecting by janitors, and work that is symbolic of degradation, that is, "something that wounds dignity." Given Hughes's concern with moral order and with occupations, he quickly turns even physically disgusting work into a discussion of degradation, noting that the janitor's physical disgust is not just a reaction to filth but to tenants who, to quote one janitor, "don't cooperate—them bastards" (pp. 343–44).

From time to time Hughes's concept has been referred to by others, but there has been, as far as we know, only one attempt to examine dirty work per se. Emerson and Pollner (1976) reported on research into the activities of psychiatric emergency teams in a regional community mental health clinic. Therapeutic work was what the teams esteemed and had been trained to do, but some of their work they called "shit work,"

> referring to cases in which they were prevented from doing anything for the clients' betterment because of the hopeless and resistant character of clients and their situations. . . . The archetypical nature of "shit work" consisted of a case in which [the emergency team] was not only unable to do for, but one in which they had to do something to a person . . . often without his consent and often in the face of his open and active opposition. (P. 218)

Emerson and Pollner argue that the work itself is not dirty but is designated as such by the workers, a conclusion not at all at variance with Hughes's position. They also draw conclusions from their data about the consequences of dirty work designations: "They function publicly to reaffirm performance criteria, to express moral distance from a particular [discrediting] performance, and to tutor an observer [such as the researcher] into the preferred interpretation of a particular transaction" (p. 243). The Emerson and Pollner paper, then, follows through on Hughes's occupational and moral-order perspective, relating observations of the work itself to that perspective. No close examination of the work itself is made.

Our own discussion is again an attempt to supplement that kind of perspective by making work itself more central. In an earlier chapter, dirty work was discussed in relation to the broader category of comfort work; here we turn to more general considerations.

Dirty work is a potential aspect of all work and all tasks. Rather than thinking of dirty work as a special class of work, it makes analytic sense to regard all work and tasks as potentially definable (by workers or onlookers) as being dirty *or* having dirty aspects. We emphasize the underlined "or" for this reason: while whole bundles of tasks may be regarded as physically or socially unpleasant or distasteful to perform (and so certain persons or classes of people are delegated to do this work part-time or totally), nevertheless, literally any arc of work can have dirty aspects—if not right now, then later under different circumstances. "Different circumstances" here can mean changed organizational conditions which make the work now more difficult or unpleasant or changed workers themselves who now find the work much less satisfying or even demeaning in their newly acquired statuses.

The bundle of tasks that comprise "the work" can become sufficiently altered, so that the work is regarded as dirty work when the proportion of satisfying versus unsatisfying tips in the direction of the unsatisfying. Hence, any arc of work, or multiplicities of arcs, can become redefined in the direction of degree of dirtiness. In fact, as everybody recognizes, even the most gratifying work has its less satisfying moments or aspects, suffered only because it has to be suffered or because the balance still tips in the direction of nondirty work. When the work itself alters, or is altered by orders from above, then the balance can, of course, tip drastically in the other direction.

The aspects of work and tasks deemed dirty are of several kinds. In the writings of Hughes and Emerson and Pollner, there is an emphasis on dirty work as dishonorable, morally shameful, discrediting to the worker's status. This seems not to exhaust what is called dirty work, regardless of the synonym used (scut work, shit work) by workers themselves—either those actually engaged in the work or others who are lucky enough to escape it. Some work is extremely routinized, boring, completely *unchallenging.* It may have been exciting when one was a novice at doing it, but it has long since become completely humdrum, even so deadening that one longs to be released from the necessity or command to do it. Whatever games one invents to jazz up these uninteresting tasks have worn thin, and the worker simply "wants out." Another type of dirty work consists of tasks so *exhausting or stressful* as to tip toward the nongratifying and so ultimately the dirty side of work. Possibly another kind consists of highly *dangerous* tasks which are not counterbalanced by personal challenge or other rewards for service, such as some jobs that soldiers must carry out because of command or contingency. Still another type of dirty work is that which is literally so *physically dirty* as to be distasteful and even horrifying or dread-producing (Hughes 1971, pp. 343–44). The blood-urine-feces handling of nursing personnel, as described earlier in this book, is an instance of this class of dirty work. That work constitutes, we should add, only a portion of their comfort work. Workers in other occupations have similar dirty, even filthy, tasks to handle—domestic workers, housewives, garbage collectors, garage mechanics, workers in industries like oil and gas, come readily to mind—but some occupations have virtually none of this particular type of dirty work. Finally, there is work that is *symbolically dirty*—socially and personally dishonorable or discrediting. (This is the Hughes and Pollner and Emerson type of dirty work.) Included in this category perhaps should be not only immoral but also illegal work and work defined as "senseless" or as harmful to clients or bystanders.

Though these several types of dirty work can be distinguished analytically, like other types they can be blurred in real life. Hence, a given set of tasks can be dull and exhausting or exhausting and symbolically dirty or dull, symbolically dirty, and filthy—the workers themselves not necessarily distinguishing among these different dimensions of their distasteful work. (We shall turn to those dimensions or types of dirty work when discussing the consequences of doing or being made to do various of them.)

Proportions of dirty work tasks can vary not only by different trajectories but by trajectory phases. The first point is obviously true; the second perhaps less so because it is more subtle. Since the total arc of envisioned work for a given trajectory carries a potential for degrees of boredom, exhaustion, necessary but filthy tasks, and so on, it follows that different sequences of its tasks, as during trajectory phases, may have different proportions of displeasing or discrediting tasks anticipated or later recognized. In fact some workers will plan on or spontaneously "make themselves scarce," disappearing during those boring, dirty, exhausting, generally nongratifying phases. (That moves the discussion into how workers minimize their share of dirty work, a topic that will be explored later.)

Different types of work may entail, for some or different workers, different proportions of dirty work. The researcher into any occupation or line of work needs to distinguish, as we have done for medical work, among different kinds of work entailed in the central activity itself. This is necessary in order to make fine analyses of how dirty work relates to the central activity. Some comfort tasks are boring to some nurses, while other comfort tasks are exhausting to other nurses, and still other comfort tasks are just plain filthy to do and are without counterbalancing rewards for some nurses. Sentimental work with certain patients may be deemed exhausting or even discrediting, and someone, if asked by a superior to do it, may demur or actually refuse the work. A staff member may glory in doing therapeutic tasks that involve physically filthy work, while glossing over certain safety tasks because these are boring or exhausting. In short, any fine-grained analysis of dirty work requires specification of what kind of dirty work is being analyzed, that is, the precise relations of the dirty work to important dimensions of the total work.

Work with clients involves their potential reaction; hence the analysis of dirty work must also include a focus both on that reaction and the worker's anticipatory or post hoc response to it. The clients may be apologetic because the task that they request or necessitate is exhausting or routine. The clients may be ashamed because their conditions—or automobile or whatever—are causing filthy work for the servicing agent. A client, in the end, may actually cause more dirty work for the agent by attempting to do his or her own work and failing at it. In turn, the servicing agents may have a clients's response in mind in doing, or deciding to do, a vastly unpleasant task, and so mask their own deeper responses to the work at hand. Simultaneously, they may be handling the client's overt, or imagined, reactions to being the cause of their having to do this scut work, shit work, or other kind of dirty work.

Dirty work can be increased or decreased by varying organizational conditions. Since work is always done in structural contexts, it follows that organizational conditions will help to make some tasks physically or psychologically easier and some more difficult. When these tasks become defined as too difficult—too exhausting, boring, symbolically discrediting—then they are no longer nondirty work. In the chapter on comfort work, we saw that routine or filthy tasks can be carried off as part of the day's customary work, providing there is adequate resource for accomplishing these tasks: sharing by other personnel, time to do the work, flexibility in when to do the tasks, adequate supplies for doing them, and the like. If any of those resources diminish sufficiently—presto, dirty work, against which the assigned staff member may complain and attribute blame against a culpable colleague, too. We especially emphasize the organizational conditions since they are potentially so changeable in many lines of work, moving the boundaries thereby of what workers will consider acceptable and not acceptable "conditions of work."

Workers' strategies for preventing, minimizing, or avoiding dirty work are related to various conditions, including organizational, ideological, and trajectory-phase ones. Everybody knows that scut work and shit work can be avoided or minimized by several different strategies, and there are common terms for these: passing the buck, delegating, trading off, cutting corners, doing the job last or first, taking revenge by doing the job badly, engaging in gallows humor, creating personal games to make the time pass faster, or parodying the work. The work can also be transvalued upwards, psychologically mitigating or eradicating its distasteful character by turning it into important and so gratifying work, as when nurses' comfort tasks are regarded as therapeutic work, especially if these require skill and experience. All these strategies, however, whether resorted to consciously or subliminally, are greatly affected by structural conditions. Some conditions are organizational, that is, they influence the resources of time, energy, supplies, space, and the like, bearing on the success or failure or even probability of using a given strategy. Ideological considerations, for instance, beliefs about the ultimate importance of certain otherwise very dirty tasks, may affect these strategies, too. And, of course, trajectory conditions will immediately impinge on the possibilities of utilizing one strategy or another for managing unwanted work. What is true of conditions bearing on workers' strategies is undoubtedly also true for those employed by well-intentioned superiors who wish to prevent or minimize the workers' dirty work.

Redefining types of dirty work from those that are not especially enhancing or discrediting identity to those that are, or vice versa, is related to arena processes (see Gerson, 6 August 1981*b*, the source of ideas used freely in the lines below). Some types of dirty tasks (routine, unpleasant, filthy, dangerous) are not particularly honoring or discrediting of identity unless so defined, either by oneself or others. Instead of thinking of definitions as formed simply by individuals or persons with whom they interact, we can profit from noting that ideological and positional debates can swirl around the kinds of tasks (and "work") that are to be regarded as degraded or honoring. Work "is dirty by definition, not only by the person doing it, but by definition of *multiple* audiences . . . some of these audiences may be likely to convert some kinds of scut work into [discrediting] work, while at the same time other audiences might be trying to convert aspects of the same . . . work into positive virtues, deserving of honor" (Gerson 1981*b*). Participants in these arenas and debates are not only representatives of various occupational and professional communities, but of other interested social worlds, which have stakes in the outcomes of the debates. This mode of looking at struggles in the definition of tasks and work gives a more processual cast to both our earlier discussion of task transvaluation upward and downward and to Hughes's concept of self-defined or other-assigned occupational dirty work.

Finally, the consequences of voluntary or involuntary engaging in dirty work will vary in accordance with all the conditions touched on in the immediately foregoing pages. So will the *range of consequences*, whether for workers and worker relations, for future work's efficiency or efficacy, for the organization itself or its organizational segments, for the implicated occupations/professions, or for the larger society. It is impossible to trace those consequences in any consistent analytic fashion unless the varieties of dirty work are related to trajectories, trajectory phases, types of implicated work, structural conditions for the arc of work, and the other relevant issues touched on above.

Information Work

Humans, as well as being talking beings, are talkative, so talk is inevitably part and parcel of their cooperative work. Chimpanzees carry out their joint tasks with only information-bearing gestures. Men and woman talk *about* their work *during* work and *after* work, and sometimes their talk is the very heart *of* the work itself. (See Johnson and Kaplan

1980 for these distinctions.) In this monograph, we have often touched on but not given separate treatment to the passing of information, which is integral to trajectory work and its component tasks, but now we shall discuss a few implications of our research for the topic of *information work* as such.

Research about people's work, including information about it or passed during the course of that work, may utilize questionnaires, interviews, and/or field observations. The use of questionnaires to gather data has long been looked upon with wariness by social scientists whose own predilection is for the alternative forms of data gathering (see the Becker and Geer exchange with Trow, 1957). Their argument is that questionnaires are likely to elicit selective, misleading, or even false reports, whereas interviews and fieldwork give a higher probability of valid data. Yet, as we all know, when people are interviewed about their work, their talk can also be misleading, not only because speakers wish to conceal the true state of affairs but because they frequently fall back on stereotypical or normative language which does not accurately reflect how they really carry out their work. For getting around these interview difficulties, there are standard methods (asking canny questions, probing, confronting, etc.), and recently Fritz Scheutze (n.d.) has proposed a form of narrative interview that makes possible a reasonably reliable separation of wheat from chaff. Besides, there are many interview situations and actual situations where people talk quite openly, truthfully, and accurately about aspects of their work. Fortunately, also, sociologists who study work are disposed toward field investigations, hence are not so plagued with validity questions bearing on the ways and whys of people's actual work. In field notes, they record what they have seen and heard people do and say while carrying out various tasks, using both sources of data for their analysis. Curiously enough, however, there has been very little focus on the passing of information as a special aspect or form of work. Of course, reference to information work is made in other terms, as in our own previous writings about the concealment of information or about what gets written into or omitted from medical charts (Glaser and Strauss 1965; Fagerhaugh and Strauss 1977), but this kind of reference does not represent a steady focus on information work as such. On the other hand, traditional approaches to information systems and information theory seem not to have been very useful for sociologists' study of work, the chief reasons being, perhaps, that organizational and situational contexts are underplayed and that the meanings of work to the workers are not an important consideration in those approaches. As E. Gerson (1981*a*) has noted, the flow of information involves reflexivity and often sentiment, each needing consideration in the analysis of information work.

Recently, F. Johnson and C. Kaplan (1980) have employed an ethnomethodological approach to the "talk in the work" of computer operators and computer users, examining closely both the interaction between these parties and their utterances while working together. This approach, while having the virtue of focusing directly on the interweaving of talk and activity, nevertheless, seems more honed in on the talk itself. For our purposes, however, it is more important to note that the approach, at least in this paper, neither reflects a very complex analysis of the talk during work nor addresses relationships between this procedural talk and talk before and after the carrying out of tasks. In addition, the sociologist of work should attack the issues of what information does not get transmitted, by whom, to whom, and why, as well as what information is sought and when. The overriding aim, then, is to illuminate how the flow of information is implied in and makes possible the organization of work discussed in monographs like ours. In Gerson's words, when commenting on "*information* or communicative *work*. . . . every kind of work involves some kind of information production/construction/consumption/use. . . . The handling and processing of information therefore is part of the task structure of every kind of work" (1981*a*, p. 7). Not to be overlooked, though, is that this information work must be related both to the arc of work itself and to the larger structural contexts that bear on all the work. We follow this dictum below, organizing the discussion around, before, during, and after the task talk; those distinctions are convenient but misleading unless related to the arc of work.

Talk during the carrying out of tasks can be varied, depending on the nature of the task and its context. We have in mind not the conversations that constitute play or are unrelated to the task itself, but talk directly required to get the task done. In this book, readers will have noted staff (and patients) doing their respective jobs—jobs that could not be done or done properly without accompanying speech. For instance, technicians request the patient to position his or her body. Or during a cardiac catheterization, the working parties feed orienting information to each other, report on procedural results, explain to each other what they are about to do or have just done, verbally work out "bugs" in their procedures, quickly make decisions when emergencies arise. They may also teach, correct, or reprimand each other, as part of getting the work done properly. Again, tasks that involve different kinds of machines will call forth quite different information from the workers, depending on what the equipment does, how safe it is, what the associated procedures are, what parts of the patient's body they deal with, and so on. It is important to recognize that all such issues will vary according to what phase in the trajectory, where in the arc of work, the tasks fall.

Information can also be linked as *microtasks* that enable a larger procedural task to get done. For instance, a postsurgical patient reports, and complains, to a nurse about his discomfort; the latter reports to the resident; the resident finds and examines the patient's X-ray film, locates a possible source for the discomfort; he then tells the nurse and informs her that she may use a given strength of morphine to relieve the patient's discomfort.

Procedural tasks involving two or more people and a series of interlocked actions can be done without any or much informational talk, especially if the procedures are routine. But the less familiar, the more serious, and the more "tricky" will almost inevitably involve transmitting necessary procedural information.

What we are emphasizing here is that the researcher must do two things: first, analyze the subspecies of talk (commands, requests, reports, reassurances) that occur while the task is being done; and second, relate these and their consequences specifically to the organizational (structural) conditions under which they occur. Both analytic jobs bear directly, precisely, and richly on how the division of labor actually operates in getting the work accomplished.

Work with clients involves them in the procedural talk. This statement is simply a reiteration of something that tends to get lost unless the researcher focuses on the clients, too—namely, that they can be an important part of the division of labor. Their contribution is easily seen in the diagnostic interviews with them, when they must report on various relevancies of their medical biographies and answer the professional questions directed at them. But, as amply illustrated in our chapters, during procedural or other staff work they may report, question, correct, complain, negotiate, and in other ways affect—and improve—the carrying out of tasks. What is true of medical work is certainly no less characteristic of that engaged in by workers in other occupations (law, police, social work): with clients seeking, demanding, offering, being asked for various items of information that are necessary to, or at least affect, the work at hand. As always, all this is to be related both to the kind of task and its structural context.

Prominent in the task-interaction of client and servicing agent are their respective attempts at negotiation and persuasion. This point probably needs little further emphasis here, except we should add that both of those activities involve work, too (try persuading an unwilling patient to have an operation or, conversely, try as a patient to negotiate pain medication with a busy or ideologically oriented nurse who believes in minimizing pain medications). The more straightforward types of talk during work are likely to strike the attention of the field observer, whereas the talk associated with persuasion and negotiation may appear descriptively in the field notes but is easily overlooked in the researcher's analysis of that talk-activity data.

Trajectory work requires an information flow before and after each task or task sequence. Another way of stating this is that tasks do not exist in isolation, since they are parts of larger chains of work. Decisions and negotiations about what tasks, in what order, to what purpose, need to be made and, as will be discussed below, are often argued about. Information may be actively sought or given by interested parties in order to get next steps, next tasks, underway. Furthermore, no task can be done without requisite resources—space, manpower, equipment, time—all requiring that people talk *beforehand* to other people: whether of the same team, the same department, different departments, the same or different echelons and specializations, even between people working in different organizations. Then *after* the tasks are done, there must be further talk in order to facilitate next steps in the arc of work. (Next steps may involve others in getting their own further work done, too, in the total arc of work.) In short, the analysis of task accomplishment must not be confined to the immediate task but should concentrate on the arc of work, the place of talk within the arc, and the integral flow of information before, after, and within the task. Need it be added that the arc of work cannot even be envisioned until the trajectory itself is envisioned—a preliminary set of tasks that involve a search for appropriate information and usually discussion, even debate, as to what that information means and will imply for future work.

Talk after the task is also varied, in kind, condition, and consequence. One general type consists of reporting. Sometimes the report is made informally, sometimes formally, and sometimes verbally but sometimes in writing. The report may simply carry the information that the task is (or is not) accomplished, but may be more elaborate: how the task was done, with what results, problems encountered, etc. However informal or sparse it may be, the report is, nevertheless, essential to the organization's system of accountability. It functions to give others necessary information so that they can do their own work in the total arc—their next tasks—and affects their decisions about what might be those next tasks. In organizations that have around-the-clock work (three shifts, as in hospitals) the changing of guard requires reports on tasks done, tasks unfinished, and "the general state of things."

Various conditions may influence form, style, substance, and selection of items included or omitted from the report. Some conditions are relatively obvious, some not. The general format of the report is set by the organizationally conceived (by superiors perhaps) function of the report; medical charts, for instance, look the same, more or less, the world over. Of course, alterations in traditional format are subject to debate, and new superiors can reshape it substantially, depending in turn on what organizational conditions further or constrain them. Style is affected not merely by personal considerations but also conceptions of audience and task. At a psychiatric hospital observed by us, the nurses' reports given at change-of-shift time were written; these were not officially required by the hospital, indeed were frowned on, but were used nevertheless. They were accompanied by the transmitting nurse's verbal commentary, which was designed to make the next shift's work easier and more efficient and to warn them against potential trouble from certain patients. The details selected for emphasis were geared to the pragmatic character of this nursing report. A striking feature of detail and style was the written and running commentary on patients' moral character, a commentary linked with what might be expected from these "difficult patients."

Questions of style move quickly, of course, into questions bearing on what is omitted or put into a report. That "depends" also: depends on time, energy, the conceived nature of the report for the arc of work; also on perception of audience and audience reaction. Much gets omitted in reporting because the listener or reader can fill in the omissions in this shorthand reporting or because the reporter is concealing mistakes or cutting of corners in doing tasks or in other ways "covering the ass" of himself or herself or of someone else. Of course, the report may be a partial or complete fabrication, too. In hospitals, it is especially noteworthy nowadays that particular kinds of audience, associated with malpractice suits or regulatory review, affect what goes into and what is omitted from reports. Equally interesting, in medical as well as other kinds of reporting, is that what is left out about tasks accomplished also relates to what information is defined as officially accountable, or in other ways important, and what is "just part of the job" but seeming not so important. Much sentimental work in hospitals goes unreported, even verbally, to anyone. Some work get done, and is deemed important, by some categories of workers but goes unreported especially to superiors or other echelons. For instance, nursing aides may not report unofficial or unmandated tasks done for or with patients, including sentimental work; sometimes no report is made because the task is not one for which the worker is accountable, but on occasion the information may be deliberately withheld because "they are not interested" or would not approve. We have even seen a deliberate, collective withholding of information by nursing aides as reprisal against their superiors.

A second general type of talk after the task is evaluative discussion of the report. While an individual listener or reader may make a judgment by himself or herself, others may be called into the evaluative process to give their respective opinions or counsel. If there are multiple recipients of a report, evaluative discussion and commentary is very probable. That discussion may even be institutionalized, as through medical case conferences, its format and style conventionalized. Also understandable in medical settings, and presumably elsewhere, is that when trajectories go strikingly and distressingly awry (cumulative mess trajectories) then evaluative discussion is found around virtually every aspect of the work, including the reporting work.

A third general type of talk after consists not of reports but of various other kinds of information transmission. A few of them are suggested by the fieldwork snippets given in Bosks's book (1979) on medical mistakes, referred to earlier. After doing their diagnostic and therapeutic tasks, we hear the physicians, both young and old, talking about the work and those who did it. Some physicians are reprimanding others for errors or sloppy work. Some are challenging others as to why they did what they did, and defenses may be made in turn. Apologies may be made, too. Explanations may be offered for how the work was done. Most of this flow of information can be subsumed under the heading of "unfinished business." In addition, Bosk's quoted field notes reflect speakers talking aloud about their own shortcomings in doing tasks, while others may disagree or agree, perhaps reassuring them too. There can be teaching after the tasks also, by superiors or more experienced colleagues. In medical settings, talk after the task may include explanations or teaching of patients by staff (such as by a respiratory therapist explaining why he did the procedure as he did, or how the machine works, or suggesting how better to breathe with the machine "next time around"). Conversely, the patient may request this information, either immediately after the task is finished or later. Perhaps one additional subspecies of commentary after the task is the passing of judgments about the competencies and motivations of associates doing a task, but behind their backs: these judgments can well affect the future decisions about whether and how to work with these associates (or even superiors).

Talk as work is another type of information work: Its primary procedural task consists in the passage of information itself. An obvious instance is the initial diagnostic interview with any client: What is wrong? Why are you here? This is what is wrong; that's why I am here. Some kinds of occupational or professional work consist mainly of talking, like psychotherapeutic work. Much sentimental work, whether with clients or colleagues, consists of talk and accompanying gestures or perhaps just listening. Explanations and teaching are also primarily talk as work: often they occur during a procedural task or afterward, but sometimes of course they occur separately.

An important variety of talk as work consists of decision making when it is the outcome of discussion, debate, negotiation, persuasion, and the like. Naturally, decision-making talk occurs before and during tasks themselves, but we are referring here to those major decisions that occur at critical junctures in the trajectory. (Several appeared in the narrative about the cumulative mess trajectory in the chapter on articulation work.) At these points, of course, the clients and their kin may either be called in or force their way into the talk, as well as into the decision-making itself: being given and requesting or demanding important informational items. Later reviews of the outcomes of decisions, and then the making of new decisions, are an inherent part of the entire decision-making process; that is, evaluation talk is periodic, sequential, and consequential.

Arena talk is a type of talk as work, but because of its great importance we shall discuss it separately. We have in mind the debates held at any and all levels of the organization about major organizational issues. These issues both affect the work and are part of the work. An arena may extend far beyond the boundaries of an organization or any of its subunits, being part of debates raging throughout an industry or even across the nation (Strauss 1978*b*). An arena debate held within a single hospital ward or among team members will reflect more than intraorganizational dynamics, since the debaters will be representative of professional, occupational, ethnic, gender, and other social worlds. Precisely who enters a particular debate, how, when, and with what impact will depend on many factors which the researcher will have to discover and bring into his or her analysis. It is important to understand, however, that among the most important factors are the ideological, for the individual paticipants qua members of social worlds represent not merely occupational or ethnic or some other "positions" but also ideological positions. The latter may be associated with occupation, ethnicity, and so on, usually with certain segments of those larger social worlds and their movements.

Kinds of information will probably vary in accordance with different types of component work (sentimental, safety, etc.). It seems reasonable to suppose that much sentimental work, for instance, may go unreported in all organizations because workers are not held accountable for it, whereas safety work may be reported carefully because it *is* organizationally (or extraorganizationally!) important. Arena debates may be frequent and severe over some issues pertaining to some types of component work, like safety or sentimental but, as in most hospitals probably, not about most comfort work. On the other hand, some aspects of comfort work, say, the giving of pain medications, may be meticulously reported but also, unlike other comfort work, may be bitterly debated. The proposition suggested at the head of this section is speculative, however, since we ourselves have no firm data on the matter; it remains to be researched.

Written reports of various kinds do, as suggested earlier, represent important information work, although this section has focused almost entirely on verbal transmission. The writings of sociologists in recent years have tended to downplay the accuracy of agency reports, pointing out both their frequently self-serving functions or deliberately misleading character as well as the deficiencies of their information-producing organizational mechanisms. *While those kinds of critique are certainly useful, they do not raise all the questions we should wish answered about written information work.* Why are the reports (reviews, etc.) required and in the particular specified form? What organizational or work strategies lie behind these requirements? How are the documents actually put together—what work goes into doing that, and who does it? How is the work learned, taught, to whom and by whom? How is the work monitored? "Improved" over time? How is the work evaluated? How does this information work fit into larger arcs of work? What is the range of consequences of doing this work, whether "successfully or unsuccessfully," for various actors in the total work drama? And what are its extraorganizational impacts? In this regard, Alfred Chandler's *The Visible Hand* (1977) is especially enlightening, dealing as it does with the rise of accounting, bills of lading, and other innovative information work that accompanied the growth of large American business firms in the nineteenth century. Imagine running a sizeable railroad system, let alone a transcontinental line, without an adequate flow and reporting of information about scheduling trains (for safety and efficiency) or flows of cash (for financial safety and organizational efficiency)! As Chandler demonstrates, the new methods of reporting and creating reports not only revolutionized a single industry but markedly altered the practices in many other industries, in the United States as well as abroad.

Clients profoundly affect the information talk. Earlier we touched on the essential contribution made by clients in the information process during procedural work done on them or their problems. This book is, of course, testimony to how clients (in this instance patients and their kinsmen) are deeply implicated in *all* kinds of work done on, around, for, and with them. The information they give and receive can be crucial, not merely pertinent; it can be of a direct or indirect nature, simple or complex in structure, technically easy or difficult to transmit, emotionally neutral or draw on immensely passionate responses, and so on. Then, there is the virtually universal issue of "keeping secrets" (by both clients and servicing agents), utilizing tactics to withhold that information as well as to control its timing, pacing, and the style of allowing or forcing its disclosure: all that occurs because the work is being done on or for clients. Of course, in a sense most work is done for someone else, hence for clients or consumers of one kind or another. Insofar as that is so, the researcher needs to take into account the special characteristics of the production, transmission, and consumption (use) of the products of relevant types of information work occurring in the trajectories under study.

Body Work

Next we wish, though only in the most sketchy fashion, to touch on an issue directly raised by our observations of medical work. An obvious feature of this work is that patients' bodies are central to that work—central in the sense that the bodies are malfunctioning and must be helped or at least managed, central also insofar as things are done to or with bodies or their parts or systems, that is, medicated, monitored, given comfort care, diagnosed, connected up with machinery, injected, pounded, manipulated, and "treated" in a multitude of other ways. Some occupations or professions, such as law or accounting, are not particularly concerned with clients' or customers' body problems. But a moment's reflection will show that clients' or customers' bodies are an important enough aspect or component of occupational work to warrant its being taken quite explicitly into account in studies of occupations and their work.

A few brief examples should underline that point. Airline pilots and cabbies are primarily concerned with managing their respective vehicles, but they are also transporting bodies—ideally with maximum safety, comfort, and efficiency. Teachers of physical skill like those used in dancing or playing the piano, may be imparting many other kinds of skills and knowledge, but work with bodies and body parts looms large in their teaching. Since most technical skills involve some proper positioning, movement, and coordination of hands, feet, and other body parts, any teaching will at least implicitly include body work. Other kinds of occupations and enterprises may involve body work on customers but not especially in their service—like the work of executioners, to choose an extreme example, or that of dress designers, who are interested less in making people's bodies look or feel good than in selling merchandise.

In all such examples, we have emphasized working with *other* persons' bodies. Analytically, it is worthwile to keep that distinct from working with one's own body (self-care, dieting, working at keeping fit). Of course, body work may also be involved when working together with other people, as in mountain climbing or building a house, where people are both doing work on or with their own bodies and with other peoples' bodies—in those examples, principally coordination and safety-body work. It is probably useful to maintain those distinctions. We have, however, in this book and in this section focused on body work with clients.

Body work is done in the context of trajectory work; said another way, different trajectories will call for different sequences and totalities of tasks; hence, the body work called for will vary by different types of trajectory. Even with medical trajectories, the surgical and the dialysis ones vary greatly in the characteristic tasks entailed, and each of these is much different from teaching someone to drive a car or to cut hair fashionably.

Other familiar points follow from thinking of body work in the context of trajectories. First, different *phases* of the same trajectory can precipitate quite different kinds of body work. Thus, when teaching someone to play the piano, the focus moves along to new parts of the body, new parts of the hand, new movements of the fingers, and so on. One of the more subtle aspects of such trajectory phasing is that previous body work is likely to leave its imprint on the body itself (or part or reactive system), like the typical dancer's foot or the advanced student's better control of responses. Hence, in later trajectory phases, certain kinds of body work are no longer necessary, but others may now be required or deemed necessary, including those that are the direct consequence of the impact of previous body work, as in countering the side effects of drugs with patients. It follows also that the different *component types of work* along an arc of work can call for various body tasks—a point again made evident by thinking of clinical safety, comfort, and diagnostic work. The *division of labor* involved in all those can vary by skills and persons doing the tasks. Even workers at higher levels in the division of labor (those making the larger decisions or doing the wider sweeps of articulation work) can be conceived of, analytically at least, as working indirectly with bodies even if not in direct contact with those bodies. And again, researchers need to observe the interplay in the division of labor of the client or customer who will be participating in the body tasks: dental technicians could not clean teeth without some effort by clients (on the face of it rather passively being worked on); even the less active customer does a small amount of work if only to keep his head still while sleeping in the chair. Like all work done within organizations, work with bodies will be affected by *organizational conditions*: resources, relationships, structures, contingencies. And, as in any organization, persons involved in the body work may disagree and debate issues because of their different positional and ideological perspectives. One additional consideration is worth touching on here: the servicing agents may be doing work on their own bodies *while* also performing tasks on the client's body, and the former may interfere with or promote the latter. All these points, though barely touched on here, are probably worth careful attention by students of work.

Clients: Objects or Participants in Work?

Throughout this book, we have witnessed consequences of one peculiarity of medical work, namely, that the work is done on the bodies of people who when sentient are responding both to the work itself and often to the workers' workmanship. Furthermore the patients are often drawn into, asked into, or move on their own initiative into the division of labor so as to accomplish the requisite tasks. The living, reacting presence of the "object" being worked on makes a significant difference in the modes and courses of work and cannot be discounted either by the workers themselves or by the social scientist who wishes to make meaningful, useful analyses of the work. This theme has been central to most of the foregoing chapters, and there is no need to repeat its details here. But for readers who are concerned with kinds of work and work relationships other than those involving medical care, a few additional thoughts on the theme should be useful.

Rather surprisingly, the distinction between tasks carried out on inanimate objects and those performed on humans seems to be implicit rather than explicit in the literature on work. Furthermore, there is a difference between tasks done on persons in their behalf (as in the professions, for clients) and tasks done on them for someone else (as when they are consumers being sold goods or services for someone else's profit, or in more extreme cases when they are tortured or killed, obviously not in their service). The literature on professions is, of course, replete with discussions pertaining to the reactions of clients but is not often focused closely or analytically on the implications of professional work as done both in the service of clients and as having to take clients' reactions to and participations in the work itself into account.

If we focus now on degrees of work "on" or "with" clients, it is useful to think of work as ranging along a continuum between two poles: (*a*) the person treated primarily as an object, as if he or she were nonexistent, and (*b*) the person explicitly regarded as a member of the working team, as if the division of labor included him or her as an essential element in getting the tasks done. In the middle ranges between these poles, the clients may be only implicitly required to help at or cooperate in the work, or at least their behaviors or psychological reactions are taken into account in carrying out the tasks. Rather obviously, the conditions making for the impersonal end of the continuum will include emergency action (no time then for frills or the human touch), when the clients' reactions are not necessary to get the work done or may impede it. At the opposite extreme, much work on and for clients involves reliance on their cooperative responses, whether the work is done on their bodies (by medical staffs, lifeguards, firemen), on their minds (psychiatrists), or on their business (lawyers); otherwise such work can be accomplished with little success or not at all. Indeed, some of that work involves their bodily and mental cooperation whether the work is done primarily on their bodies, minds, or business.

To dwell on this continuum may seem banal, but these distinctions, we believe, are a first step in thinking about what may be involved in any work under scrutiny by an analyst, leading to a better understanding of why work gets done efficiently, effectively, effortlessly, cooperatively—or the opposite. After all, the various participants in the work may have different ideas about which part of the continuum is or should be operative. E. C. Hughes's (1971, p. 346) well-known remark that the client's emergency often seems merely routine to the professional is simply one instance of how conflict can occur between client and servicing agent because of their differing definitions, which assume quite divergent accounts of involvement.

Conditions that profoundly and specifically affect which parts of the continuum are operative, for whom, and with what consequences can understandably be usefully discussed under the rubrics of trajectory, ideology and organization.

Trajectory work will vary in its emphases on the responding or cooperating clients. Different kinds of trajectories will embody tasks which differentially minimize or maximize the humanness or objectness of the client. Thus, a lawyer's management of a difficult criminal trial will entail his client's cooperation in the matter of giving information, acting as witness in the trial itself, and perhaps concurrence with plea bargaining or agreeing to plead guilty. By contrast, lawyers who handle routine delinquency or criminal cases, process their clients through the customary plea-bargaining mechanism whereby the clients are treated with relative impersonality (Skolnik 1966).

Trajectory phases will also involve different degrees of client as object or participant. For instance, in presurgical phases, the patient involvement is high; in the operating room, the patient is maximally treated as an object (either nonsentient or under a local anesthetic to minimize reaction); in the recovery room, the patient is still pretty much treated as an object; in postoperative phases, the patient's responses to or actual involvement in the trajectory work will vary depending on the type of surgery and the degree of severity of the recovery period.

Different component types of work will involve different degrees of work on or with the patient. Thus, in medical work, we have seen that in sentimental work the "with" element is maximal. It is also very high with comfort work. Some safety work may not involve the patient in the requisite division of labor though it may certainly involve the patient's response. Articulation work at operative levels may, under certain conditions, very much involve working with patients, but work on higher policy levels may not involve their involvement or response. Error work—preventing, monitoring, rectifying, etc.—may under certain conditions be carried out quite independent of client response or participation but under other conditions be responsive to clients' reactions and involve them in the error work itself. Component types of work—whether in medicine, law, or whatever—will, then, vary in their respective foci or emphases on client responsiveness and participation.

Ideological positions can profoundly affect whether the client is managed as an object or is worked with. This point is relatively self-evident if one considers that the very definition of the trajectory, the arc of work, the relationship of tasks, the issue of who is to do those tasks—when, where, and how—may all be affected by the ideological positions of the participants. Who will regard the client more or less or not at all as an object can lead to cooperation or conflict between staff and client and among staff itself.

A particularly striking feature of work with clients is that ideological issues are more complex because clients also have ideologies pertaining to the work done for, on, and with them. Like other ideological positions, theirs can be aggressively asserted and so quite plainly affect the trajectory work. Or their positions can, like those of the recognized workers themselves, enter more covertly into carrying out tasks.

Organizational conditions inevitably affect the degree of objectness or humanness with which clients are regarded and their responses or contributions to work taken into account. Thus, constraints of time, skill, experience, equipment, personnel, and other resources bear rather crucially on the working "on" or "with" issue. This point has been amply if often implicitly illustrated throughout this book. We would only remind our readers that organizational conditions also include the presence, experience, and other resources of classes of persons who, like the patient's relatives, may be overlooked by the participants themselves, as well as by researchers, but can be important organizational elements in work.

Teamwork within Organizational Contexts

A team of experienced mountain climbers manages to scale the heights of Mount Everest. A team of dedicated, technologically skilled, and innovative men develop a motorless, man-propelled plane that wins a coveted prize for crossing the English Channel. Several prisoners team up to plan and successfully carry out their collective escape from prison. A number of engineers employed by a business corporation are assigned to a specific project and at the end of many months, through teamwork, accomplish the goals outlined for the project. The famous, mammoth enterprise leading to the landing of men on the moon was accomplished through countless numbers of teams whose work interlocked and was articulated in dazzlingly complex ways.

These examples help to make several points First, *much work is carried out through teams*—whether they are called that or not—the work itself being in the service of a project or an enterprise. Second, *this team work may utilize or run afoul of organizations.* This is true even if the team is not actually an integral part of an organization. However, many if not most teams operate within organizations. It will make a considerable difference in the character of the team and how it works together whether the teamwork occurs within an organization or not. (As the title of this section signals, we are interested here in the situation where teams are actually part of organizational functioning.) Third, a *very great deal of work of organizations gets accomplished through the formation and operation of teams* (the treatment of patients in hospitals, the development of engineering plans and projects in industry are instances.) Standard repetitive work draws on teams accustomed to working together and on relatively conventional modes of articulating the work of multiple teams. Problematic or innovative work gets done by supplementing or even circumventing conventional teams with alternative new modes of teamwork.

Teamwork itself involves an organization of effort, of work, one implication of which is that its organization will be profoundly affected by the following two sets of conditions. To begin with, the nature of the project or enterprise (call it "trajectory") will quite obviously comprise a set of conditions influencing (1) the types of sequencing, timing, and articulating of tasks; (2) the composition of the teams doing these tasks; (3) how team members are recruited; (4) the envisioned and operative divisions of labor; (5) the resources drawn upon, and so on. Besides, when a team is part and parcel of an encompassing organization, as are the teams that treat patients in hospitals, then organizational properties themselves will bear decisively upon how the trajectory itself is conceived, managed, and shaped and how the work of implicated teams is organized, maintained, evaluated, reviewed, reorganized, and articulated. In more concrete terms, who will be available to be on the team, what resources will be allocated to or drawn upon or seized upon, which organizational rules must be taken into account or followed or circumvented, which authorities must be persuaded, negotiated with, satisfied, neutralized, or placated—all these and many other kinds of considerations bear upon the work of any operative team as it succeeds or fails to get "its" work done. Teamwork, in short, is being carried out within a *thick context of organizational possibilities, constraints, and contingencies.*

In addition, students of work cannot afford to ignore the fact that much work that is accomplished through teamwork also takes place *within a larger matrix of linked organizations or organizational settings.* This is merely another way of stating that activities carried out within an organization cannot profitably be studied while ignoring the extraorganizational conditions that impinge on those activities "within" the organization. When thinking of teams and their specific project or trajectory work, it is easy to lose sight of those larger conditions. Just as a team of research biologists cannot get its work done without linkages to the laboratory, the university or institute, the funding agencies, and other research teams attached to other organizations, so, few teams pursuing other kinds of goals in other kinds of organizations can operate independent of those larger organizational matrixes. These considerations of organizational embeddedness (intraorganizational and interorganizational) are what make the management and shaping of trajectories—of projects, enterprises—different for teams which operate either formally outside or inside of organizations. The former certainly are related to organizations with which they must deal or whose services they utilize, but their tasks are not so complexly woven with the related organizations' goals, projects, requirements, internal battles, and debates, as are those of teams which are formally within an organization. The same is true of the linkages between *this* team's work and other teams' work in carrying out a larger project in which all play some part. Medical work as analyzed in this book exemplifies clearly the kinds of points raised in the above paragraphs, suggesting as well how students of work and organizations need to think in terms of linkages among trajectory work, teamwork, and intra- and extraorganizational contexts.

Negotiations and Negotiative Work

Seen or at least glimpsed throughout this book, as part of the texture of getting work done, is the phenomenon of negotiation. Negotiation enters into how work is defined, as well as how to do it, how much of it to do, who is to do it, how to evaluate it, how and when to reassess it and so on. Even under the most coercive conditions—where work is ordered by the harshest or most authoritative of regimes—tasks, sequences of tasks, arcs of work, even entire projects or trajectories will be subject to negotiation. Negotiation takes place around all the topics considered in this chapter (dirty work, error work) and around all types of work (sentimental, safety) involved in a major line of activity.

The negotiation can, of course, be of various kinds, such as making a deal (an explicit compromise), trading off, reaching an informal agreement (say to respect each other's turf), or reaching more formal agreements signified by contracts and other signed arrangements. Within industries, it is notable, too, that competition cannot proceed without certain kinds of what historians of industry call "cooperation" or "collaboration" or "alliance" or "federation," or "making agreements." Whether intraorganizational or interorganizational, negotiations can, of course, be coercive in nature as well as happily cooperative. They almost always will occur in connection with the persuasion and manipulation of situations, persons, or resources. Negotiations are linked even with displays or actual use of force. No matter—negotiation is a necessary cement for organizational action. Elsewhere we have termed this cement "negotiated order" (Strauss 1978*a*), but having written so much about it already, and so explicitly, we shall not discuss it further except to emphasize that to negotiate *is* to work.

Some negotiation feels more like actual work to the negotiating parties and some negotiating involves doing a great number of sequential or simultaneous, and well-articulated, tasks in order to carry out the negotiation successfully, but negotiating is always work: *negotiative work*. The most complicated unquestionably takes place when the representatives of multiple worlds and organizations are intersecting, for then at first nothing is routinized and virtually everything must be "worked out," later to be reassessed, reordered, in a word, reworked. Since those complex intersections are likely to lead to further segmentation within the organizations and social worlds of the respective participants, the negotiative work spawns further negotiations. Inevitably, the new segmentation leads to alterations of lines, modes, styles, and arcs of work, with all the attendant negotiations. It is no wonder that negotiative contexts—the conditions for negotiating—become so complicated and so interrelated.

Chapter 10

Division of Labor

Sociologists and economists recognize the classic origins of the term "division of labor" in the writings of theorists like Adam Smith, Durkheim, and Marx. Contemporary theorists have added to the older perspectives on this concept (Clemente 1972, Labovitz and Gibbs 1964, Rushing 1968). Eliot Freidson (1975) has reviewed recent literature and then offered his own suggestions for conceptualizing this important phenomenon. In both the classic and contemporary writings, including Freidson's, since *work* itself is neither the major concern nor intently looked at, this leaves open certain questions about the division of labor which are raised by our own study. Freidson's paper provides a useful transition to our questions.

In his review, Freidson makes quite clear that whatever their differences, the various perspectives on the division of labor are primarily concerned with its *occupational* aspects. How does the totality of work get divided up among the various occupations? That is the core of the issue. For instance, in the "ecological approach to the division of labor in our own day," Labovitz and Gibbs made "an important distinction between two general ideas associated with the concept—first, occupational differentiation as such, designated as the *degree* of the division of labor; second, the *basis* on which a person's occupation in the division of labor is determined" (Freidson 1976, p. 306). But ten years later these distinctions are blurred. "The numbers of occupational roles and the distribution of the work force through them become the accepted best representation of the division of labor as such" (cf. Clemente 1972 and Freidson 1975, p. 307). Freidson distinguishes three basic approaches to the question of the relation between social organization and division of labor: (1) the Adam Smith–derived "free-market" principle of the organization of labor; (2) the Max Weber principle of rational-legal bureaucratic rationalization of work; and (3) an approach that was prominent before the industrial revolution, "but which has continued to show vitality. I refer to circumstances in which the worker himself excercises control over his work and sets the organization of the division of labor. Historically, guilds, crafts, and professions have exercised such control in at least some segments of the economy" (p. 310). Freidson comments that all three foci for organization are probably present, "though with varying degres of importance in any historical moment." How can those logically incompatible types of social organization coexist in reality? Freidson asks. Here he begins to develop his own interactionist approach to the division of labor issue.

> They can co-exist because, as formal models, they are principles and plans for human activities and as such are in a sense separate from the work activities they purport to order. They are diffused when translated into work. In and of themselves, the concrete work activities of the division of labor are interactive and emergent in character. Individuals and groups are engaged in a continuous process of conspiracy, evasion, negotiation, and conflict in the course of coping with the varying circumstances and situations of their work, in some sense shaping the terms, conditions, and content of their work no matter what the formal mode of organization being used to justify, control, or conceptualize their activities. (P. 310)

After emphasizing the emergent side of the equation, Freidson quickly warns that there are constraints on the workers' freedom of choice. Like any classical Chicago-style interactionist (Fisher and Strauss 1978), Freidson is opting for a position (the judgment is ours) that balances between extreme freedom and extreme constraint. However, having arrived at this point of advising us that the social organization of the division of labor lies somewhere between those poles, he ends with neither discussion of what his position implies nor analysis of the work processes themselves. He simply points to the roles of negotiation and choice:

> Among the individuals on the factory shop floor or on the hospital ward, and among the groups engaged in negotiating legislation and formal plans for controlling work, there are boundaries set on what will be considered legitimate to negotiate, how the negotiation will take place, and what bargains can be struck. . . . It is in that practical variety where we see the division of labor as, ultimately, a process of social interaction whereby the participants create their own specialized jobs and work relationships. (P. 311)

Freidson is quite right in emphasizing negotiative aspects in the division of labor. But what tasks are negotiated, when, what is given in mutual exchange, how much there is to give in the situation, all these are dependent on the structural context within which the negotiation goes on. (For instance, in the experimental mood of psychiatric reform during the 1950s, at a state mental hospital, Bucher and Schatzman [1964] reported that nurses were profferred and persuaded to take psychiatric therapeutic roles on wards where ideologically committed staff believed everybody should do therapy rather than only the psychiatrists and psychologists. Patients were also profferred the right to decide which among them were sufficiently fit to go home on given weekends. But more is involved than just bargaining: on the same psychiatric wards, Bucher and Schatzman noted that the physicians were forbidden by staff consensus from carrying out their traditional, legally guaranteed, work of prescribing drugs; that task was now allocated to staff members acting in concert.) When, indeed, researchers scrutinize work itself, rather than being primarily concerned with the division of labor employed to get that work done, then they are likely to unearth some of the complexities and operating mechanisms of the actual division of labor.

Using Glaser's study (1976) of home building again, we can note in his monograph that certain conditions will enhance or decrease the likelihood that a patsy will vigorously enter the division of labor or with passivity accept the official division of labor: "they build, I only pay." An assertive patsy is backed by knowledge, skill, experience at home building, and an appropriate ideology. In Glaser's book, we see the patsy doing the research necessary for proper choice of contractors and of construction materials. We see him also negotiating with city officials, with subcontractors, and with workers on site. The patsy is doing error work, supervisory work, and above all both high-level and operational-level articulation work. He even undertakes to do a certain number of the construction tasks. Furthermore, he has a choice of how much or little of all this work to engage in. So it is not just a matter of electricians doing electrical tasks, roofers doing roofing tasks, patsys doing the initial work of selecting and purchasing the site, finding the contractor, and getting the financing. If we were to follow the entire course of the trajectory of "building a house," we would see that the division of labor would vary by phase and by unexpected contingencies affecting task consequences and their articulation. An analytic focus on *work* itself is needed—quite as with mistakes at work—to develop the concept of "division of labor" in new directions. Especially is this true when the trajectories are uncertain, and new classes of workers or work are appearing, tasks are undergoing continual revision, and external contingencies stemming from government or industry are affecting the work.

A distinction should be made between arc of work, its implicated tasks, and the persons who will do those tasks and that work. In repetitive and standard arcs of work, conventional categories of persons will, with great probability, do the tasks: persons varying by skill, education, occupational title, ethnicity, gender, age, or social class. Of course, tasks get divided up or allocated in terms of political considerations (i.e., by jurisdictional, legal, and power considerations), but analytically the prior consideration is one of task structure. We do need to know the place of occupational and other statuses in task allocation and indeed in trajectory definition itself, but only as an analytic instrument for understanding the central issue of how the work is done and what goes into getting it (all or some of it) done.

Departures from official, even legally sanctioned, divisions of labor are commonly recognized and are epitomized in the story by a sociologist, Harvey Smith, who when studying a hospital was given its official table of organization by its director, but was later asked "would you like to see how this place really works?" The director then reached into his desk drawer and gave Smith the "informal" but operational table of organization. The distinctions made by social scientists some years ago between formal and informal organization grew out of the realization that official status and job allocation were not necessarily coterminous.

Different trajectories with their implicated arcs of work entail different divisions of labor to get the constituent tasks done. Insofar as the mix and articulation of tasks varies, so will the divisions of labor.

The division of labor may, therefore, be different during *different phases of the trajectory*, each successive one perhaps necessitating new types of labor or relying on different skills of the same workers. The skills and actions are the essential elements, not the class of worker as such.

The division of labor called for may vary considerably by the *component type of work* being performed as part of the total trajectory work. Thus in medical work, different workers (or the same worker employing different skills) may be called on to handle safety work, error work, and sentimental work. Again, it is the variation in labor—not the laborer—that is the essential ingredient in getting tasks accomplished.

The division of labor may perforce also vary depending on the *"level" of operation* called for during each phase and by component type of work. In safety work, for instance, different skills or personnel are utilized for discerning a safety error, calling for its rectifications, rectifying it, and monitoring the rectification.

Not only do the skills and personnel vary during a trajectory with its phases, its component work types, and task levels, but so do the *relationships of the labor which is embodied in worker skills.*

Analysis of the division of labor requires detailed scrutiny of *how those relationships shift* with phase, level, and work type, and also *how the relationships fare between the instances of shifting.* For example, when a cardiac patient is brought into the surgical recovery room, an observer can note that the immediate tasks consist of making a multitude (perhaps ten to twenty) connections between the patient's body parts or apertures and various machines. Two or three nurses or technicians will be busy making the connections at which they are skilled—one, two, or more of them—while a physician will be making others; meanwhile perhaps four other technicians and nurses will be standing at the foot of the bed awaiting their turns to make their respective connections. Notable in this division of labor is how jobs are done simultaneously and sequentially, but involve only a single worker performing one job at a time; that is, no task is likely to engage the cooperative effort of two or more workers. In later phases of working on the same patient two or more physicians and nurses or nurses and technicians, may work together on a common task.

We would emphasize that all five points noted above are directed at understanding how *labor*—not laborers—is related to the trajectory tasks. *Labor and its relationship to the tasks is the salient issue,* rather than the types of worker. Of course, as noted earlier, it is undeniable that workers with different occupational or professional titles, having associated training, skills, and status will be assigned or lay successful claim to different tasks. The basis of allocation, claim, and jurisdictional control, as the sociological and economic literature bearing on those issues makes clear, may not necessarily be related to the relative competence of workers in getting particular tasks done efficiently or effectively. But, in turn, these varied jurisdictional and allocational issues should not be allowed to obscure the main aim when analyzing an actual division of labor: how the labor is accomplished, how tasks are articulated, how the labor of workers is related during their performance of tasks.

Paradoxically, one can even conceive of *symbolic work being accomplished while the "actual" task is being done*, by virtue of the particular bases of jurisdictional participation or control. For instance, if professional power is the main allocational basis, then more than pure competence may be involved when a physician legally performs a task that a more skilled nurse or medical technician could do. Indeed, those personnel may be bystanders restlessly or angrily observing an incompetent performance but powerless to intervene because of the symbolic (even legalized) work that sustains the superordinate professional's status. Even when the physician's competence is not in question, we might suspect that his or her doing the actual task is simultaneously sustaining the professional right to do that task.

Intersections of types of laborers (by occupational title), in getting partial or total arcs of work done, involve intersections of representatives from different social worlds or subworlds. For instance, they may variously represent the communities of nursing, medicine, law, bioengineering, machine industry, and given medical specialties. Each of those representatives is trained or experienced in salient activities characteristic of his or her respective community and brings that training and experience into the arc of work. Whether the work goes smoothly or conflictfully is not just because personalities conflict or can work in harmony but, first and foremost, because the *divergent lines of work characteristic of those different social worlds* mix harmoniously or only with great tension and discord. *The greater the discrepancy in social world perspective and activity, the more obviously will there be a need for explicit negotiation* among workers in order to get the joint tasks accomplished with any efficiency. If the workers have labored together previously and are now accustomed to working together, then they will have done the negotiative work previously, and only new contingencies will bring about any awareness among them that negotiative work is again necessary.

Flexibility in the division of labor varies by different types of work entailed in the arc of work. Certain types of work (in medicine: machine, safety, comfort, etc.) are formulated more distinctly, even to being spelled out in legal or other official documents. Only lawyers argue cases in court; in hospitals, only surgeons open and close the body. But some aspects of the total arc involve types of work not spelled out so clearly in terms of who shall do them—or who only may do them. In terms of probability, nurses will certainly engage much more in comfort work than physicians, social workers, or respiratory therapists; on the other hand, none of the staff ever know when they will get drawn into, or feel they should do, some bit of comfort work for a patient. Different categories of staff are involved with different safety tasks, yet realistically there can be much overlap in their actual safety work. Sentimental work, of course, is so implicit in the total arc, that everyone may engage in one or another subtype of it, albeit nurses are more likely to engage in some and physicians in others. What is true of medical work cannot be so different in other industries or lines of work: the analytic challenge for the researcher is to discover what types of work make up the total bundle and then—if interested in the division of labor—to check out its variations by type of work.

The relative invisibility or nonacountability of tasks can affect the official or customary division of labor. In this book, readers will have noted that the performance of tasks by staff, patients, and kin can be invisible, either because not actually observed or because not reported. This is characteristic of all subtypes of medical work. The phenomenon of invisibility implies not so much a blurring of the official division of labor as the nonaccountability of certain tasks. It also implies that a task may get done by someone who is dissatisfied with how somebody else did it or who realizes the task has not been done at all but should be done. Most often in this ad hoc division of labor, no official report is made of work accomplished. In all lines of work, whether medical or other, it seems probable that those subtypes of work that are less clearly spelled out or have generally lower priority will be less accountable. Hence, there will be less clarity, more flexibility in, the division of labor.

When tasks are performed under new or somewhat uncustomary conditions or when they are new tasks, then the division of labor along usual lines may not obtain. Under the first condition, various persons may do the task, depending on "circumstance": whoever just happens to be there or is less tired or is willing to do the work, and so on. When a task is quite new, certain persons may be allocated to do it because of such factors as being available, being willing to undertake the new challenge or the dirty work, or having the most transferable skill or previous experience. Around the new task structures, thereby, ensue considerable debate and negotiation, before the division of labor settles into some semblance of regularity and relative permanence. Even then, there may be much latitude for persons to negotiate the boundaries—expanding or contracting them—to fit their own desires, aspirations, energies, and goals.

Task structures change at different rates of speed, so that some may rest on stable divisions of labor while others may be changing fast enough to open up and make the division of labor more flexible. This phenomenon has been apparent in this book. For instance, in the history of ICN development there has been (and is now in many hospitals) a transition period during which respiratory therapists seek to convince nurses and physicians that their own skills are actually greater and their responsibility equal to the nurses' for many specific tasks that pertain to respiratory care. During the transition period, both cadres of workers are engaged in those tasks, but the respiratory therapists do not invade other parts of the nurses' job territory. As the transition period begins to close, the division of labor becomes less blurred, less overlapping. Examples aside, there is also the phenomenon that *the more segments of the total arc of work which are in flux, then correspondingly the more task structures there will be which entail a fluid division of labor.*

In fast-changing or developing or expanding industries, a high proportion of task structures are changing continuously, even explosively. This means that, more than in stable industries, a great proportion of trajectories and their associated arcs of work are unpredictable, subject to unforeseen contingencies, more difficult to standardize—standardize either the task structures themselves of who is to do the tasks. There is an inevitable movement, of course, or work that travels from a novel, somewhat amiguous and fluid condition into a more standard, relatively rationalized and routinized condition. Even SOP work, however, as we have seen, can have its contingent (hence standard division of labor shattering, if only temporary) moments. So *it is characteristic of fast-changing industries to have a more apparent mix of SOP and novel arcs of work, with divisions of labor to match.*

Fast-changing industries also produce new specializations, new segments of their total work forces—produced from within the industries but also drawn into them—which both disturb the previous divisions of labor and expand them. Expansion, too, contributes to the fluidity of the division of labor, bringing about uncertainties about who should be working at given tasks. This brings the sociologist's analysis into the well-known realm of jurisdictional debates, fights, negotiations, ideologies of legitimacy and efficiency, and the like.

Fast-changing industries are also subject to new customer requirements and demands. We shall have more to say about this in a later section, suffice to say here that social movements (feminists, natural birth, holistic medicine) impinge upon definitions of work and component tasks, affecting not only how they should be done but who will do them. The arenas for debate multiply and the arguments and negotiations within those arenas, of course, affect the arrangements of divisions of labor—so much so that they may not only be different in different work organizations (firms, hospitals) but within the same organization itself.

The sources of structural impact on divisions of labor come also from within the industry in the form of ideational, technological, organizational, and other intraindustry changes: all these contribute to ambiguities, uncertainties, overlapping terrains, and ad hoc task fulfillment in the total divisions of labor. Intraorganizational changes, of course, also profoundly affect changes of division of labor within an organization.

Summing up, then: given this array of conditions for fluidity in the division of labor, it is easy to see why certain industries (for example, health or computer) look so different, including the instabilities of their divisions of labor. In more stable industries, the task structures change slowly, even if the specific persons doing the tasks change relatively rapidly, the division of labor then being affected primarily by turnover, death, rotation, vacations, new recruitment, training, retraining, and the like. More rapidly changing industries—or firms or sections of firms—look different even to the naked eye. To the researcher looking very closely at their work, they can look different in still other ways. One way is in the complexity of organization of their divisions of labor—or if not complexity at least ambiguity.

Two additional points have been suggested by Berenice Fisher (New York University) in a personal communication. First, she has pointed out some similarities between John Dewey's general argument about the primacy of activity and ours about the primacy of work in the division of labor. But the content of this book should have made clear the differences between activity as such and the narrower kind of activity called work, with its implicated tasks. Second, although we have emphasized the primacy of trajectories and the arc of work in the division of labor, we should also emphasize that the ideologies and conceptions of workers (especially powerful or influential workers) constitute conditions that affect definition of the work and its associated tasks. The work of definings is not at all uncolored or unaffected by those considerations, no matter how rational the working out may be in its operational aspects.

Temporal Order and Temporal Matrix

Anyone who works in an organization thinks—has to think—of his or her work, and of the organization itself, in temporal terms. Those who write about work in organizations inevitably include or touch on such matters as scheduling, timing, pacing, and frequency in their descriptions. Sometimes they do so in their analyses, too, although analysis is usually implicit, explicit analyses being far less frequent.

Two of the most focused discussions of time and work or organizations are by Moore (1963) and Zerubavel (1979). Moore's discussion is rather general, as suggested by his title (*Man, Time, and Society*), but he does consider specific issues like employers' "inventories of time" and sequential ordering of activities and various temporal strategies of administrators. He also notes phenomena like the competition among voluntary organizations for members' time and their temporal strategies for keeping membership at a maximum by using convenient times for meetings, for instance. Zerubavel's book about time in hospitals highlights matters like staff rotation, the three-shift daily movement of staff, and scheduling. It is not our purpose, however, to review studies of time and organization extensively, but rather to point out as an introduction to our own discussion that analytic emphases have been mainly on such temporal matters as noted above, and others such as worker slowdown (Roy 1952), "time off" (Dalton 1959), controlling pace of work (Jackall 1978), as well as testing points and other organizational career junctures (Roth 1963, Wager 1959, Becker and Strauss 1956).

One of the most explicit discussions of temporal aspects of work and organization is in a previous book by one of us (Glaser and Strauss 1968). We shall quote from this before drawing out the fuller implications of the perspective outlined in it. In the earlier discussions, about work and "temporal order," we noted with respect to the care given to the dying by staff and kin:

This work has important temporal features. For instance, there are prescribed schedules governing when the patient must be fed, bathed, turned in bed, given drugs. There are times when tests must be administered. There are crucial periods when the patient must be closely observed or when crucial treatments must be given or actions taken to prevent immediate deterioration—even immediate death. Since there is a division of labor, it must be organized in terms of time. For instance, the nurse must have the patient awake in time for the laboratory technician to administer tests, and the physician's visit must not coincide with the patient's bath or with the visiting hours of relatives. When the patient's illness grows worse, the pace and tempo of the staff's work shifts accordingly: meals may be skipped and tests may be less frequent, but the administration of drugs and the reading of vital signs may be more frequent. During all this work, calculated organizational timing must consider turnover among staff members or their absence on vacations or because of illness.

With rare exceptions, medical services include both recovering and dying patients. Even on intensive care units or on cancer services, not all patients are expected to, or do, die. On any given service, the temporal organization of work with dying patients is greatly influenced by the relative numbers of recovering and dying patients and by the types of recovering patients. For instance, on services for premature babies, babies who die usually do so within 48 hours after birth; after that, most are relatively safe. The "good preemie" does not stay very long on the service, but moves along to the normal babies' service. Hence the pace and the kind of work in the case of a premature baby vary in accordance with the number of days since birth, and when a baby begins to "turn bad" a few days after birth—usually unexpectedly—the pace and the kind of work are greatly affected.

The temporal ordering of work on each service is also related to the predominant types of death in relation to the normal types of recovery. As an example, we may look at intensive care units: some patients there are expected to die quickly, if they are to die at all; others need close attention for several days, because death is a touch-and-go matter; while others are not likely to die but do need temporary round-the-clock nursing. Most who die here are either so heavily drugged as to be temporarily comatose or are actually past consciousness. Consequently, nurses or physicians do not need to converse with these patients. When a patient nears death he may sometimes unwittingly compete with other patients for nurses' or physicians' attention, several of whom may give care to the critically ill patient. When the emergency is over, or the patient dies, then the nurses, for instance, return to less immediately critical patients, reading their vital signs, managing treatments, and carrying out other important tasks.

Each type of service tends to have a characteristic incidence of death, which also affects the staff's organization of work. Closely allied with these incidences are the tempos of dying that are charactertistic of each ward. On emergency services, for example, patients tend to die quickly (they are accident cases, victims of violence, or people stricken suddenly and acutely). The staff on emergency services, therefore, is geared to perform urgent, critical functions. Many emergency services, especially in large city hospitals, are also organized for frequent deaths, especially on weekends. At such times, recovering (or non-sick) patients sometimes tend to receive scant attention, unless the service is organized flexibly to handle both types of patients.

The already complex organization of professional activity for terminal care is made even more so by several other matters involving temporality. For one, what may be conveniently termed the "experiential careers" of patients, families, and staff members are highly relevant to the action around dying patients. Some patients are familiar with their diseases, but others are encountering their symptoms for the first time. The patient's knowledge of the course of his disease, based on his previous experience with it, has an important bearing on what happens as he lies dying in the hospital. Similarly, some personnel are well acquainted with the predominant disease patterns found on their particular wards; but some, although possibly familiar with other illnesses, may be newcomers to these diseases. They may be unprepared for sudden changes of symptoms and vital signs; taken by surprise at crucial junctures, they may make bad errors in timing their actions. More experienced personnel are more likely to be able to take immediate appropriate action at any turn in the illness.

Experiential careers also include the differing experiences that people have had with hospitals. Some patients return repeatedly to the same hospital ward. When a familiar face appears, the staff may be shocked at the patient's deterioration, thinking "*Now* he is going to die," and may therefore react differently than they would to someone new to the ward. Likewise, the extent of the patient's familiarity with the ways of hospitals or of a particular hospital influence his reactions during the course of dying. In short, both the illness careers and the hospital careers of all parties in the dying situation may be of considerable importance, affecting both the interaction around the dying patient and the organization of his terminal care.

One other type of experience is highly relevant: the differing "personal careers" of the interactants in the dying situation—the more personal aspects of the interaction. . . . An aspect of the effect of personal career on the dying situation is in the conception of time. Recognizing his approaching death, an elderly patient who has had a long and satisfying life may welcome it. He may also wish to review that life publicly. His wife or nurse, however, may refuse to listen, telling him that he should not give up hope of living, or even cautioning him against being "so morbid." On the other hand, other patients may throw the staff into turmoil because they will not accept their dying. Nonacceptance sometimes signifies a patient's protest against destiny for making him leave "unfinished work." These various time conceptions of different patients in the dying situation may run counter not only to each other, but also to the staff's work time concepts; as, for instance, when a patient's personal conception prevents the nurse from completing scheduled actions.

One further class of events attending the course of dying is of crucial importance for the action around the dying patient. These events are the characteristic work required by medical and hospital organization, which occurs at critical junctures of the dying process. That the person is actually dying must be recognized if he is to be treated like a dying person. At some point, everyone may recognize that there "is nothing more to do." As dying approaches its conclusion, a death watch usually takes place. When death has ended the process, there must be a formal pronouncement, and then an announcement to the family. At each point in time, the staff's interrelated actions must be properly organized.

Taken all together, then, the total organization of activity—which we call "work"—during the course of dying is profoundly affected by temporal considerations. Some are evident to almost everyone, some are not. The entire web of temporal interrelationships we shall refer to as the *temporal order*. It includes the continual readjustment and coordination of staff effort, which we term the *organization of work*. . . .

In general, sociological writing about groups, organizations, and institutions tends to leave their temporal features

> unanalyzed. When they are handled explicitly, the focus is on such matters as deadlines, scheduling, rates, pacing, turnover, and concepts of time which may vary by organizational, institutional, or group position. The principal weakness of such analyses stems from an unexamined assumption that the temporal properties worth studying involve only the work of organizations and their members. For instance, the work time of personnel must be properly articulated—hence deadlines and schedules. Breakdowns in this temporal articulation occur not only through accident and poor planning, but also through differential valuation of time by various echelons, personnel, and clientele. But from our analysis the temporal order of the organization appears to require much wider range of temporal dimensions. We have assumed in this book that, for instance, people bring to an organization their own temporal concerns and that their actions there are profoundly affected by those concerns. Thus, woven into our analysis were experiential careers (hospital, illness, and personal), as well as the patient's and the families' concepts of time. In our analysis, we have attempted to show how temporal order in the hospital refers to a total, delicate, continuously changing articulation of these various temporal considerations. Such articulation, of course, includes easily recognizable organizational mechanisms but also less visible ones, including "arrangements" negotiated by various relevant persons.

Next we shall discuss the implications both of these quoted materials and those presented throughout the present book.

An organization can be conceived as a temporal matrix. Any organization—including the hospitals as sites for the work discussed in this book—embodies multiple lines of work, each of which has a biography. We say "biography" because past, present, and future are involved. Lines of work, of course, include the procedural and the conceptual, and in complex organizations there are many varieties of each. In addition, it is useful to think of other biographies being implicated in such organizations. Here is a list of a few of them. (*A*) Every kind of technology (in hospitals, these would include machine, drug, and surgical technologies) is at a different phase of its biography: some have just been invented and marketed, while others are phasing out, having lost competitive battles with newcomers; others are midstream in their temporal careers. (*B*) Occupations, too, have their "life histories," so that where a plurality of occupations and professions are found in a given organization, they will be at different phases of their histories. (*C*) Employees, too, will be at varying points in their different personal biographies. (*D*) So will be their clients whom they service or the customers to whom they market. (*E*) The organization itself and each of its subunits will have their own biographies. (*F*) And the organization as an institutional form will have a unique biography. Together these constitute the *temporal matrix* of an organization. In turn, each component of the matrix is affected in its development by more macroscopic temporal conditions: movements of impinging industries, larger social movements, and industrywide or nationwide or international trends.

Components of the temporal matrix intersect with each other, yielding temporal intersections and interactional nodes, which point to two main features of a temporal matrix. First, every biography crosscuts other biographies (for instance, technological with personal, occupational with technological). Those temporal intersections must be discovered for the organization under study by the interested researcher. Second, the intersections give rise to temporal interactional nodes, that is, clusters of interactions. Empirically these look to the observer just like any set of interactions, but viewed as the products of *temporal* intersections, they take on other colorations. Thus, the work situation in front of our eyes involves not merely a young black nurse and a young Spanish-American respiratory therapist and a middle-aged Jewish cardiologist, but three representatives of evolving occupations, as well as representatives of intensely personal biographies, and doubtless gender and ethnic and other "social movement" temporal intersections.

The work drama (Hughes's term, 1971) *is profoundly affected by the temporal images of the actors.* This propositon is simply the corollary of the preceding one, translated into the perspectives of the participants themselves. We have in mind the temporal images of, for instance, the patient who nears the end of his anticipated dying trajectory, the nurse who is close to retirement from her occupation, the bioengineer who is a missionary for his aspiring specialization, the physician who is downhearted because his specialty is losing ground to other specialties. Their temporal images are carried into interaction; the observer needs, therefore, to sense them and elicit them when interviewing. Otherwise he or she cannot understand the fuller import of interactions and their outcomes.

The temporal matrix consists of a set of conditions leading to observable or discoverable consequences. In any organizational setting that is rapidly changing—like an ICN (see chap. 9)—some consequences are known by the participants and others can be traced by a persistent observer. Where the temporal matrix seems frozen, as in rather stable organizational settings, the matrix nevertheless constitutes a set of conditions having consequences discoverable by a perceptive observer. The linkages between temporal conditions and their consequences are only less apparent. Types of consequences can be distinguished as follows.

The temporal conditions can impinge, first of all, on the temporal categories mentioned when reviewing the Moore and Zerubavel books, namely, sequence, pacing, scheduling, and so on. Empirically, it is possible to note how the particular biographical phase of technological product (say, a new type of machine) can alter scheduling, pacing, duration. Thus, when dialysis sessions were shortened from six to five hours, because of improved equipment, there occurred considerable changes in the temporal order of a dialysis ward (Wolfram Fischer 1983). Scheduling was speeded up. The numbers of patients dialyzed each day could then be increased, but this in turn altered the pacing of staff work. Even the temporal ordering of patients' lives was affected, for some could now arrange for dialysis in the evenings, thus allowing them to work during the daytime. In short, elements in the temporal matrix can operate in such fashions as to produce various temporal junctures and disjunctures in work and organization. These need to be discovered by the interested researcher.

Second, various types of work (safety, sentimental, etc.) can be affected differentially by components of the temporal matrix. A new technological biography, for instance, can have terrifying consequences for the safety of clients and/or employees, while having highly exciting progressive impact on occupational/professional knowledge, and may raise all sorts of bioethical or other sentimental-work issues for the workers, the worked-upon, and the bystanding public, too.

Third, it follows that there are consequences for the relationships among workers and between them and clients or customers. Probably this point is by now so apparent as to constitute a truism, but again researchers need to discover the most consequential of those linkages.

All of the above (temporal matrix, intersections, nodes, images, and their consequences) constitute the temporal order of an organization. We should not think of temporal order as a separate type of social order, but as a concept that can foster a deeper grasp of how work and institutions are organized. It is crucial to understand also that elements of temporal order—not just schedules and pacing, but even technological and personal biographies—are arguable, negotiable, manipulatable. It would be a mistake to conceive of them as inflexibly grounded in organizational rules or moving along through an inherent determinism. To underscore this point, recollect the closing lines of the material quoted earlier: "temporal order . . . refers to a total, delicate, continuously changing articulation of these various temporal considerations. Such articulation . . . includes . . . 'arrangements' negotiated by various relevant persons." Like all other human products, temporal order is partly a human construction, partly the outcome of structural constraints. Although we have not in this book made temporal order and temporal issues central to our analysis—except in the key chapter on trajectory—they are to be seen or glimpsed on various of its pages.

Industries and Interorganizational Transactions

In this section we shall explore implications of our approach for future research on relationships among organizations and for the industries with which they are associated. The organizations referred to here are those which, like hospitals and most others studied by specialists of "organizations," are producing goods or services. These organizations do not stand in splendid isolation, although until recently they were traditionally treated that way in organizational theory and research. They are related to each other in patterned modes (Strauss 1982*a*) and contextually related to one or more industries. Our exploration below will be more extensively programmatic than in the preceding sections. It will also be critical of two alternative approaches, namely, the resource dependence perspective on organizations and the ecological perspective on organizations. Our approach, of course, emphasizes the primacy of lines of work in and among organizations, linking them with conceptions of social worlds and arenas; to that, we shall add a discussion of the related phenomenon of industries.

The External Control of Organizations: A Resource Dependence Perspective, by Pfeffer and Salancik (1978), is part of a now overwhelming criticism of predominant types of organizational theory that for some years have been focused on individual organizations. The emphasis in their new, and influential, approach is on moving the focus of organizational studies toward an outside environment which necessarily must impinge on any organization. Most organizational theorists "give only token consideration to the environmental context of organizations." Moreover, most organizational writings are about how organizations operate, taking their existence for granted, but the resource dependence approach conceives organizational existence as "constantly in question, and . . . survival . . . as problematic." Organizational survival is, then, at the heart of this approach, and organizations are viewed as surviving "to the extent that they are effective," the key to that being "their ability to acquire and maintain resources." To obtain those resources, an organization depends on transactions with other organizations, whether the latter are public or private, small or large, bureaucratic or organic in nature. In struggling for survival, an organization can achieve some measure of success in shaping its destiny despite the external controls that emanate from an environment composed of other organizations. So, the constraining environment does not wholly or crudely determine an organization's behavior, but interacts with it through the "focal" organization's perception of the environment.

From our standpoint, there are several notable features of the resource dependence perspective. First, despite an emphasis on the "interconnectedness of organizations," Pfeffer and Salancik are avowedly concerned with the focal organization itself. They are not really directing our gaze away from the individual organization so much as referring us to how other organizations relate to the organization under study. Second, they are centrally concerned with the focal organization's survival, hence, with conditions and strategies making for its success or failure, that is, for "effective performance." Third, the environment seems to consist, for them, mainly of other organizations—other firms, government agencies, interest group organizations. Presumably each of those is also resource dependent on others, but the mechanics and consequences of that interdependence are not central to Pfeffer and Salancik's approach. (An appropriate metaphor here is that these theorists are directing us not how to study an interstellar system so much as the fate of individual stars, taken one by one.) Fourth, there is understandably therefore no focus on organizations' being embedded in or straddling industries (the term does not appear in the index of the Pfeffer and Salancik book), nor on a corresponding necessity to study industries as a context for understanding even the single, focal organization. Fifth, these theorists have a conception of any organization as composed of a coalition of interest groups—they are reacting against older conceptions of "the" organization as having a relatively homogeneous structure, an organization with clear goals rationally planned and sought after—but they do not direct our attention to the negotiation and internal debate that necessarily attend the formation and maintenance of internal coalitions. In our terminology, they focus neither on internal arenas nor on the relations of those to external arenas, *each* embodying governmental, occupational, ethnic, and various other social movement ideologies, debates, and operational positions. While they think of "the environment" outside as impinging on an organization, constraining it, challenging it, they do not conceive of elements in that environment as literally inside the organization itself, in the form of workers carrying the outside into the work of the organization—"work" being not merely the production of goods or services but decisions about what goods or what services and how, when, where, how much to produce and market.

In general, this listing of features of the resource dependency perspective suggests that it is not so radically different from those it is designed to supplant. The vision offered us fails to come to grips with either the struggles within an organization's internal arenas (with their accompanying debates, ideologies, and inevitable processes of negotiation, persuasion, manipulation, and coercion) or with issues pertaining to the organization's (or its parts) relationships with a multiplicity of powerful arenas and their implicated social worlds, whose argumentative outcomes profoundly affect the internal structure and functioning of the organization. Nor is the organization put into a potentially changing structural context—as with the ICU in chapter 9—which can profoundly impinge on the organization. Nevertheless, this perspective's fuller attention to an environmental context composed of other organizations is certainly a great improvement over traditional organizational theory's bemusement with the internal dynamics of "an" organization's efficiency or lack of efficiency.

The ecological perspective (Brittain and Freeman 1980) on organizations is exemplified by the writings of J. Freeman, M. Hannan, N. Tuma, and J. Brittain (Hannan and Freeman 1974, 1978*a*, 1978*b*; Hannan, Freeman, and Tuma 1978; Brittain and Freeman 1980). Their basic criticism of traditional organizational theorists is that they "have largely ignored the broader social system of which organizations are a part and the patterned ways in which populations of organizations expand in repsonse to changes of that broader system" (Brittain and Freeman 1980, p. 291). This broader system is conceptualized in the most recent paper as an industry, where industry is defined as "a set of organizations that may be divided into populations characterized by different organizational forms but are interrelated on the basis of characteristic resources and basic usage technologies." Each industry is distinguishable from others "in terms of the 'resource space' it occupies." And the designation of industry "implies neither a multiplicity of form nor a particularly significant interaction among forms, except as the interdependence among forms is related to the defining resources" of money, market segments, people, energy, space, and physical substances. The overlap among the organizational populations within an industry is much greater than their overlap across industries. Another key concept is that of niche: "Any particular combination, or set of combinations, of resource utilization that distinguishes one organizational population from another is what we will call a 'niche.' An industry, then, may include a number of distinct niches, filled to varying degrees by specific organizational populations" (p. 293).

Proponents of the ecological perspective understandably focus on the appearance, development, and disappearance of organizations (quite like their counterparts in ecological biology who are concerned with the evolution and decline of biological forms). The development of new organizational forms, and the expansion of organizational populations, for instance, "can be studied as the intersection of two processes." As industries develop, they open new niches, and "organizations and the individuals who populate them will move into these niches in ways that reflect both past histories of organizational growth/decline and personal careers" (p. 337). Brittain and Freeman illustrate those propositions by an examination of the fast-expanding semiconductor industry, which is characterized by rapid technological change and marked expansion of its products and services.

Notable features of this ecological perspective include the following. First, the perspective takes as its basic unit entire populations of organizations, not single organizations or their environments (in the sense discussed by organizational theorists like Pfeffer and Salancik). Second, a central focus is the expansion and contraction of organizational populations within industries, including the evolution, development, and decline of their organizational forms. Third, there is an emphasis on availability of and changes in resources, as well as competition for those resources among organizations. ("Selection in organizational ecology is based on differential advantage among organizational forms in competition for scarce resources" in high density organizational populations. However, under conditions of low density, competition may not be so severe: a chief factor in successful competition then may be the "timely arrival" of the new organization in the industry itself.) Fourth, organizational strategies will vary in accordance with different conditions within the industry: whether there is a high or low density of organizations, whether there is much uncertainty of resource possibilities, and so on. Fifth, the organizational forms are profoundly affected in their internal characteristics by their embeddedness in the organizational population itself, that is, by factors like an industry's expansion or contraction.

As an approach to the study and understanding of organizations, the ecological perspective represents an improvement over its competitors. It focuses attention away from the individual organization except as the organization is affected by its location within industries. And it firmly directs our gaze at what is transpiring within industries so that we can then look at individual organizations, their characteristics, and strategies. However, like other organizational theorists, the ecological people are basically still caught up in the centrality of competitive processes. This means that they, at least until now, have far less concern for cooperation and conflict among or within organizations than those economists and historians who study industries and industrial firms have. Nor are they yet drawn to examine either the vital intersections between organizations and impinging arenas and social movements (occupational, ethnic, mass, etc.) or the ideological features that profoundly affect negotiation, persuasion, coercion, and other strategies or processes within and among organizations. Utilizing the ecological approach, researchers can probably fruitfully examine lines of work within and among organizations, but the ecologists have not addressed that central organizational issue either.

We have discussed the ecological and the resource dependence perspectives in order to contrast our own perspective on organizations and industries, as implied by the kinds of materials presented in this book on medical work. We have not here, of course, made organizations or industries our central concerns, but we did move carefully from health industry (indeed supra-industry) conditions to work, and in closing chapters in the reverse direction as well. What then are some implications of this approach to work for the research on organizations and industries?

The core concept with which we begin is that of social world. Ostensively defined, social worlds include occupational worlds (medicine, physics), ethnic worlds, leisure worlds (ski, tennis), industrial worlds (chemical, oil), and so on. There would be no social worlds unless there were similar or common activities that lay at their core and people who performed them (Strauss 1978*b*). For performing those activities, there are internally developed or borrowed technologies, plans to do them, other activities, and ideologies affecting how they are done. Every social world of any complexity has its subdivisions or "segments," and in fact one feature of complex worlds is their relatively rapid change, giving rise to segmentation processes (Strauss 1983). Likewise, every social world (and its segments) is characterized by intersection processes, wherein it exchanges, negotiates, conflicts, and so on with other social worlds and subworlds. In addition every social world and subworld is characterized by their engaging in debates; that is, they participate both in internal and external debates about their activities (and other activities that may affect them): their nature, legitimation (Strauss 1982*b*), technology, siting—how, when, where, who. Every complex world also has its characteristic organizations; indeed, like hospitals, they are embedded in one or more worlds, though some organizations straddle many worlds, universities and hospitals for instance. "It is possible to conceptualize 'society as a whole' as consisting of a mosaic of social worlds, which both touch and interpenetrate. . . . The manner and consequences of these interpenetrations (or *intersections*) is one of the major areas for research on social worlds" (Gerson 1978, p. 22).

It follows that industries can be conceived of as social worlds organized around the production of a group of related goods or services. "Clearly the characteristics of these worlds will vary according to a number of criteria, but the common characteristic of organization around a core production activity, to which all other activities in the social world can be oriented defines a specialized class of social worlds" (Gerson 1978, p. 23; see also Becker 1982; Kling and Gerson 1978). Industries do appear to differ in accordance as they vary around a number of dimensions. These include: size, technology, products, geographic situation, organizational forms, market structure, public visibility, governmental regulation, governmental subsidy, structural interests, segmentation, financing, type of integration, accessibility to entry, the composition of the labor force, and so on.

Among the questions that a researcher would wish to raise about the industry under study (and/or any of its firms or associations) is its intersections with governments (especially those involving regulations, subsidies, and relevant legislation), with various interest groups (like those of the environmentalists), and with social movements (occupational, gender, ethnic). The researcher would also wish to know what its segmentation patterns are and how they relate to the organization and change of central production patterns (i.e., lines of work). A particularly important intersection for industrial worlds, of course, pertains to markets: "what is the pattern of markets in which the world [and its organizations] is engaged, and how do these 'map' onto the pattern of intersections among sub-worlds?" (Gerson 1978, p. 24)

Where do "organizations" fit into this conceptualization of industries? A glance at a few books written by economists or historians about industries and industrial firms shows very quickly that—quite as the ecologists say—firms, associations, industrial bureaus do occupy specialized niches within the total industry; that is, they do not all engage in producing the same product, use exactly the same resources, deal with exactly the same markets. Furthermore, like nonindustrial organizations, these firms and associations may straddle or be parts of two or more social worlds (industries) and so, affected by different sets of intersections and segmentations. (For instance, a vertically integrated paper company intersects differently with segments of lumber and chemical industries than does a firm that is not vertically integrated.) Any organization's characteristics, then, are linked in very complex ways with its location in a contextual social world or worlds and, of course, also with intersections between it and salient other organizations in these and related worlds. Internally, the specific lines of work, indeed the characteristic arcs of work, engaged in will be tightly linked with the structural conditions discussed above; in turn, as illustrated by chapter 9 on the ICN and the ICU, quite possibly the former will affect those larger conditions.

Hallmarks of our approach to organizations and their work, we might add, include two other emphases. First, there is the crucial importance of arenas, both internal and external. Second, there is the centrality of ideological positions taken by workers, whether they be floor nurses or the directors of large corporations. Those ideologies are not merely legitimating of lines and modes of work (Strauss 1982*b*) but profoundly affect the choice of intra- and extraorganizational strategies (cf. Chandler 1977). On occasion, the individual or concerted strategies of powerful corporations can even affect the strategies of entire industries (McConnell 1953; Kling and Gerson 1978) and thereby significantly affect large markets, government agencies, even national policy. It is not at all necessary for researchers to adopt the "natives' view" of these managerial-organizational strategies as basically rational: they may be well thought out and carried out, but deeply ideological in coloration. Just as a team climbing Mt. Everest displays an amazing technology and technical organization but also carries its full complement of ideological baggage, so do industrial (and other) organizations. A social world–work approach to organizations enjoins us to look for these ideological underpinnings, especially as they appear in arena debates and disputes which can be so crucial to the directions of organizational work and to the fates of organizations themselves.

The Sociology of Work—But What Work?

Most work goes on within or in connection with organizations. And a great proportion of work is done by people who have various occupational or professional titles. So it is not surprising that sociologists and other social scientists who write about work do not separate their analyses or commentaries or critiques of work from considerations of work-place and occupations/professions. Indeed, most writings that comprise the "sociology of work" turn out, on scanning, really to be about occupations or professions and the organizations worked in. (Even a short list of some of the best-known books and articles in this subfield of sociology will make that point: for instance, Hughes's *Sociological Eye*, Freidson's *Professional Dominance*, Becker, Geer, Hughes, and Strauss's *Boys in White*, Sutherland's *Professional Thief*, Smigel's *Wall Street Lawyer*.) Not incidentally, of course, there are descriptions and analyses of work done by members of professions, occupations, and by organizational members, but intense focus on the work itself—its task sequences, its organization, its many variants and their conditions and consequences, its articulation, its evaluative processes—is far less usual. The literature of the "sociology of medicine" is quite representative of emphases in the more encompassing field which, in fact, is traditionally called—all in one breath—"the sociology of work and occupations," a linkage exemplified by the journal by that name.

Those observations are perhaps not so startling, at least not at this point in the book. A more unconventional observation is that work which is not linked with work places or which is not paid work has generally not been regarded as work, as Freidson (1976, Wadel 1979) and various women reformers and scholars have remarked, by official agencies such as the U.S. Census Bureau, by the general public, or even by social scientists. We shall carry the line of argument still further, following through the implications of our data and their conceptualization. We suggest that studies of work, done from whatever disciplinary perspective, should include *any enterprise*, even when those engaged in the enterprise do not think of it as involving work. We have in mind not only enterprises like some touched on in this book (dying with grace, living as decently as possible despite an intrusive illness), but the thousand and one lines of action that anyone can quickly imagine, if one thinks of lines of action as lines of *work*: escape from a prisoner-of-war camp, a political campaign, a fund-raising campaign by unpaid volunteers, or further out on the margins of what seems at first blush nonwork: going through therapy, keeping a marriage going, raising a child properly, making a quilt or doing a puzzle, learning to ski or skate.

Any or all of those activities may be fun (one's paid work can be fun, too), but they also involve some, even tremendous, amounts of work. Each can usefully be conceived of as a trajectory, with its arc of work and implicated tasks. Most of the analyses done in this book are surely relevant—substantive issues aside—to these enterprises, are they not? A genuine sociology of work can be germane to many activities not now studied by students of work. So we have given one answer to the question asked in the title of this section: The Sociology of Work—But What Work?

Appendix: Methodological Note

The research reported on in this monograph took about five years, beginning with an exploratory phase (1977) and ending with the final writing (1981–82). It involved a team of four researchers working in close concert. The research style utilized on that project has been extensively described in previous publications written or co-authored by the senior author of this monograph (*Psychiatric Ideologies and Institutions*, 1964; *Awareness of Dying* [with B. Glaser], 1965; *Time for Dying* [with B. Glaser], 1968; *Discovery of Grounded Theory* [with B. Glaser], 1967; *Anguish* [with B. Glaser], 1970; "Discovering New Theory from Previous Theory," 1970; *Politics of Pain Management* [with S. Fagerhaugh], 1977; *Field Research* [with L. Schatzman], 1973; *Theoretical Sensitivity* [with B. Glaser], 1978). There is no need to retrace that ground. However, there is at least one feature of the research reported on here that is rather special, and another that is rather usual. We shall address these for what light they may shed on our research report as well as for whatever the discussion might add for readers who are interested in methodological issues as such. In our discussion, we shall assiduously avoid the customary "we did this and this" anecdotal style, which really adds very little to cumulative methodological knowledge, however enlightening it might be about the situational context within which the researchers gathered the data.

First, a few details about the research project: exploratory interviewing and field observation were carried on for several months in 1976. The project received USPH funding through the years 1977–81. The research design called generally for field observation on diverse hospital wards—

selected at first by selective sampling (Schatzman and Strauss 1973) and later by theoretical sampling (Glaser and Strauss 1967, Glaser 1978) and also on various kinds of wards in several different kinds of hospitals to maximize certain structural conditions: a city-county hospital, a large urban community hospital, a military hospital, a university hospital, two small urban hospitals, a suburban community hospital.

The fieldwork was intensive and was carried out by three members of the research team. In addition, a great number of open-ended interviews were conducted with hospital personnel selected in accordance with concepts and hypotheses that emerged over the course of the study. Other but substantially fewer interviews were done with persons who represented special interests arising also from our emergent research: for instance, hospital architects, hospital administrators, medical equipment innovators, designers, and researchers. The resulting data were analyzed along the lines discussed in the above-mentioned books. The research ultimately led in some directions not at all foreseen when writing the original research proposal. Thus, we began with the idea that there would be at least one monograph and several articles, presumably about the impact of medical equipment on patient care and perhaps on the health occupations. We did not anticipate either the themes and shape of this particular monograph nor three others that will be published respectively on: (1) clinical safety, (2) the work of kin, and (3) major issues in the health policy arena as seen from our perspective on the prevalence of chronic illness and the accompanying explosion of medical technology.

We turn now to the two special attributes of the research project itself. First, the experiential history of the senior author, which it is necessary to know in order to understand essential features of the research itself. That experiential history begins in 1957 when Strauss spent three months observing and talking with residents and interns at the University of Kansas medical school, collecting minor background data for what later became *Boys in White* (Becker, Geer, Hughes, and Strauss 1961). From 1958–60, he did fieldwork at two mental hospitals. His education in medical matters became considerably deeper during the several years of field research (1960–64) that culminated in three books about death and dying, later, (1972–74) to be added to by reading, talking about, and analyzing the field notes of his research associate, Shizuko Fagerhaugh, pertaining to the handling of pain in hospitals. Relevant to all this is that after the study on dying, around 1969, Strauss *finally* became aware that all of the patients whom he had been observing in hospitals, whether they were dying or not, were there because they suffered from one form or another of chronic illness. So he sent research students into clinics and into the homes of clinic patients to interview them. His conceptions of chronic illness, and of the profound implications of the prevalence of chronic illness, took shape from reading these interviews (see Strauss and Glaser 1975). In 1972, he had a heart attack, followed by a long period of gradual recuperation. Those years gave him further data to mull over.

But he had for a long time, ever since the middle 1960s, sensed that the cutting edge of medicine was its technology, which led to changes in medical work and in the character and composition of the health occupations/professions. It eventually dawned on him around 1974 that the "acute care" given in hospitals was nothing more than one pole of a continuum pertaining to chronic illness, another pole being the management of chronic illness at home by the sufferers and their kinsmen. Hence, it was not only interest in technology that prompted his seeking funds to study technology in the hospital—technology employed for intervening in the courses of chronic illnesses.

Consequently, when exploratory work for the "medical machinery" research began, it rested on a large amount of detailed observation about hospitals, of work and interactions there, of hospital personnel and their respective occupations or professions. The research was also underpinned by several important concepts developed in the earlier writings. This experiential grounding—personal as well as research—meant that the research team could move rather quickly into their theoretical sampling, comparative analysis, coding, and the memo writing in which conceptual densification and integration were at least begun.

After the first months of exploratory work, however, *the* unexpected contingency that really affected the work style and outcome of the project—far more than the particular research itself—was the choice of research associates and their evolution as a research team. The team members were women, middle-aged, and married. They were all Strauss's former students and gifted fieldworkers: two of them (Suczek and Wiener) were sociologists, and the third (Fagerhaugh) was a sociologically trained research nurse. The sociologists had had minimal experience with "medical research"; the nurse was steeped in it. She provided much needed ballast for the ship, coming through with medically oriented and professionally oriented information when required, quite aside from the observations gathered by all three during their respective months in the field. (Strauss did only a little fieldwork around special issues like sentimental work.) The team met weekly almost from the project's inception. (For a time, three students in the Graduate Program in Sociology of the University of California, San Francisco, Diane Beeson, Roberta Lessor, and Irma Zuckermann, participated in the team sessions, most helpfully, and also did some fieldwork for us. During the third year a visiting professor from the University of Bielefeld, West Germany, Fritz Schuetze, was also a full working member of the team.) The initial team meetings were probably like those in many other group projects: planning sessions, reports on recent fieldwork or interviewing, reports on documentary search, preliminary analyses of data, and blue-skying conceptualization. Meanwhile preliminary coding and memo writing were going on, principally but not exclusively by Strauss.

However, much to our surprise the weekly meetings began to take on a life of their own, began to turn into verbal-coding and memo-building sessions. After a couple of years of this, there were a few meetings for which summarizing memos were prepared, typed, and discussed; so that later memos were built systematically atop of these major memos. Before Fritz Schuetze left for Germany, near the end of the project's third year, a number of meetings were devoted to thinking through the formulation that constitutes the core chapter of this book—on trajectory—as well as some of the muddier aspects of our thinking about what came to be termed "sentimental work."

It may interest readers to know also that no commitment was made to the basic theme of this book until all of the transcribed tapes of the team-meeting memos had been scrutinized, along with a number of other typed memos and a minor amount of actual coding of data. In this sense there was a radical departure from the intensive coding described and advocated in *Discovery of Grounded Theory* (Glaser and Strauss 1967) and in *Theoretical Sensitivity* (Glaser 1978). We certainly could have followed the counsel given in those books but the analytic mode that emerged, like topsy, from this particular research team's experience with its weekly meetings seemed generally to be exciting and satisfying, even seductive, while still seeming adequate to what we wished to accomplish. Even so, we were surprised that we were not forced back to doing a great deal more coding and memo writing. Of course, in this as in other publications, including the papers published earlier (Wiener, Strauss, Fagerhaugh, and Suczek 1979; Strauss 1980; Strauss, Fagerhaugh, Suczek, and Wiener 1980, 1981, 1982*a*, *b*; Fagerhaugh, Strauss, Suczek, and Wiener 1980) considerable coding, memo writing, and other focused thinking went on during the writing, with the usual surprises of additional discovery then.

Perhaps more important for us to emphasize about the team's work—in line with earlier comments about Strauss's previous experiences informing the whole project—is how the personal experiences of each project member enriched both the data collection and the analysis. We emphasize this particularly because of firmly held canons, widespread among social scientists, about the biased subjectivity of personal experience, which ought therefore to be carefully screened out of research like potential impurities from drinking water. Strauss had a bout of severe illness during the fourth year of this project: his experiences became usable data. Carolyn Wiener's mother had a hospitalization that yielded useful data, as did her own experiences with two minor illnesses. Barbara Suczek had had a longstanding and severe problem with her eyes, and her numerous experiences with her physicians and with a period of hospitalization afforded additional data. Shizuko Fagerhaugh—a nurse, after all—helped to guide her brother through a difficult surgery and her mother through many complicated dealings with medical people around back and eye problems. In addition, Barbara Suczek was involved in extensive kin work with other family members when her sister-in-law went into fateful emergency surgery. Finally, one of this researcher's teaching colleagues was, during three long years of our project, dying from a lung disease; he and his wife expressed themselves freely to her about their extraordinarily independent and resourceful management of his trajectory, which culminated finally in his death.

The point of this long recital of the researcher's fortuitous experiences is that they afforded both additional insight into our formally acquired "research data," *and* material which we decided to use as data since they are "perfectly good data, so why not?" Some of those data are utilized, including quotations as field notes, in this monograph; others have been used in papers about patient work and kin work, as well as in the other books spawned by the project. What we have done is something in the spirit of people like Robert Park and Everett Hughes, both of whom poured their own living experiences into their constructions of sociological theory, albeit neither explicitly wrote research papers or monographs (though Hughes did write one, on French Canada). In this regard we have also followed the spirit of the philosophical movement called "pragmatism," which lies solidly behind the interactionist tradition in which we work and which had as one of its major figures John Dewey who wrote books with such titles as *Experience and Nature* and *Art as Experience*. Or to paraphrase the words of Richard Wohl, a social historian, colleague, and diseased friend: "Be like a good tailor, use every last piece; don't waste *any*-thing!"

Perhaps a few words might be useful concerning our use of illustrative data in this monograph, since we do not follow the practice of frequently quoting chunks of material drawn from interviews or field notes, as is the standard practice in qualitative-research publications. Back in 1967, one of us published (with Barney Glaser) a book on method, the *Discovery of Grounded Theory*, which among other things was, and is, a forceful argument for theoretical formulation based on the qualitative analysis of data. Then and now, much that passes for analysis is relatively low-level description or is a labeling of data with Goffman's or some other theorist's concepts and schemes. Then and now, many quite esteemed and excellent monographs use a great deal of data—quotes or field note selections. This procedure is very useful when the behavior being studied is relatively foreign to the experiences of most readers or when the factual assertions being made would be under considerable contest by skeptical and otherwise relatively well-informed readers. Most of these monographs are descriptively dense, but alas theoretically thin. If you look at their indexes, there are almost no new concepts listed, ones that have emerged in the course of the research; furthermore, the linkages made by the author among the phenomena represented by his or her concepts are often not especially numerous, nor are variations specified by noting the relevant conditions, consequences, associated strategies, etc. Sometimes the monographs can have exciting ideas, but these may not be well integrated.

In our monographs, and in writings by people whom we have trained, we attempt to analyze data closely (beginning with line-by-line analysis of interviews, field notes, and documents), so as to construct an integrated and dense theory. So the interview and field note quotations tend to be brief, and often are woven in with the analysis within the same or in closely related sentences. Longer quotes (especially from field notes) are used for case illustrations—and there are several in this book—or when the events and actions described in the field notes might help the reader visualize them better in tandem with the analytical points being made, especially when the events or actions might otherwise be difficult to grasp (as with the vignettes in the sentimental work chapter). And, since many readers may be quite unfamiliar with what goes on in hospitals, the illustrative material is used sometimes to fill that gap, though generally our own words should handle that problem. Our inclusion of the cumulative-mess trajectory case is the only instance of very extensive quoting; sometimes we do this when presenting case histories. In general, however, we think twice about loading a theoretically oriented monograph with too many chunks of descriptive material and are fairly deliberate about those that are included. Understandably in this style of presentation—where the basic analysis shapes the organization of both the monograph and its descriptive elements—the predominant forms of quotation are the short quote and the precise quote.

References

Andreopolus, S., ed. 1974. *Primary Care: Where Medicine Fails.* Sun Valley Forum on National Health. New York: John Wiley & Sons.

Arms, S. 1975. *Immaculate Deception.* Boston: Houghton Mifflin.

Becker, H. 1982. *The Art World.* Berkeley: University of California Press.

Becker, H., and Geer, B. 1957. "Participant Observation and Interviewing: A Comparison." *Human Organization* 16:28–32.

Becker, H.; Geer, B.; Hughes, E. C.; and Strauss, A. L. 1961. *Boys in White: Student Culture in Medical School.* Chicago: University of Chicago Press.

Becker, H., and Strauss, A. 1956. "Careers, Personality, and Adult Socialization." *American Journal of Sociology* 62:253–63.

Benoliel, J. Q. 1975. "Childhood Diabetes: The Commonplace in Living Becomes Uncommon." In A. Strauss and B. Glaser, *Chronic Illness and the Quality of Life*, pp. 89–98. St. Louis: C. V. Mosby Publishing Co.

Bosk, C. 1979. *Forgive and Remember: Managing Medical Failure.* Chicago: University of Chicago Press.

Bradley, R. A. 1974. *Husband-Coached Childbirth.* Rev. ed. New York: Harper & Row.

Braudel, F. 1980. "History and the Social Sciences." *On History.* Chicago: University of Chicago Press. Originally published in 1958.

Brittain, J., and Freeman, J. 1980. "Organizational Proliferation and Density Dependent Selection." In *Organizational Life Cycle*, pp. 291–341. Edited by J. Kimberly et al. San Francisco: Jossey-Bass.

Bucher, R., and Schatzman, L. 1964. "Negotiating a Division of Labor among Professionals in the State Mental Hospitals." *Psychiatry* 27:266–77.

Burns, T., and Stalker, G. M. 1961. *The Management of Innovation.* London: Tavistock.

Chandler, A. 1977. *The Visible Hand.* Cambridge, Mass.: Belknap Press, Harvard University Press.

Clemente, F. 1972. "The Measurement Problem in the Analysis of an Ecological Concept: The Division of Labor." *Pacific Sociological Review* 15:30–40.

Dalton, M. 1959. *Men Who Manage.* New York: John Wiley & Sons.

Davis, M. Z. 1980. "The Organizational, Interactional, and Care-Oriented Conditions for Patient Participation in Continuity of Care: A Framework for Staff Interaction." *Social Science and Medicine* 14:39–47.

Duff, R. S., and Hollingshead, A. B. 1968. *Sickness and Society.* New York: Harper & Row.

Emerson, R., and Pollner, M. 1976. "Dirty Work Designations: Their Features and Consequences in a Psychiatric Setting." *Social Problems* 23:243–54.

Ephron, N. 1978. *San Francisco Chronicle,* December 4, p. 19.

Fagerhaugh, S., and Strauss, A. 1977. *Politics of Pain Management: Staff-Patient Interaction.* Menlo Park: Addison-Wesley Publishing Co.

Fagerhaugh, S.; Strauss, A.; Suczek, B.; and Wiener, C. 1980 "The Impact of Technology on Patients, Providers, and Care Patterns." *Nursing Outlook* 28:666–72.

———. Forthcoming. *Safety, Danger and Risk in the Technologized Hospital.*

Fischer, W. 1983. *Time and Chronic Illness, A Study on the Constitution of Temporality.* Rehabilitation, University of Bielefeld, West Germany.

Fisher, B., and Strauss, A. 1978. "The Chicago Tradition: Thomas, Park and Their Successors." *Symbolic Interaction* 1:5–23.

Fox, H. A. 1979. Comment at conference on Technological Approaches to Obstetrics: Benefits, Risks, Alternatives, San Francisco, California, February 3–4.

Fox, R. C. 1959. *Experiment Perilous.* New York: Free Press.

Freidson, E. 1970. *Professional Dominance: The Social Structure of Medical Care* New York: Atherton.

———. 1976. *Doctoring Together: A Study of Professional Social Control.* New York: Elsevier.

Freundenberger, H. J. 1974. "Staff Burnout." *Journal of Social Issues* 30:159–65.

Futterman, E., and Hoffman, L. 1973. "Crisis and Adaptation in the Families of Fatally Ill Children." In *The Child in His Family,* 2:127–43. Edited by E. J. Anthony and C. Koupernik. New York: John Wiley & Sons.

Garfinkel, H. 1967. *Studies in Ethnomethodology*. Englewood Cliffs, N.J.: Prentice-Hall.
Gerson, E. 1976. Personal communication on division of labor, Tremont Research Institute, San Francisco.
———. 1977. "Rationalization and Varieties of Technical Work." Tremont Research Institute, San Francisco.
———. 1978. "The Unit of Analysis in Symbolic Interaction Research." Tremont Research Institute, San Francisco.
———. 1981*a*. Memo on Human Information Systems. 16 July. Tremont Research Institute, San Francisco.
———. 1981*b*. Memo on Dirty Work and Scut Work. 6 August. Tremont Research Institute, San Francisco.
———. Forthcoming. "Scientific Work Organization: The Population Realignment in Biology, 1880–1925." Tremont Research Institute, San Francisco.
Gerson, E., and Strauss, A. 1975. "Time for Living." *Social Policy* 6:12–18.
Glaser, B. 1976. *Experts Versus Laymen: A Study of the Patsy and the Subcontractor*. New Brunswick, N.J.: Transaction Books.
———. 1978. *Theoretical Sensitivity*. Mill Valley: Sociology Press.
Glaser, B. G., and Strauss, A. 1965. *Awareness of Dying*. Chicago: Aldine Publishing Co.
———. 1967. *Discovery of Grounded Theory: Strategies for Qualitative Research*. Chicago: Aldine Publishing Co., 1967.
———. 1968. *Time for Dying*. Chicago: Aldine Publishing Co.
———. 1971. *Status Passage: A Formal Theory*. Chicago: Aldine Publishing Co.
Goffman, E. 1963*a*. *Behavior in Public Places*. New York: Free Press.
———. 1963*b*. *Stigma: Notes on the Management of Spoiled Identity*. Englewood Cliffs, N.J.: Prentice-Hall.
Hall, P., and Hall, D.-A. S. 1982. "The Social Conditions of the Negotiated Order." *Urban Life* 11:328.
Hall, R. 1980. "Theoretical Trends in the Sociology of Occupations." *Sociological Quarterly* 24:5–24.
Hamil, E. M. 1976. "People Power." *National League of Nursing Publication* 20-1623:3–8.
Hannan, M., and Freeman, J. 1974. "Environment and the Structure of Organizations." Paper presented at annual meeting of American Sociological Association, Montreal, September.
———. 1978*a*. "Internal Politics of Growth and Decline." In *Environments and Organizations*, 177–99. Edited by M. Meyer et al. San Francisco: Jossey-Bass.
———. 1978*b*. "The Population Ecology of Organizations." In *Environments and Organizations*, 131–76. Edited by M. Meyer et al. San Francisco: Jossey-Bass.

Hannan, M.; Freeman, J.; and Tuma, N. 1978. "Organizational Ecology." Mimeographed report, Stanford University.

Hoffman, J. 1974. "Nothing Can Be Done: Social Dimensions of the Treatment of Stroke Patients in a General Hospital." *Urban Life and Culture* 3:50–70.

Hughes, E. C. 1951. "Mistakes at Work." *Canadian Journal of Economics and Political Science* 17:320–27.

———. 1971. *The Sociological Eye*. Chicago: Aldine, 1971.

Jackall, R. 1978. *Workers in a Labyrinth*. Montclair: Allanheld, Osman.

Johnson, F., and Kaplan, C. 1980. "Talk-in-the-Work: Aspects of Social Organization of Work in a Computer Center." *Journal of Pragmatics* 4:351–65.

Kassenbaum, G., and Bauman, B. 1965. "Dimensions of Sick Role in Chronic Illness." *Journal of Health and Human Behavior* 6:16–27.

Klaus, M. 1979. Comment at conference on Technological Approaches to Obstetrics: Benefits, Risks, Alternatives, San Francisco, California, February 3–4.

Kling, R., and Gerson, E. 1978. "Patterns of Segmentation and Intersection in the Computer World." *Symbolic Interaction* 1:24–43.

Labovitz, S., and Gibbs, J. 1964. "Urbanization, Technology, and the Division of Labor: Further Evidence." *Pacific Sociological Review* 7:3–9.

Lamaze, F. 1970. *Painless Childbirth: The Lamaze Method*. Chicago: Contemporary Books.

Latour, B., and Woolgar, S. 1979. *Laboratory Life: The Social Construction of Scientific Facts*. Beverly Hills: Sage Publications.

Leboyer, F. 1975. *Birth without Violence*. New York: Alfred A. Knopf, 1975.

Lorber, J. 1981. "Good Patients and Problem Patients: Conformity and Deviance in a General Hospital." In *The Sociology of Health and Illness*, pp. 395–404. Edited by P. Conrad and R. Kern. New York: St. Martins Press.

Mayo, L. 1956. "Problems and Challenge." In *Guides to Action on Chronic Illness*. New York: National Health Council of New York.

McConnell, G. 1953. *The Decline of Agrarian Democracy*. Reprint 1969. New York: Atheneum.

Millman, M. 1977. *The Unkindest Cut*. New York: Morrow.

Moore, W. 1963. *Man, Time, and Society*. New York: John Wiley & Sons.

Mundinger, M. O. N. 1973. "Primary Nurse—Role Evolution." *Nursing Outlook* 21:643–45.

National Institute of Child Health and Human Development. 1979. *Antenatal Diagnosis*. Report of a Consensus Development Conference, March 5–7, 1979. Publication No. NIH 79-1973. Bethesda.

Neutra, R. 1979. Comment at conference on Technological Approaches to Obstetrics: Benefits, Risks, Alternatives, San Francisco, California, February 3–4.

Olesen, V., and Whittaker, E. 1968. *The Silent Dialogue.* San Francisco: Jossey-Bass.
Parsons, T. 1951. *Social System.* New York: Free Press.
Pfeffer, J., and Salancik, G. 1978. *The External Control of Organizations: A Resource Dependence Perspective.* New York: Harper & Row.
Plough, A. 1981. "Medical Technology and the Crisis of Experience: The Costs of Clinical Legitimation." *Social Science and Medicine* 15F:89.
Redman, B. 1976. *The Process of Patient Teaching in Nursing.* 3d ed. St. Louis: C. V. Mosby Publishing Co.
Reichle, M. 1975. "Psychological Stress in the Intensive Care Unit." *Nursing Digest* 3:12–14.
Reif, L. 1975. "Ulcerative Colitis: Strategies for Managing Life." In A. Strauss and B. Glaser, *Chronic Illness and the Quality of Life*, pp. 81–88. St. Louis: C. V. Mosby Publishing Co.
Riemer, J. 1976. "Hard Hats' Mistakes at Work: The Social Organization of Error in Building Construction Work." *Social Problems* 23:255–67.
Roth, J. 1963. *Timetables.* Indianapolis: Bobbs-Merrill.
———. 1972. "Some Contingencies of the Moral Evaluation and Control of Clientele: The Case of the Hospital Emergency Service." *American Journal of Sociology* 77:836–49.
Roy, D. 1952. "Quota Restriction and Goldbricking in a Machine Shop." *American Journal of Sociology* 57:427–42.
Rushing, W. 1968. "Hardness of Material as Related to Division of Labor in Manufacturing Industries." *Administrative Science Quarterly* 13:229–45.
Russell, L. B. 1979. *Technology in Hospitals: Medical Advances and Their Diffusion.* Washington, D.C.: Brookings Institute.
Schatzman, L., and Strauss, A. 1973. *Field Research.* Englewood Cliffs, N.J.: Prentice-Hall.
Schuetze, F. N.d. "Die Technik Narrativer Interviews." University of Kassel, West Germany.
Simonton, O. C. 1974. Management of the Emotional Aspect of Malignancy. Symposium on New Dimensions of Rehabilitation for Handicapped, University of Florida, Gainsville, Florida, Department of Health and Rehabilitation Services, June 14–16. Mimeographed.
Skolnik, J. 1966. *Justice without Trial.* New York: John Wiley & Sons.
Smigel, E. 1964. *The Wall Street Lawyer.* New York: Free Press.
Star, S. L., and Gerson, E. M. Forthcoming. "Management of Anomalies in Scientific Research, I: Varieties of Anomaly; II: Properties of Artifacts."
Stelling, J., and Bucher, R. 1973. "Vocabularies of Realism in Professional Socialization." *Social Science and Medicine* 7:661–75.
Stinson, R., and Stinson, P. 1979. "On the Death of a Baby." *Atlantic Monthly* 244:64–72.

Strauss, A. N.d. "Awareness Contexts."
———. 1978*a*. *Negotiations*. San Francisco: Jossey-Bass.
———. 1978*b*. "A Social World Perspective." In *Studies in Symbolic Interaction*, 1:119–28. Edited by N. K. Denzin. Greenwich, Conn.: JAI Press.
———. 1980. "Chronic Illness." *Social Sciences and Medicine, Medical Geography* 14D:351–53.
———. 1982*a*. "Interorganizational Negotiation." *Urban Relations* 11:350–67.
———. 1982*b*. "Social Worlds and Legitimation Processes." In *Studies in Symbolic Interaction*, 4:171–90. Edited by N. K. Denzin. Greenwich, Conn.: JAI Press.
———. 1984. "Social Worlds and Their Segmentation." In *Studies in Symbolic Interaction*, 5:123–39. Edited by N. K. Denzin. Greenwich, Conn.: JAI Press.
Strauss, A.; Fagerhaugh, S.; Suczek, B.; and Wiener, C. 1980. "Gefühlsarbeit, Ein Beitrag zur Arbeits- und Berufssoziologie." *Kölner Zeitschrift für Soziologie und Sozialpsychologie* 32:629–51.
———. 1981. "Patients' Work in the Technologized Hospital." *Nursing Outlook* 29:404–12.
———. 1982*a*. "Sentimental Work in the Technologized Hospital." *Sociology of Health and Illness* 4 (3):254–78.
———. 1982*b*. "The Work of Hospitalized Patients." *Social Science and Medicine* 16:977–86.
———. 1970. *Anguish: The Case History of a Dying Trajectory*. San Francisco: Sociology Press.
Strauss, A., and Glaser, B. 1975. *Chronic Illness and the Quality of Life*. St. Louis: C. V. Mosby Publishing Co.
Strauss, A.; Schatzman, L.; Bucher, R.; Ehrlich, D.; and Sabshin, M. 1964*a*. "The Hospital and Its Negotiated Order." In *The Hospital in Modern Society*. Edited by E. Freidson. New York: Free Press of Glencoe.
———. 1964*b*. *Psychiatric Ideologies and Institutions*. New York: Free Press of Glencoe.
Sutherland, E. 1937. *The Professional Thief*. Chicago: University of Chicago Press.
Thomas, L. 1974. *The Living Cell*. New York: Bantam Books.
Trow, M. 1957. "Comment on 'Participant Observation and Interviewing: A Comparison." *Human Organization* 16:33–35.
Wadel, C. 1979. "The Hidden Work of Everyday Life." In *Social Anthropology at Work*. Edited by S. Wallman. London: Academic Press.
Wager, W. 1959. "Career Patterns and Role Problems of Airline Pilots in a Major Airline Company." Ph.D. diss., Department of Sociology, University of Chicago.

Wiener, C.; Fagerhaugh, S.; Strauss, A.; and Suczek, B. 1980. "Patient Power: Complex Issues Need Complex Answers." *Social Policy* 11 (September–October): 31–38.

Wiener, C.; Strauss, A.; Fagerhaugh, S.; and Suczek, B. 1979. "Trajectories, Biographies, and the Evolving Medical Scene: Labor and Delivery and the Intensive Care Nursery." *Sociology of Health and Illness* 1:261–83.

Zerubavel, E. 1979. *Patterns of Time in Hospital Life*. Chicago: University of Chicago Press.

Author Index

Subject Index